Contents

Dedication

To our long-suffering wives – Jill Hansel and Olivia Barnes

Acknowledgements

We would like to thank Jean Wright, Grant Weston and David Bloomer of Parthenon Publishing for their enthusiasm and highly professional work in organizing this Atlas. We are especially grateful to Andrew Tan and Lynda Payne for being meticulous in preparing the figures, tables and illustrations. We are also indebted to our colleagues within Imperial College and the Royal Brompton Hospital for expert advice: Onn Min Kon, Mike Polkey, Ed Erin, Rachel Tennant, Bryan Corrin, David Hansell and Simon Ward.

THE ENCYCLOPEDIA OF VISUAL MEDICINE SERIES

An Atlas of
CHRONIC OBSTRUCTIVE PULMONARY DISEASE
COPD

Trevor T. Hansel
BSc, MBBCh, MSc, FRCPath, PhD

Medical Director
National Heart and Lung Institute Clinical Studies Unit
Royal Brompton Hospital, London

Peter J. Barnes
DM, DSc, FRCP, FMedSci

Professor and Head of Thoracic Medicine
National Heart and Lung Institute
Imperial College School of Medicine, London

Foreword by
Bartolome R. Celli, MD

Professor of Medicine, Tufts University
Chief of Pulmonary and Critical Care Division
St. Elizabeth's Medical Center
Boston, MA

The Parthenon Publishing Group
International Publishers in Medicine, Science & Technology

A CRC PRESS COMPANY
BOCA RATON   LONDON   NEW YORK   WASHINGTON, D.C.

Published in the USA by
The Parthenon Publishing Group Inc.
345 Park Avenue South, 10th Floor
New York
NY 10010
USA

Published in the UK and Europe by
The Parthenon Publishing Group
23–25 Blades Court
Deodar Road
London SW15 2NU
UK

Library of Congress Cataloging-in-Publication Data
Hansel, T.T. (Trevor T.), 1956-
    An atlas of chronic obstructive pulmonary disease / Trevor T. Hansel, Peter J. Barnes.
      p. ; cm. – (The encyclopedia of visual medicine series)
    Includes bibliographic references and index.
    ISBN 1-84214-004-3 (alk. paper)
      1. Lungs--Diseases, Obstructive--Atlases. 2. Lungs--Diseases, Obstructive--Handbooks,
manuals, etc. I. Title: Chronic obstructive pulmonary disease. II. Barnes, Peter J., 1946-
III. Title. IV. Series.
    [DNLM: 1. Pulmonary Disease, Chronic Obstructive--Atlases. WF 17 H249a 2003]
RC776.O3H365 2003.
616.2'4--dc21   2003056356

British Library Cataloguing in Publication Data
Hansel, Trevor T.
    An atlas of chronic obstructive pulmonary disease. - (The
    encyclopedia of visual medicine series)
    1. Lungs - Diseases, Obstructive - Atlases
    I. Title II. Barnes, Peter J., 1946-
    616.2'4

ISBN 1-84214-004-3

First published in 2004

Composition by The Parthenon Publishing Group
Printed and bound by Butler & Tanner Ltd, Frome and London, UK

Foreword

It is a rare occurrence that new books about a chronic disease provoke excitement. However, the chronic disease in question is chronic obstructive pulmonary disease (COPD) and the book is an atlas that gathers the most important information to be provided about that disease, and presents it in an easy-to-read and extraordinarily clear manner. To view COPD in its proper perspective, it is necessary to recognize that the disease is reaching epidemic proportions around the world. In the United States alone, the death rate from COPD has increased 13% in men and 185% in women between 1987 and 2000. Similar increases in the developed, and, more worrisome yet, in the developing countries have led the medical community to pay more attention to this once-forgotten killer.

This atlas represents an exciting addition to the field of COPD. It summarizes our current knowledge without sacrificing details and depth. Superb clear figures provide the reader with tools that complement the content of the well-written chapters. This atlas is produced and edited by two persons who have spent a significant amount of time thinking and investigating all of the different aspects of COPD. Indeed, Trevor Hansel and Peter Barnes have been able to present not only all of the issues of COPD that pertain to those health-care providers interested in clinical medicine, but also provide insightful information to those interested in more basic mechanisms. The chapters dealing with pathophysiology and current and future pharmacological agents are a clear example of how much the basic understanding of cellular and biochemical mechanisms can contribute to the overall approach to the diagnosis and, above all, treatment of chronic disease. The same depth is appreciated in the first chapter dealing with the definition, epidemiology and causation of COPD. The body of chapters devoted to the clinical aspects, smoking cessation, pulmonary rehabilitation, oxygen and surgery provides the clinician with a coherent series. All of the recent advances are presented with carefully selected graphs and flow charts that make the reading of all of the chapters easy to grasp.

Importantly, this atlas comes at a time when we need to use the current interest in the disease to further mobilize the medical community and society as a whole if we are to decrease the dreadful projections currently being discussed. There are important obstacles to be overcome. The first is to raise awareness among the larger medical community about the importance of early diagnosis of the disease. Indeed, several studies show that COPD remains largely under-diagnosed. Health-care providers will seldom think of COPD as the disease to diagnose when confronted with patients reporting dyspnea or cough. This is surprising when the diagnosis is easily confirmed with a simple spirometry. The second is also to increase awareness in the general public. Indeed, patients with COPD systematically under-rate the extent and severity of their symptoms and their disease. When we add to that lack of awareness the frequent misunderstanding that the disease is largely irreversible and untreatable, the result is a generalized nihilistic attitude that needs to be changed. Trevor Hansel and Peter Barnes provide us with a highly unique tool to enhance our capacity to face the challenge. This atlas is extremely well done; it is relatively brief and full of visual tools, which in most cases are presented adjacent to the written material. This has the unique virtue of making this book an almost interactive experience.

Trevor Hansel and Peter Barnes need to be commended for an excellent book. In the name of all of us, our thanks for a well-thought out product that should become a favorite not only of the cognoscenti but also of physicians in training and all those interested in this fascinating disease.

Bartolome R. Celli, MD
Professor of Medicine, Tufts University
Chief of Pulmonary and Critical Care Division
St. Elizabeth's Medical Center
Boston, MA

1

Introduction: definitions, burden and causation

THE GLOBAL TOBACCO EPIDEMIC

Cigarette smoking is the most common form of addiction world-wide and by far the most important cause of chronic obstructive pulmonary disease (COPD), as well as a spectrum of non-respiratory diseases (Figure 1.1). Particularly deleterious are the effects of cigarette smoke on the respiratory and cardiovascular systems, as well as the carcinogenic actions of cigarette smoke in causing a range of malignancies.

The World Health Organization (WHO) has been active in promoting international and national awareness of the dangers of smoking. A previous Director-General of WHO, Dr Gro Harlem Brundtland, has called for tougher measures to control smoking, including large tax increases, total advertising bans, phasing out of cigarette vending machines, support for legislation on liability and compensation, and strict legislation to prevent damage from passive inhalation of cigarette smoke. The WHO's Framework Convention on Smoking Control (FCSC) is a public health treaty that embodies these principles, and was considered by the World Health Assembly in May 2003[1].

The major health hazards internationally concern consumption: too little for the poor and too much in the case of the prosperous. Hence, the deleterious effects of smoking on health, together with the

Figure 1.1	Smoking-related diseases

Lung
COPD: chronic bronchitis, obstructive bronchiolitis, emphysema
Respiratory tract infections, sinusitis and pneumonia
Lung cancer

Cardiovascular
Arteriosclerosis and atheroma
Thromboembolic disease
Peripheral vascular disease
     Intermittent claudication
     Buerger's disease (thromboangiitis obliterans)
Aortic aneurysm
Malignant hypertension
Coronary heart disease: myocardial ischemia and infarction
Heart failure and arrhythmias
Cerebrovascular disease: stroke and subarachnoid hemorrhage

Malignancies
Cancer of lung and most other organs
     Oropharynx, esophagus, stomach, pancreas, bowel
     Kidney, bladder, uterine cervix

Gastrointestinal
Chronic gingivitis, stomatitis and laryngitis
Peptic ulcer and gastroesophageal reflux disorder

Reproductive
Sexual dysfunction in men, infertility
Effects on pregnancy, fetus and child

Other conditions
Premature facial wrinkling
Osteoporosis in females
Graves' disease, cataracts, retinal disorders and sleep disturbance

dangers of excess intake of food and alcohol and lack of exercise, comprise major preventable risks in industrialized societies. The scale of the smoking epidemic is vast, and the WHO has noted that almost a billion men and 250 million women in the world are daily smokers. Many of these individuals will die prematurely from smoking-related diseases. Of especial concern is that 35% of men in developed countries smoke, but the figure is almost 50% in developing nations, and nearly two-thirds of Chinese men smoke. However, smoking rates have declined in some high-income countries, decreasing from 80% to 39% in UK men from 1948 to 1998[2].

The importance of chronic obstructive pulmonary disease has only recently been recognized by the formulation of international treatment guidelines. The WHO and the US National Institutes of Health have formed a Global Initiative for Chronic Obstructive Lung Disease (GOLD), and have formulated a 'Global Strategy for the Diagnosis, Management and Prevention of COPD'. The 20 members of the Gold Expert Panel have participated in a series of workshops, and have provided an evidence-based management strategy. The report was released in 2001, with an update in July 2003, and is available in pamphlet form and on the internet (www.goldcopd.com)[3,4].

DEFINITION OF CHRONIC OBSTRUCTIVE PULMONARY DISEASE

A working definition of COPD is given within the GOLD Global Strategy as:

'A disease state characterized by airflow limitation that is not fully reversible. The airflow limitation is usually progressive and associated with an abnormal inflammatory response of the lungs to noxious particles or gases.'

COPD is a complex disease, and this brief definition does not detail risk factors such as cigarette smoke, does not describe the symptoms of COPD, and does not describe the range of pathological processes and diseases encompassed within COPD. In addition, the name 'COPD' is inaccurate since chronic obstructive airway disease may occur in association with more severe asthma, tuberculosis, bronchiectasis and cystic fibrosis. Gordon Snider has suggested that the classification and terminology of COPD should be reviewed by an international expert panel[5].

The following are key features of COPD (Figure 1.2):

- COPD is defined physiologically as chronic airflow limitation reflected by a reduction in

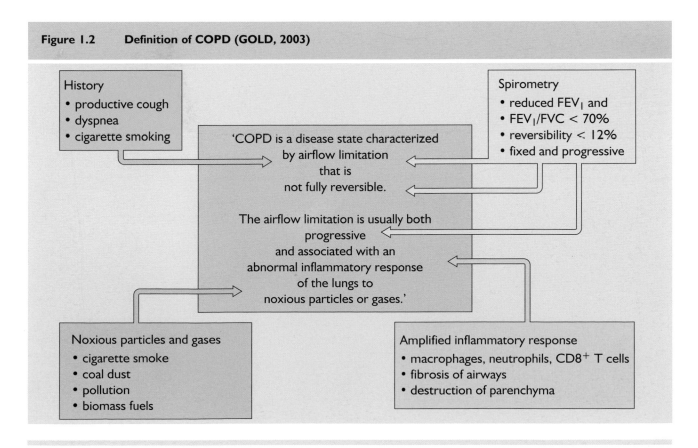

Figure 1.2   Definition of COPD (GOLD, 2003)

History
- productive cough
- dyspnea
- cigarette smoking

Spirometry
- reduced FEV_1 and
- $FEV_1/FVC < 70\%$
- reversibility $< 12\%$
- fixed and progressive

'COPD is a disease state characterized by airflow limitation that is not fully reversible.

The airflow limitation is usually both progressive and associated with an abnormal inflammatory response of the lungs to noxious particles or gases.'

Noxious particles and gases
- cigarette smoke
- coal dust
- pollution
- biomass fuels

Amplified inflammatory response
- macrophages, neutrophils, $CD8^+$ T cells
- fibrosis of airways
- destruction of parenchyma

Figure 1.3   Classification of severity of COPD (GOLD 2001 and 2003 update)

Stage		Symptoms	Lung function	
GOLD, 2003	GOLD, 2001		FEV$_1$/FVC	FEV$_1$ (% predicted)
0: At risk	0	chronic productive cough	normal	normal
I: Mild	I	with or without symptoms	< 70%	> 80%
II: Moderate	IIA	with or without symptoms	< 70%	50–80%
III: Severe	IIB	with or without symptoms	< 70%	30–50%
IV: Very severe	III	*dyspnea, cough, sputum respiratory failure or right heart failure	< 70%	*< 30%

*Patients have very severe COPD if they have either a post-bronchodilator FEV$_1$ of < 30%, or FEV$_1$ < 50% predicted with respiratory failure or clinical signs of right heart failure. From Global Initiative for Chronic Obstructive Lung Disease (GOLD) global strategy (2001 and 2003 update).

maximum expiratory flow and slow forced emptying of the lungs.

- Airway obstruction is not fully reversible (< 12%), in contrast to the > 12% reversibility and variability in the airflow obstruction in asthma.

- Extensive airflow limitation occurs before the patient is aware of symptoms, such as exertional dyspnea, due to the slowly progressive nature of the airflow obstruction and various coping maneuvers.

- The abnormal inflammatory response involves macrophages, neutrophils and CD8+ T cells and may result in structural changes and fixed narrowing of the airways, with destruction of the lung parenchyma. The definition encompasses the concept that COPD is a chronic inflammatory disease.

- Noxious particles or gases generally consist of long-term cigarette smoke in developed countries. COPD may also be caused by exposure to

mineral dusts, fumes from indoor biomass fuels in developing countries, as well as outdoor air pollution[6].

CLASSIFICATION OF SEVERITY OF COPD

Expert panels have given varying classifications of the severity of COPD in terms of the percentage predicted forced expiratory volume in 1 second (FEV$_1$) that the patient can achieve on spirometry. These classifications are used for purposes of simplicity, but are arbitrary and not clinically validated.

There have been considerable differences in four of these classification systems:

- The American Thoracic Society (ATS) guidelines of 1995 suggested: mild (stage I) is FEV$_1$ > 50%, moderate (stage II) is FEV$_1$ 35–49%, severe (stage III) is FEV$_1$ < 35%[7].

- The European Respiratory Society (ERS) consensus statement on optimal assessment and

Figure 1.4   Diseases included within COPD

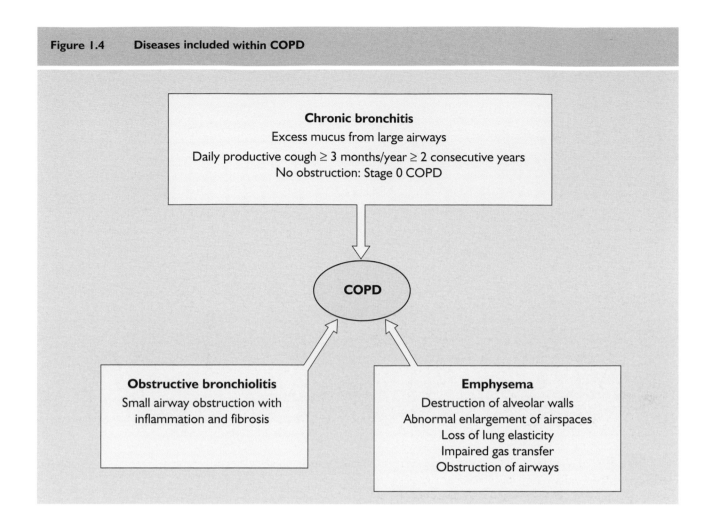

management of COPD recommended: mild ≥ 70%, moderate 50–69%, severe < 50%[8].

- The British Thoracic Society (BTS) guidelines of 1997 proposed: mild (60–80%), moderate (40–60%), severe (< 40%)[9].

- The Global Initiative for Chronic Obstructive Lung Disease (GOLD, 2003) strategy has proposed a novel classification (Figure 1.3): mild (> 80%), moderate (50–80%), severe (30–50%) or very severe (< 30%)). The GOLD strategy suggests that patients with normal spirometry but a chronic productive cough should be in 'Group 0: at risk', although a 15-year study found that Gold Stage 0 does not identify patients that proceed to airways obstruction[10]. There is also the need to validate the parameters for 'Stage I: mild COPD' in terms of presence of FEV_1/FVC at < 70% with FEV_1 > 80%.

DISEASES ENCOMPASSED WITHIN COPD

The pathology of COPD can involve chronic bronchitis, obstructive bronchiolitis, emphysema, pulmonary vascular disease, and systemic complications[11] (Figure 1.4).

Chronic bronchitis

Chronic (simple) bronchitis is defined by a productive cough on most days for at least 3 months for at least 2 consecutive years, which cannot be attributed to other pulmonary or cardiac causes. The original clinical definition arose from the British Medical Research Council (MRC) in 1965[12,13]. Chronic bronchitis is a consequence of mucus hyperplasia, resulting in hypersecretion of mucus, and is not necessarily related to airway obstruction. In addition, the term 'chronic bronchitis' can also be used to describe histopathological features (see Chapter 2).

Figure 1.5   Prevalence of COPD

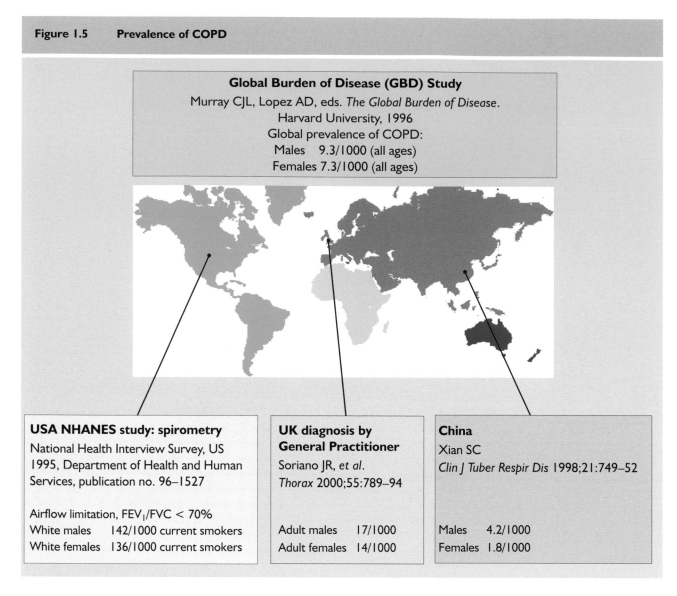

Global Burden of Disease (GBD) Study
Murray CJL, Lopez AD, eds. *The Global Burden of Disease.*
Harvard University, 1996
Global prevalence of COPD:
Males   9.3/1000 (all ages)
Females 7.3/1000 (all ages)

USA NHANES study: spirometry
National Health Interview Survey, US
1995, Department of Health and Human
Services, publication no. 96–1527

Airflow limitation, FEV$_1$/FVC < 70%
White males   142/1000 current smokers
White females   136/1000 current smokers

**UK diagnosis by
General Practitioner**
Soriano JR, *et al.*
Thorax 2000;55:789–94

Adult males   17/1000
Adult females   14/1000

China
Xian SC
Clin J Tuber Respir Dis 1998;21:749–52

Males   4.2/1000
Females   1.8/1000

Prevalence data for COPD in adults from the Global Burden of Disease Study, the USA, UK and China. See text for details.

Obstructive bronchiolitis

Obstructive bronchiolitis is due to obstruction of the peripheral airways as a result of an inflammatory response, with a type of fibrosis involving airway remodelling. Airway remodelling, loss of alveolar attachments and elastic recoil, and excess mucus are all believed to contribute to obstruction and collapse of small airways.

Emphysema

Emphysema is a pathological diagnosis characterized by destruction of alveolar walls, resulting in abnormal and permanent enlargement (dilatation) of airspaces and loss of lung elasticity, with consequent obstruction of peripheral airways.

Respiratory failure

Chronic hypoxia occurs late in COPD and may result in pulmonary hypertension and right heart failure (*cor pulmonale*). Respiratory failure can be defined as an arterial blood partial pressure of oxygen (PaO_2) < 8.0 kPa (60 mmHg), with or without partial pressure of CO_2 ($PaCO_2$) > 6.7 kPa (50 mmHg) while breathing air at sea level.

| Figure 1.6 | Leading causes of mortality world-wide |

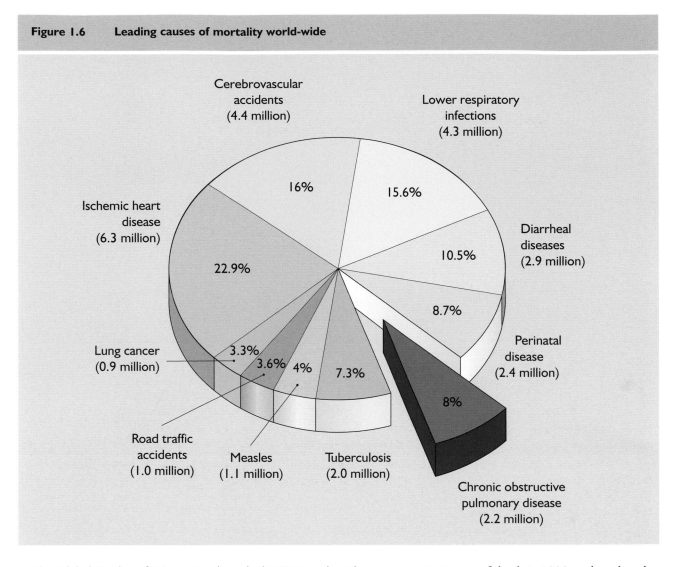

The Global Burden of Disease Study ranked COPD as the 6th most important cause of death in 1990, and predicted that it will be the 3rd most common cause of death by 2020. Adapted from Murray CJL, Lopez AD. *Lancet* 1997;349:1498–504.

THE BURDEN OF COPD

Prevalence of COPD

Prevalence data for COPD are derived mostly from industrial countries, and tend to be an underestimate of the true picture, because COPD is generally not diagnosed until it is clinically obvious. Epidemiological studies have also been hampered by debate over the definition of COPD. Nevertheless, there is consensus that there has been a world-wide increase in COPD, reflecting increases in cigarette smoking, especially in developing countries.

The prevalence of COPD is illustrated in Figure 1.5:

- The Global Burden of Disease Study run by the World Bank and the World Health Organization used data from published and unpublished studies, as well as informed estimates by experts, to derive a world-wide all-ages prevalence of just under 1%[14,15].

- The National Health and Nutrition Examination Survey (NHANES), conducted in the USA between 1988 and 1994, measured the prevalence of COPD, by evidence of airflow limitation, at approximately 14% of current smokers[16].

- The UK General Practice Research Database used physician-based diagnosis in 525 practices serving 3.4 million patients, and found a prevalence in adult males of 1.7% and in adult females of 1.4%[17].

- Data from China are based on a survey of three regions, which found a prevalence at < 0.5%[18].

Global mortality

COPD is a major health problem world-wide with a high prevalence and cost; it is a leading cause of morbidity and mortality in the adult population. As the major cause of COPD is cigarette smoking, the epidemiology of COPD largely reflects the demographics of cigarette smoking. There are marked differences in mortality and morbidity between countries and these may reflect classification differences. Figures are generally greatly underestimated because COPD is not diagnosed until it is clinically apparent and moderately advanced, and death from COPD may be due to secondary complications such as heart failure. According to the Global Burden of Disease Study, COPD was the sixth most common cause of death in the world in 1990 and will rise to the third most common by 2020[19,20] (Figures 1.6 and 1.7).

Figure 1.7	World-wide mortality: 1990–2020

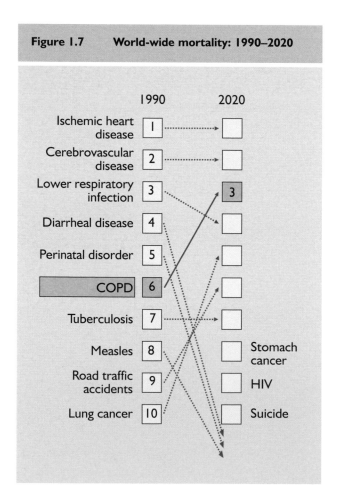

The ten world-wide leading causes of mortality in 1990 (Global Burden of Disease Study). Murray CJL, Lopez AD, *Lancet* 1997;349:1269–76.

Figure 1.8	World-wide causes of lost DALYs: 1990–2020

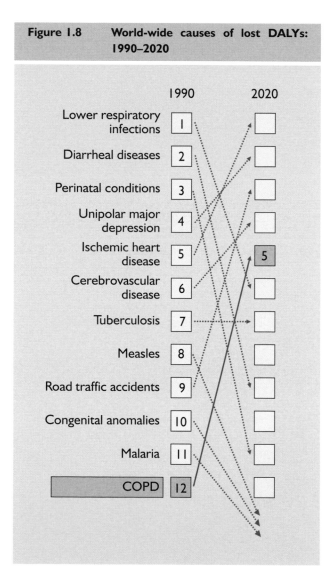

Leading causes of disability-adjusted life years (DALYs) lost world-wide, 1990–2020 (projected). Based on data from the Global Burden of Disease Study (Murray CJL, Lopez AD. *Science* 1996;274: 740–3). DALYs are the sum of years of life lost because of premature mortality and years of life lived with disability.

Social burden

The amount of disability may be quantified as disability-adjusted life years (DALY, the sum of years lost because of premature mortality and years of life lived with disability, adjusted for the severity of disability). In terms of lost DALYs, COPD was ranked 12th in 1990 and is predicted to rise to 5th ranking by 2020[14,21] (Figure 1.8). DALYs have proved very useful in providing an assessment of the social burden of a disease.

Economic burden

The economics of tobacco control have been studied by the World Bank together with the WHO, and they have noted that tax increases are the single intervention most likely to reduce demand for tobacco, but tax is less than half of the total price in lower income countries[22]. A study on the health-care costs of smoking in The Netherlands has suggested that there would only be a short-term decrease in health-service costs, and eventually there would be increased health-service costs[23]. In Germany, smoking-related health-care costs have been estimated at 16.6 billion Euros, or 6% of total German health-care costs[24,25].

COPD is a very costly public health problem due to its high prevalence and serious clinical consequences. Direct costs of COPD are due to hospital admissions and expensive treatments such as long-term oxygen, whereas indirect costs include loss of working capacity and poor quality of life[26,27]. The economic burden of COPD has been studied in the USA[28], UK[29], The Netherlands[30] and Sweden[31]. The *Confronting COPD in North America and Europe* survey of the economic costs of COPD in seven countries (Canada, France, Italy, The Netherlands, Spain, UK, USA) has demonstrated high but variable costs of COPD (Figure 1.9)[32].

| Figure 1.9 | The economic burden of COPD |

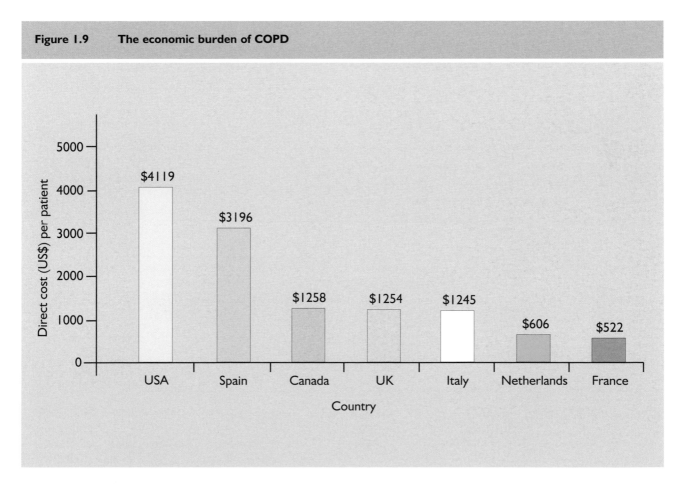

Data from the *Confronting COPD in North America and Europe* survey of the economic impact of COPD. Adapted from Wouters EFM. *Respir Med* 2003;97(Suppl C):S3–14

UK epidemiology

In the UK, 15–20% of middle-aged men and 10% of women report chronic cough and sputum production, so most chronic smokers develop mucus hypersecretion or chronic simple bronchitis. COPD is diagnosed in approximately 4% of men and 2% of women over 45 years in the UK, and approximately 6% of deaths in men and 4% in women are due to COPD. In the UK, COPD is the third most common cause of death, and is the only common cause of death that is increasing. COPD is a very common cause of hospitalization, and the mortality of patients who are hospitalized with COPD is almost 15%, which exceeds that of myocardial infarction. Despite decreases in the numbers of smokers, there have been few changes in the prevalence of COPD over the last 30 years in the UK, in contrast to an increase in asthma.

THE CAUSES OF COPD

There are several causative or risk factors involved in COPD, which can be classified into host factors and environmental exposures[3,6,33].

Host factors (Figure 1.10)

Genetic factors

Complex genetic-environment factors are involved in the pathogenesis of COPD and a number of reviews have addressed this area[34,35], although the Framingham Study suggests that, in the general population, genetic factors contribute modestly to loss of lung function[36], with FEV_1 most influenced by a locus on chromosome 6[37]. However, the fact that only 10–20% of heavy smokers develop COPD may be largely determined by as yet unidentified genetic factors[38,39]. Siblings of patients with severe COPD have increased risk of airways obstruction, suggesting a recessive model of inheritance[40,41]. There appear to be ethnic differences in susceptibility to the effects of cigarette smoking, as only 5% of oriental subjects who smoke develop COPD.

- A clearly established genetic risk factor for COPD is the ZZ allele of the α_1-antitrypsin (α_1-AT) or α_1-protease inhibitor (α_1-PI) gene (piZ phenotype)[42], but α_1-AT deficiency accounts for less than 1% of cases of COPD in Northern Europe[43]. Short-term augmentation therapy with intravenous α_1-AT in patients with α_1-AT deficiency causes[44] decreased sputum leukotriene B_4, and weekly infusions may slow the annual decline in FEV_1 in severe hereditary α_1-AT deficiency[43,45]. In addition, rapid decline of FEV_1 has been associated with the MZ allele of the α_1-AT gene[46], and studies in mice exposed to tobacco smoke have shown that α_1-AT expression determines the pattern of emphysema[47].

- There is also an association with a polymorphism of the tumor necrosis factor (TNF)-α promoter gene (TNF2) that is associated with greater inducibility of TNF-α in a Taiwan population[48,49], although this has not been confirmed in Caucasian populations[46,50]. TNF-α-308 promoter gene (TNF allele 2) is partly associated with the appearance of emphysema on computed tomography (CT) scan[51].

- There are no major risks from α_1-antitrypsin TAQ 1 polymorphisms nor α_1-antichymotrypsin mutations[52], but weak associations with vitamin D-binding protein exist[53].

- A polymorphism in the gene for an enzyme, microsomal epoxide hydrolase, which is responsible for metabolism of reactive epoxide intermediates, and which may be generated in tobacco smoke, has been associated with a four- to five-fold increased risk of COPD and emphysema[54]. An association has been confirmed in the Lung Health Study[46].

- Associations have been described for the polymorphisms of antioxidant glutathione-S-transferase and rapid decline in lung function[55]. In this study, there was no association between heme oxygenase-1 alleles and the rate of decline of lung function in smokers.

- Matrix metalloproteinase (MMP) polymorphisms in MMP1 and MMP12 have been associated with rapid decline in lung function[56]. Polymorphism of tissue inhibitor of metalloproteinases-2 (TIMP-2), that may downregulate activity, have been associated with COPD[57].

- In severe early-onset COPD, a genome-wide analysis has demonstrated significant linkage of FEV_1/FVC to chromosome 2q[58].

- In continuing smokers, an IL4RA (interleukin-4 receptor-α) polymorphism together with certain IL-13 polymorphisms may be associated with accelerated rate of decline in lung function[59].

Figure 1.10   Risk factors for COPD: host factors

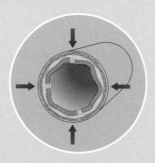

Airway hyperresponsiveness (AHR):
'Dutch hypothesis'

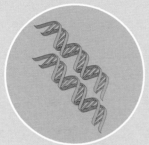

Genetic factors:
α_1-antitrypsin deficiency

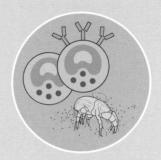

Atopy:
mast cell coated with IgE and
allergen (house dust mite)

Host factors

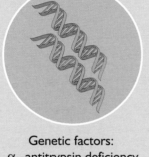

Premature baby:
small for dates
low birth weight
impaired lung growth

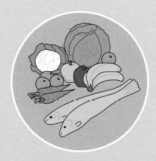

Diet deficient in
antioxidant vitamins (A, C and E),
fish oil and protein

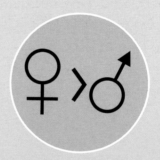

Gender controversial

Many genetic factors may be involved in susceptibility to COPD, although the best documented is α_1-antitrypsin deficiency, which is a recessive trait in North Europeans. The 'Dutch hypothesis', that there is a relationship between airway hyperresponsiveness (AHR) and atopy with increased risk of developing COPD, remains controversial. Mast cells are shown coated with IgE, degranulating in response to a house dust mite. Impaired lung growth predisposes to COPD, as occurs in premature babies. Elderly smokers commonly have diets deficient in antioxidant vitamins A, C and E. Females may be predisposed compared to males.

Atopy and airway hyperresponsiveness

There has been considerable debate about the influence of atopy and airway hyperresponsiveness on the development of COPD. The 'Dutch hypothesis' proposed that atopy and IgE underlie the development of COPD[60–62]. This hypothesis claims that asthma and COPD are two extremes of the same basic process, while the recent GOLD global strategy stresses the differences between the clinical features, pathology and pharmacology of these diseases[3]. COPD itself may result in increased airway responsiveness to histamine or methacholine due to geometric factors related to fixed airway narrowing[61]. Nevertheless, there is increased bronchodilator responsiveness among first-degree currently smoking and ex-smoking relatives of patients with early onset COPD[63]. Airways responsiveness is associated with the development of chronic respiratory symptoms[62,64,65], mortality from COPD increases with more severe atopy and airway hyperresponsiveness to histamine[66,67], and bronchodilator reversibility is associated with increased survival in COPD patients[68].

Nutrition and lung growth

Low dietary intake of antioxidant vitamins (A, C and E) has sometimes been found to be associated with increased risk of COPD[69–71], although a more recent study found vitamin C and magnesium to be important[72]. There is some evidence that a diet rich in fish oil is associated with a lower prevalence of COPD[73,74], although this was not confirmed in another study[75]. However, there are beneficial effects of flavonoids (especially catechins) in solid fruits and vegetables[76,77], and alcohol consumption has also been found to be protective in heavy smokers[78,79].

Early nutrition may be important and small-for-dates babies have an increased risk of development of COPD in later life[80]. Patients with emphysema are more likely to have had a low birth weight[81] and be underweight in adult life, and those with chronic bronchitis are more likely to be obese[82]. Cachexia with dramatic weight loss can itself be part of the clinical features of severe COPD[83,84].

Gender

It is controversial whether females are more susceptible to the effects of cigarette smoking, although a range of studies have found greater prevalence of COPD in women[85–89]. There is evidence that adolescent females exposed to smoking may achieve lower maximal lung function[87], but there are different patterns in lung function development between males and females[90]. However, effects on females may be underestimated since males tend to smoke more, often start earlier, and have a greater degree of inhalation[91]. In developing countries, women may have greater exposure to air pollution from burning cooking fuels[92,93].

Environmental factors (Figure 1.11)

Cigarette smoking

Cigarette smoking is by far the most common cause of COPD world-wide, accounting for more than 95% of cases in industrialized countries, but it is very relevant that some patients with COPD are non-smokers[94]. Usually, there is a smoking history of more than 20 pack-years, and active smoking causes both mucus hypersecretion and chronic airflow obstruction. Cessation of smoking decreases respiratory symptoms[95] and reduces the rate of decline in lung function[96–99]. Pipe and cigar smokers have a higher risk of COPD than non-smokers, although rates are lower than for cigarette smokers. Passive smoking is associated with COPD, possibly via effects on lung growth during fetal development and childhood[87,100,101]. Smoking during pregnancy may also be a risk factor for COPD for the child, as this may affect lung growth[102].

The number of marijuana (cannabis) smokers is increasing in western society, and this may become a major cause of COPD in the future. Although marijuana cigarettes are generally smoked less than nicotine cigarettes, marijuana smoking involves a larger inhalation volume and a longer breath hold[103]. Early studies suggested that marijuana smoking may not be associated with an accelerated decline in FEV_1[104,105], although a serious bullous lung disease has been reported in young people[106]. The clinical picture and inflammatory lung changes in marijuana smokers are similar to those in nicotine cigarette smokers[107,108].

Air pollution: outdoor and indoor

Air pollution, particularly sulfur dioxide and particulates (black smoke or particulate matter of $\leq 10\,\mu m$ [PM_{10}]), is associated with chronic simple bronchitis

Figure 1.11   Risk factors for COPD: environmental factors

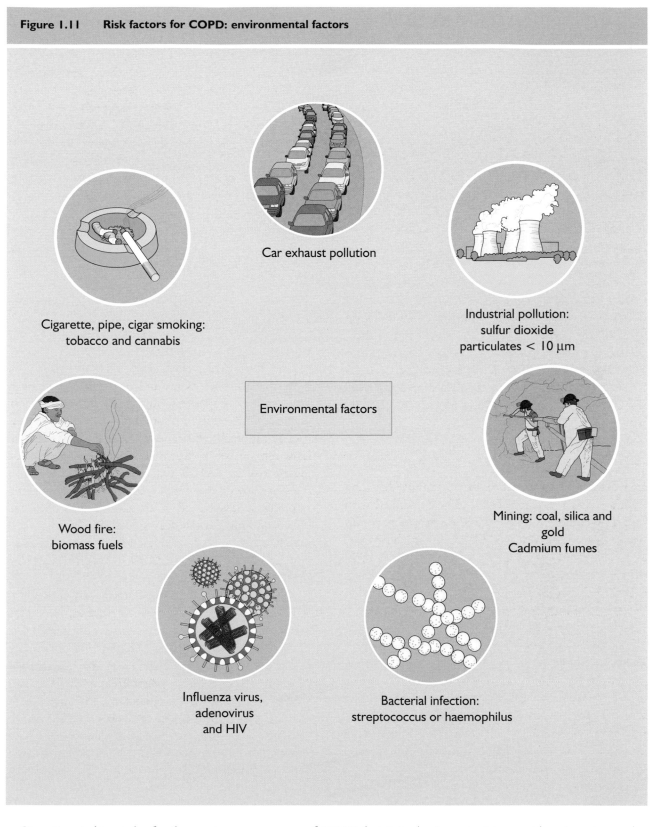

Car exhaust pollution

Industrial pollution:
sulfur dioxide
particulates < 10 μm

Cigarette, pipe, cigar smoking:
tobacco and cannabis

Environmental factors

Wood fire:
biomass fuels

Mining: coal, silica and
gold
Cadmium fumes

Influenza virus,
adenovirus
and HIV

Bacterial infection:
streptococcus or haemophilus

Cigarette smoking is by far the most common cause of COPD, but it is also important to consider pipe, cigar and cannabis smoking. Indoor air pollution from the burning of biomass fuels in poorly ventilated homes may be a factor, especially for women in some communities, while air pollution from exhaust and industrial emissions is more relevant in industrialized societies. Occupational exposure to coal and silica dust may interact with cigarette smoking, while bacterial and viral infections may also contribute.

and COPD[109,110]. There may be interactions between cigarette smoking and air pollution. In places where there is heavy air pollution, this may be as important a risk factor as cigarette smoking. Indoor air pollution from biomass fuel, which is burned for cooking and heating in poorly ventilated homes, may be an important risk factor for COPD in developing countries and this may account for the relatively high rates of disease amongst women[92,111–116].

Occupational dusts and chemicals

Occupational exposure to dusts (coal, silica, quartz), isocyanate fumes, and solvents may be important and these noxious agents may interact with cigarette smoke to cause COPD[117–121]. The importance of occupational dust exposure to miners of coal and gold may be underestimated[122,123]. Exposure to cadmium and welding fumes may also be associated with emphysema[124].

Infection

Chest infections during the first year of life are associated with COPD in later life[80,125], and infections in childhood may play a role[126]. There is also evidence that certain latent virus infections (such as adenovirus) may cause amplification of inflammation in emphysema and predispose to the development of COPD[127–129]. Human immunodeficiency virus (HIV) seropositive smokers have increased susceptibility to emphysema[130–134]. The Lung Health Study has noted that illnesses of the lower respiratory tract promote FEV_1 decline in current smokers[135], and exacerbation frequency also contributes to rate of lung function decline[136].

THE FUTURE

COPD is a common disease but has been neglected in terms of research on molecular and pathophysiological mechanisms, as well as development of novel modes of treatment. It has been proposed that there is the need to raise the profile of COPD, in efforts to prevent the causes of COPD, to alter the natural history, and implement measures to minimalize suffering[137]. Nevertheless, further advances in our understanding of COPD continue to be made[138], and the National Heart Lung and Blood Institute has convened a workshop to propose needs and opportunities for future clinical research in COPD[139].

REFERENCES

1. Twombly R. Tobacco use a leading global cancer risk, report says. *J Natl Cancer Inst* 2003;95:11–12

2. Peto R, Darby S, Deo H, *et al*. Smoking, smoking cessation, and lung cancer in the UK since 1950: combination of national statistics with two case-control studies. *Br Med J* 2000;321:323–9

3. National Institutes of Health (NIH), National Heart Lung and Blood Institute (NHLBI), World Health Organisation (WHO). Global Initiative for Chronic Obstructive Lung Disease (GOLD) : Global Strategy for the Diagnosis, Management, and Prevention of Chronic Obstructive Pulmonary Disease NHLBI/WHO Workshop Report. www.goldcopd.com/workshop/index.html. 2001 and update in 2003

4. Fabbri LM, Hurd SS, for the GOLD Scientific Committee. Editorial: Global strategy for the diagnosis, management and prevention of COPD: 2003 update. *Eur J Respir* 2003;22:1–2

5. Snider GL. Nosology for our day. Its application to chronic obstructive pulmonary disease. *Am J Respir Crit Care Med* 2003;176:678–83

6. Anto JM, Vermeire P, Vestbo J, *et al*. Epidemiology of chronic obstructive pulmonary disease. *Eur Respir J* 2001;17:982–94

7. American Thoracic Society: Standards for the diagnosis and care of patients with chronic obstructive pulmonary disease. *Am J Respir Crit Care Med* 1995;152:S77–120

8. Siafakas NM, Vermeire P, Pride NB, *et al*. Optimal assessment and management of chronic obstructive pulmonary disease (COPD). The European Respiratory Society Task Force. *Eur Respir J* 1995;8:1398–420

9. British Thoracic Society. BTS guidelines for the management of chronic obstructive pulmonary disease. *Thorax* 1997;52(Suppl 5)

10. Vestbo J, Lange P. Can GOLD Stage 0 provide information of prognostic value in chronic obstructive pulmonary disease? *Am J Respir Crit Care Med* 2002;166:329–32

11. Barnes PJ. Chronic obstructive pulmonary disease. *N Engl J Med* 2000;343:269–80

12. Medical Research Council. Definition and classification of chronic bronchitis for clinical and epidemiological purposes. *Lancet* 1965;i:775–9

13. Definitions of emphysema, chronic bronchitis, asthma, and airflow obstruction: 25 years on from the CIBA symposium. *Thorax* 1984;39:81–5

14. Murray CJ, Lopez AD. Evidence-based health policy-lessons from the Global Burden of Disease Study. *Science* 1996;274:740–3

15. *The Global Burden of Disease: A Comprehensive Assessment of Mortality and Disability from Diseases, Injuries and Risk Factors in 1990 and projected to 2020.* Cambridge, MA: Harvard University Press, 1996

16. National Center for Health Statistics. Current estimates from the National Health Interview Survey, United States, 1995. Department of Health and Human Services, Public Health Service, Vital and Health Statistics 1995;96:1527

17. Soriano JB, Maier WC, Egger P, *et al.* Recent trends in physician diagnosed COPD in women and men in the UK. *Thorax* 2000;55:789–94

18. Chen XS. Analysis of basic data of the study on prevention and treatment of COPD. *Chin J Tuber Respir Dis* 2003;21:749–52

19. Murray CJ, Lopez AD. Mortality by cause for eight regions of the world: Global Burden of Disease Study. *Lancet* 1997;349:1269–76

20. Murray CJ, Lopez AD. Alternative projections of mortality and disability by cause 1990–2020: Global Burden of Disease Study. *Lancet* 1997;349:1498–504

21. Lopez AD, Murray C.C. The global burden of disease, 1990–2020. *Nat Med* 1998;4:1241–3

22. Jha P, Chaloupka FJ. The economics of global tobacco control. *Br Med J* 2000;321:358–61

23. Barendregt JJ, Bonneux L, van der Maas PJ. The health care costs of smoking. *N Engl J Med* 1997;337:1052–7

24. Ruff LK, Volmcr T, Nowak D, Meyer A. The economic impact of smoking in Germany. *Eur Respir J* 2000;16:385–90

25. Loddenkemper R, Sybrecht GW. Health care costs of smoking. *Eur Respir J* 2000;16:377–8

26. Sullivan SD, Ramsey SD, Lee TA. The economic burden of COPD. *Chest* 2000;117:5–9S

27. Strassels SA. Economic consequences of chronic obstructive pulmonary disease. *Curr Opin Pulm Med* 1999;5:100–4

28. National Heart LaBI. Morbidity & mortality: chartbook on cardiovascular, lung, and blood diseases. Bethesda, MD: US Department of Health and Human Services, Public Health Service, National Institutes of Health. Available from URL: www.nhlbi.nih.gov/nhlbi/seiin/other/cht-book/htm 1998

29. National Health Service Executive. *Burdens of Disease: A Discussion Document.* London: Department of Health, 1996

30. Rutten-van Molken MP, Postma MJ, Joore MA, *et al.* Current and future medical costs of asthma and chronic obstructive pulmonary disease in The Netherlands. *Respir Med* 1999;93:779–87

31. Jacobson L, Hertzman P, Lofdahl CG, *et al.* The economic impact of asthma and chronic obstructive pulmonary disease (COPD) in Sweden in 1980 and 1991. *Respir Med* 2000;94:247–55

32. Dahl R, Lofdahl C-G (Guest editors). The economic impact of COPD in North America and Europe: analysis of the confronting COPD survey. *Respir Med* 2003;97(Suppl C):S1–90

33. Altose MD. Approaches to slowing the progression of COPD. *Curr Opin Pulm Med* 2003;9:125–30

34. Hoidal JR. Genetics of COPD: present and future. *Eur Respir J* 2001;18:741–3

35. Sandford AJ, Silverman EK. Chronic obstructive pulmonary disease. 1. Susceptibility factors for COPD the genotype–environment interaction. *Thorax* 2002;57:736–41

36. Gottlieb DJ, Wilk JB, Harmon M, *et al.* Heritability of longitudinal change in lung function. The Framingham study. *Am J Respir Crit Care Med* 2001;164:1655–9

37. Joost O, Wilk JB, Cupples LA, *et al.* Genetic loci influencing lung function: a genome-wide scan in the Framingham Study. *Am J Respir Crit Care Med* 2002;165:795–9

38. Sandford AJ, Weir TD, Pare PD. Genetic risk factors for chronic obstructive pulmonary disease. *Eur Respir J* 1997;10:1380–91

39. Barnes PJ. Molecular genetics of chronic obstructive pulmonary disease. *Thorax* 1999;54:245–52

40. McCloskey SC, Patel BD, Hinchliffe SJ, *et al.* Siblings of patients with severe chronic obstructive pulmonary disease have a significant risk of airflow obstruction. *Am J Respir Crit Care Med* 2001;164:1419–24

41. Kurzius-Spencer M, Sherrill DL, Holberg CJ, *et al.* Familial correlation in the decline of forced expiratory volume in one second. *Am J Respir Crit Care Med* 2001;164:1261–5

42. Dowson LJ, Guest PJ, Stockley RA. Longitudinal changes in physiological, radiological, and health status measurements in alpha(1)-antitrypsin deficiency and factors associated with decline. *Am J Respir Crit Care Med* 2001;164:1805–9

43. The Alpha-1-Antitrypsin Deficiency Registry Study Group. Survival and FEV1 decline in individuals with severe deficiency of alpha1-antitrypsin. *Am J Respir Crit Care Med* 1998;158:49–59

44. Stockley RA, Bayley DL, Unsal I, *et al.* The effect of augmentation therapy on bronchial inflammation in alpha1-antitrypsin deficiency. *Am J Respir Crit Care Med* 2002;165:1494–8

45. Seersholm N, Wencker M, Banik N, *et al.* Does alpha1-antitrypsin augmentation therapy slow the annual decline in FEV1 in patients with severe hereditary alpha1-antitrypsin deficiency? Wissenschaftliche Arbeitsgemeinschaft zur Therapie von Lungenerkrankungen (WATL) alpha1-AT study group. *Eur Respir J* 1997;10:2260–3

46. Sandford AJ, Chagani T, Weir TD, *et al.* Susceptibility genes for rapid decline of lung function in the lung health study. *Am J Respir Crit Care Med* 2001;163:469–73

47. Takubo Y, Guerassimov A, Ghezzo H, *et al.* Alpha1-antitrypsin determines the pattern of emphysema and function in tobacco smoke-exposed mice: parallels with human disease. *Am J Respir Crit Care Med* 2002;166:1596–603

48. Huang S, Su C, Chang S. Tumor necrosis factor alpha gene polymorphism in chronic bronchitis. *Am J Resp Crit Care Med* 1999;156:1436–9

49. Sakao S, Tatsumi K, Igari H, *et al.* Association of tumor necrosis factor alpha gene promoter polymorphism with the presence of chronic obstructive pulmonary disease. *Am J Respir Crit Care Med* 2001;163:420–2

50. Higham MA, Pride NB, Alikhan A, *et al.* Tumour necrosis factor-a gene promoter polymorphism in chronic obstructive pulmonary disease. *Eur Respir J* 2000;15:281–4

51. Sakao S, Tatsumi K, Igari H, *et al.* Association of tumor necrosis factor-alpha gene promoter polymorphism with low attenuation areas on high-resolution CT in patients with COPD. *Chest* 2002;122:416–20

52. Benetazzo MG, Gile LS, Bombieri C, *et al.* Alpha 1-Antitrypsin TAQ I polymorphism and alpha 1-antichymotrypsin mutations in patients with obstructive pulmonary disease. *Respir Med* 1999;93:648–54

53. Schellenberg D, Pare PD, Weir TD, *et al.* Vitamin D binding protein variants and the risk of COPD. *Am J Respir Crit Care Med* 1998;157:957–61

54. Smith CA, Harrison DJ. Association between polymorphism in gene for microsomal epoxide hydrolase and susceptibility to emphysema. *Lancet* 1997;350:630–3

55. He JQ, Ruan J, Connett JE, *et al.* Antioxidant gene polymorphisms and susceptibility to a rapid decline in lung function in smokers. *Am J Respir Crit Care Med* 2002;166:323–8

56. Joos L, He JQ, Shepherdson MB, *et al.* The role of matrix metalloproteinase polymorphisms in the rate of decline in lung function. *Hum Mol Genet* 2002;11:569–76

57. Hirano K, Sakamoto T, Uchida Y, *et al.* Tissue inhibitor of metalloproteinases-2 gene polymorphism in chronic obstructive pulmonary disease. *Eur Respir J* 2001;18:748–52

58. Silverman EK, Palmer LJ, Mosley JD, *et al.* Genomewide linkage analysis of quantitative spirometric phenotypes in severe early-onset chronic obstructive pulmonary disease. *Am J Hum Genet* 2002;70:1229–39

59. He J-Q, Connett JE, Anthonisen NR, Sandford AJ. Polymorphisms in the IL13, IL13RA1, and IL4RA genes and rate of decline in lung function in smokers. *Am J Respir Cell Mol Biol* 2003;28:379–85

60. Orie NGM, Sluiter HJ, De Vreis K, *et al.* The host factor in bronchitis. In Orie NGM, Sluiter HJ, eds. *Bronchitis, an international symposium*. Assen, Netherlands: Royal Vangorcum, 1961

61. Pride N. Smoking, allergy and airways obstruction: revival of the 'Dutch hypothesis'. *Clin Allergy* 1986;16:3–6

62. Vestbo J, Prescott E. Update on the 'Dutch hypothesis' for chronic respiratory disease. *Thorax* 1998;53:S15–19

63. Celedon JC, Speizer FE, Drazen JM, *et al.* Bronchodilator responsiveness and serum total IgE levels in families of probands with severe early-onset COPD. *Eur Respir J* 1999;14:1009–14

64. Xu X, Rijcken B, Schouten JP, *et al.* Airways responsiveness and development and remission of chronic respiratory symptoms in adults. *Lancet* 1997;350:1431–4

65. Tashkin DP, Altose MD, Connett JE, Kanner RE, Lee WW, Wise RA. Methacholine reactivity predicts changes in lung function over time in smokers with early chronic obstructive pulmonary disease. The

Lung Health Study Research Group. *Am J Respir Crit Care Med* 1996;153:1802–11

66. Hospers JJ, Postma DS, Rijcken B, *et al.* Histamine airway hyper-responsiveness and mortality from chronic obstructive pulmonary disease: a cohort study. *Lancet* 2000;356:1313–17

67. Vestbo J, Hansen EF. Airway hyperresponsiveness and COPD mortality. *Thorax* 2001;56(Suppl 2): 11–14

68. Hansen EF, Phanareth K, Laursen LC, *et al.* Reversible and irreversible airflow obstruction as predictor of overall mortality in asthma and chronic obstructive pulmonary disease. *Am J Respir Crit Care Med* 1999;159:1267–71

69. Britton JR, Pavord ID, Richards KA, *et al.* Dietary antioxidant vitamin intake and lung function in the general population. *Am J Respir Crit Care Med* 1995;151:1383–7

70. Morabia A, Sorenson A, Kumanyika SK, *et al.* Vitamin A, cigarette smoking, and airway obstruction. *Am Rev Respir Dis* 1989;140:1312–16

71. Shahar E, Folsom AR, Melnick SL, *et al.* Does dietary vitamin A protect against airway obstruction? The Atherosclerosis Risk in Communities (ARIC) Study Investigators. *Am J Respir Crit Care Med* 1994;150:978–82

72. McKeever TM, Scrivener S, Broadfield E, *et al.* Prospective study of diet and decline in lung function in a general population. *Am J Respir Crit Care Med* 2002;165:1299–303

73. Shahar E, Folsom AR, Melnick SL, *et al.* Dietary n-3 polyunsaturated fatty acids and smoking-related chronic obstructive pulmonary disease. *N Engl J Med* 1994;331:228–33

74. Sharp DS, Rodriguez BL, Shahar E, *et al.* Fish consumption may limit the damage of smoking on the lung. *Am J Respir Crit Care Med* 1994;150:983–7

75. Tabak C, Smit HA, Rasanen L, *et al.* Dietary factors and pulmonary function: a cross sectional study in middle aged men from three European countries. *Thorax* 1999;54:1021–6

76. Tabak C, Arts IC, Smit HA, *et al.* Chronic obstructive pulmonary disease and intake of catechins, flavonols, and flavones: the MORGEN Study. *Am J Respir Crit Care Med* 2001;164:61–4

77. Watson L, Margetts B, Howarth P, *et al.* The association between diet and chronic obstructive pulmonary disease in subjects selected from general practice. *Eur Respir J* 2002;20:313–18

78. Durak I, Avci A, Kacmaz M, *et al.* Comparison of antioxidant potentials of red wine, white wine, grape juice and alcohol. *Curr Med Res Opin* 1999;15:316–20

79. Garshick E, Segal MR, Worobec TG, *et al.* Alcohol consumption and chronic obstructive pulmonary disease. *Am Rev Respir Dis* 1989;140:373–8

80. Barker DJ, Osmond C, Law CM. The intrauterine and early postnatal origins of cardiovascular disease and chronic bronchitis. *J Epidemiol Community Health* 1989;43:237–40

81. Hagstrom B, Nyberg P, Nilsson PM. Asthma in adult life – is there an association with birth weight? *Scand J Prim Health Care* 1998;16:117–20

82. Guerra S, Sherrill DL, Bobadilla A, *et al.* The relation of body mass index to asthma, chronic bronchitis, and emphysema. *Chest* 2002;122:1256–63

83. Agusti AGN, Noguera A, Sauleda J, *et al.* Systematic effects of chronic obstructive pulmonary disease. *Eur Respir J* 2003;21:347–60

84. Wouters EF, Creutzberg EC, Schols AM. Systemic effects in COPD. *Chest* 2002;121(Suppl 5):127–30S

85. Feinleib M, Rosenberg HM, Collins JG, *et al.* Trends in COPD morbidity and mortality in the United States. *Am Rev Respir Dis* 1989;140:S9–18

86. Xu X, Weiss ST, Rijcken B, *et al.* Smoking, changes in smoking habits, and rate of decline in FEV1: new insight into gender differences. *Eur Respir J* 1994;7:1056–61

87. Gold DR, Wang X, Wypij D, *et al.* Effects of cigarette smoking on lung function in adolescent boys and girls. *N Engl J Med* 1996;335:931–7

88. Prescott E, Bjerg AM, Andersen PK, *et al.* Gender difference in smoking effects on lung function and risk of hospitalization for COPD: results from a Danish longitudinal population study. *Eur Respir J* 1997;10:822–7

89. Silverman EK, Weiss ST, Drazen JM, *et al.* Gender-related differences in severe, early-onset chronic obstructive pulmonary disease. *Am J Respir Crit Care Med* 2000;162:2152–8

90. Schwartz J, Katz SA, Fegley RW, Tockman MS. Sex and race differences in the development of lung function. *Am Rev Respir Dis* 1988;138:1415–21

91. Prescott E, Bjerg AM, Andersen PK, *et al.* Importance of detailed adjustment for smoking when comparing morbidity and mortality in men and women in a Danish population study. *Eur J Publ Health* 1998;8:166–9

92. Dennis RJ, Maldonado D, Norman S, *et al.* Woodsmoke exposure and risk for obstructive airways disease among women. *Chest* 1996;109:115–19

93. Behera D, Jindal SK. Respiratory symptoms in Indian women using domestic cooking fuels. *Chest* 1991;100:385–8

94. Birring SS, Brightling CE, Bradding P, *et al.* Clinical, radiologic, and induced sputum features of chronic obstructive pulmonary disease in nonsmokers: a descriptive study. *Am J Respir Crit Care Med* 2002;166:1078–83

95. Kanner RE, Connett JE, Williams DE, *et al.* Effects of randomized assignment to a smoking cessation intervention and changes in smoking habits on respiratory symptoms in smokers with early chronic obstructive pulmonary disease: the Lung Health Study. *Am J Med* 1999;106:410–6

96. Scanlon PD, Connett JE, Waller LA, *et al.* Smoking cessation and lung function in mild-to-moderate chronic obstructive pulmonary disease. The Lung Health Study. *Am J Respir Crit Care Med* 2000;161:381–90

97. Murray RP, Anthonisen NR, Connett JE, *et al.* Effects of multiple attempts to quit smoking and relapses to smoking on pulmonary function. Lung Health Study Research Group. *J Clin Epidemiol* 1998;51:1317–26

98. Pride NB. Smoking cessation: effects on symptoms, spirometry and future trends in COPD. *Thorax* 2001;56 (Suppl 2):7–10

99. Anthonisen NR, Connett JE, Murray RP. Smoking and lung function of lung health study participants after 11 years. *Am J Respir Crit Care Med* 2002;166:675–9

100. Cook DG, Strachan DP, Carey IM. Health effects of passive smoking. 9. Parental smoking and spirometric indices in children. *Thorax* 1998;53:884–93

101. Cook DG, Strachan DP. Health effects of passive smoking.10. Summary of effects of parental smoking on the respiratory health of children and implications for research. *Thorax* 1999;54:357–66

102. Morgan WJ. Maternal smoking and infant lung function. Further evidence for an in utero effect. *Am J Respir Crit Care Med* 1998;158:689–90

103. Vilagoftis H, Schwingshackl A, Milne CD, *et al.* Protease-activated receptor-2-mediated matrix metalloproteinase-9 release from airway epithelial cells. *J Allergy Clin Immunol* 2000;106:537–45

104. Tashkin DP, Simmons MS, Sherrill DL, Coulson AH. Heavy habitual marijuana smoking does not cause an accelerated decline in FEV$_1$ with age. *Am J Respir Crit Care Med* 1997;155:141–8

105. Van Hoozen BE, Cross CE. Marijuana. Respiratory tract effects. *Clin Rev Allergy Immunol* 1997;15:243–69

106. Johnson MK, Smith RP, Mirison D, Laszlo G, White RJ. Large lung bullae in marijuana smokers. *Thorax* 2000;55:340–2

107. Roth MD, Arora A, Barsky SH, Kleerup EC, Simmons M, Tashkin DP. Airway inflammation in young marijuana and tobacco smokers. *Am J Respir Crit Care Med* 1998;157:928–37

108. Fligiel SE, Roth MD, Kleerup EC, Barsky SH, Simmons MS, Tashkin DP. Tracheobronchial histopathology in habitual smokers of cocaine, marijuana, and/or tobacco. *Chest* 1997;112:319–26

109. Abbey DE, Burchette RJ, Knutsen SF, *et al.* Long-term particulate and other air pollutants and lung function in nonsmokers. *Am J Respir Crit Care Med* 1998;158:289–98

110. Viegi G, Sandstrom T, eds. Air pollution effects in the elderly. Proceedings of a workshop held in Pisa, Italy, on March 12–14, 2001. *Eur Respir J* 2003; 21(Suppl 40):1–95S

111. Dossing M, Khan J, al Rabiah F. Risk factors for chronic obstructive lung disease in Saudi Arabia. *Respir Med* 1994;88:519–22

112. Perez-Padilla R, Regalado J, Vedal S, Pare P, Chapela R, Sansores R, *et al.* Exposure to biomass smoke and chronic airway disease in Mexican women. A case-control study. *Am J Respir Crit Care Med* 1996;154:701–6

113. Amoli K. Bronchopulmonary disease in Iranian housewives chronically exposed to indoor smoke. *Eur Respir J* 1998;11:659–63

114. Pandey MR. Prevalence of chronic bronchitis in a rural community of the Hill Region of Nepal. *Thorax* 1984;39:331–6

115. Pandey MR. Domestic smoke pollution and chronic bronchitis in a rural community of the Hill Region of Nepal. *Thorax* 1984;39:337–9

116. Smith KR. National burden of disease in India from indoor air pollution. *Proc Natl Acad Sci USA* 2000;97:13286–93

117. Hendrick DJ. Occupational and chronic obstructive pulmonary disease (COPD). *Thorax* 1996;51: 947–55

118. Heederik D, Kromhout H, Burema J, *et al.* Occupational exposure and 25-year incidence rate of

non-specific lung disease: the Zutphen Study. *Int J Epidemiol* 1990;19:945–52

119. Post WK, Heederik D, Kromhout H, *et al.* Occupational exposures estimated by a population specific job exposure matrix and 25 year incidence rate of chronic nonspecific lung disease (CNSLD): the Zutphen Study. *Eur Respir J* 1994;7:1048–55

120. Humerfelt S, Gulsvik A, Skjaerven R, Nilssen S, Kvale G, Sulheim O, *et al.* Decline in FEV1 and airflow limitation related to occupational exposures in men of an urban community. *Eur Respir J* 1993;6:1095–103

121. Humerfelt S, Eide GE, Gulsvik A. Association of years of occupational quartz exposure with spirometric airflow limitation in Norwegian men aged 30–46 years. *Thorax* 1998;53:649–55

122. Oxman OD, Guyatt GH. Guidelines for reading literature reviews. *Can Med Assoc J* 1988;138:697–703

123. Oxman AD, Muir DC, Shannon HS, *et al.* Occupational dust exposure and chronic obstructive pulmonary disease. A systematic overview of the evidence. *Am Rev Respir Dis* 1993;148:38–48

124. Davison AG, Fayers PM, Taylor AJ, *et al.* Cadmium fume inhalation and emphysema. *Lancet* 1988;1:663–7

125. Strachan DP, Seagroatt V, Cook DG. Chest illness in infancy and chronic respiratory disease in later life: an analysis by month of birth. *Int J Epidemiol* 1994;23:1060–8

126. Barker DJ, Osmond C. Childhood respiratory infection and adult chronic bronchitis in England and Wales. *Br Med J* 1986;293:1271–5

127. Matsuse T, Hayashi S, Kuwano K, *et al.* Latent adenoviral infection in the pathogenesis of chronic airways obstruction. *Am Rev Respir Dis* 1992;146:177–84

128. Meshi B, Vitalis TZ, Ionescu D, *et al.* Emphysematous lung destruction by cigarette smoke. The effects of latent adenoviral infection on the lung inflammatory response. *Am J Respir Cell Mol Biol* 2002;26:52–7

129. Retamales I, Elliott WM, Meshi B, *et al.* Amplification of inflammation in emphysema and its association with latent adenoviral infection. *Am J Respir Crit Care Med* 2001;164:469–73

130. Diaz PT, Clanton TL, Pacht ER. Emphysema-like pulmonary disease associated with human immunodeficiency virus infection. *Ann Intern Med* 1992;116:124–8

131. Diaz PT, King MA, Pacht ER, *et al.* Increased susceptibility to pulmonary emphysema among HIV-seropositive smokers. *Ann Intern Med* 2000;132:369–72

132. Diaz PT, King MA, Pacht ER, *et al.* The pathophysiology of pulmonary diffusion impairment in human immunodeficiency virus infection. *Am J Respir Crit Care Med* 1999;160:272–7

133. Diaz PT, King MA, Pacht ER, *et al.* Increased susceptibility to pulmonary emphysema among HIV-seropositive smokers. *Ann Intern Med* 2000;132:369–72

134. Beck JM, Rosen MJ, Peavy HH. Pulmonary complications of HIV infection. Report of the Fourth NHLBI Workshop. *Am J Respir Crit Care Med* 2001;164:2120–6

135. Kanner RE, Anthonisen NR, Connett JE. Lower respiratory illnesses promote FEV(1) decline in current smokers but not ex-smokers with mild chronic obstructive pulmonary disease: results from the lung health study. *Am J Respir Crit Care Med* 2001;164:358–64

136. Donaldson GC, Seemungal TA, Bhowmik A, *et al.* Relationship between exacerbation frequency and lung function decline in chronic obstructive pulmonary disease. *Thorax* 2002;57:847–52

137. Partridge MR. Patients with COPD: do we fail them from beginning to end? *Thorax* 2003;58:373–5

138. Tobin MJ. Chronic obstructive pulmonary disease, pollution, pulmonary vascular disease, transplantation, pleural disease and lung cancer in AJRCCM 2002. *Am J Respir Crit Care Med* 2003;167:356–70

139. Croxton TL, Weinmann GG, Senior RM, Wise RA, Crapo JD, Buist AS. Clinical research in chronic obstructive pulmonary disease: needs and opportunities. *Am J Respir Crit Care Med* 2003;167:1142–9

2

The pathophysiology of COPD

CONTENTS

Tobacco smoke

Amplified inflammation

Cells and their actions
Macrophages
T cells
Neutrophils
Eosinophils
Epithelial cells
Fibroblasts

Inflammatory mediators
Leukotriene B_4
IL-8 and chemokines
TNF-α
TGF-β_1
IL-13
Endothelin-1

Oxidative stress
Reactive oxygen species
Impaired antioxidant defenses
Mechanisms of oxidant damage

Protease–antiprotease imbalance

Fibrosis

The pathology of COPD
Chronic bronchitis
Obstructive bronchiolitis
Emphysema
Pulmonary vascular disease
Systemic extrapulmonary effects

Asthma compared with COPD

SUMMARY

Oxidants, inflammation, repair, fibrosis, proteolysis and tissue remodelling

Following chronic exposure to oxidants in cigarette smoke and other inhaled noxious agents, patients with COPD have an amplified inflammatory response in the airways and lung parenchyma (Figure 2.1). Epithelial cell injury and macrophage activation cause release of chemotactic factors that recruit neutrophils from the circulation. Macrophages and neutrophils then release proteases, with involvement of matrix metalloproteinases (MMPs) and neutrophil elastase (NE) which break down connective tissue. Cytotoxic CD8+ T cells may also be involved in this inflammatory cascade. Over many years of injury, cycles of inflammation and repair occur which may result in resolution, but which can be associated with proteolysis, fibrosis, and both airway and parenchymal remodelling.

Pathology at five sites

At five separate anatomical sites, different pathological events occur, with distinct physiological sequelae, that result in varying clinical manifestations (Figure 2.2):

- *Chronic bronchitis*: chronic inflammation of the central airways results in mucus hyper-secretion, and a chronic productive cough

- *Obstructive bronchiolitis*: inflammation of the peripheral airways results in local airway wall fibrosis and remodelling and manifests as obstructive airways disease

- *Emphysema*: proteolytic destruction, together with remodelling, occurs in the respiratory bronchioles and alveoli. Lung parenchymal destruction and remodelling cause various types of emphysema; in advanced cases, impaired gas exchange results in hypoxic respiratory failure

- *Pulmonary vascular disease and cor pulmonale*: destruction of the pulmonary capillary bed and inflammation of pulmonary arterial vessels cause pulmonary arterial hypertension and, in turn, right-sided heart failure. This heart disease arising from lung pathology is known as *cor pulmonale*

- *Systemic disease*: extrapulmonary inflammatory disease occurs in advanced COPD, causing cachexia and loss of fat-free mass, with respiratory and peripheral muscle weakness.

Figure 2.1   Inflammatory mechanisms in COPD

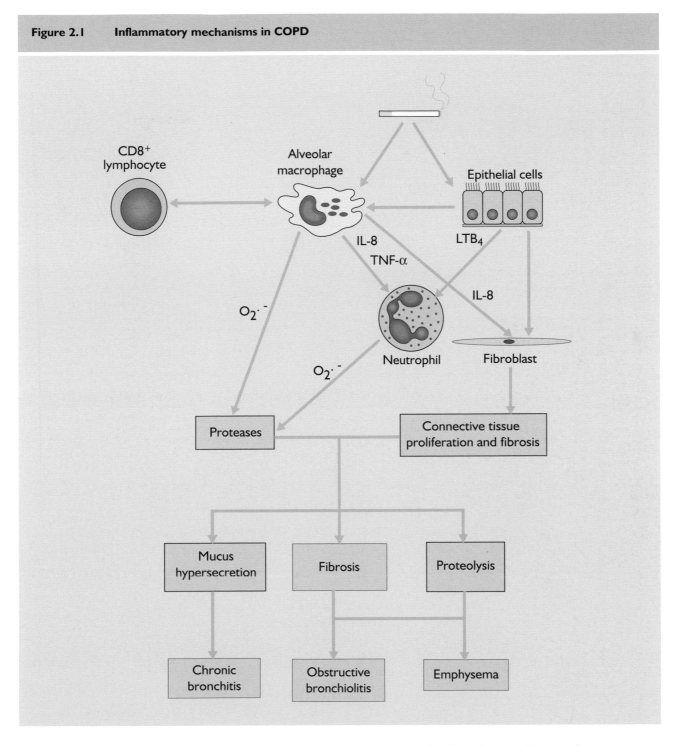

Oxidants within cigarette smoke, as well as other irritants, activate epithelial cells and macrophages in the respiratory tract to release neutrophil chemotactic factors, including interleukin-8 (IL-8) and leukotriene B_4 (LTB$_4$). In addition, tissue macrophages and neutrophils are a potent source of oxidants ($O_2\cdot^-$) and proteases, the latter being normally inhibited by a panel of endogenous protease inhibitors. The role of the increased numbers of CD8+ T lymphocytes remains obscure. Mucus hypersecretion in the large airways is manifest as chronic bronchitis, while fibrosis and remodelling of the small airways causes obstructive bronchiolitis. Proteolysis, fibrosis and remodelling are prominent features in the pathology of emphysema. Vascular endothelial cells, pneumocytes and mast cells may also contribute to the pathogenesis of COPD.

Figure 2.2   **Pathophysiology of COPD**

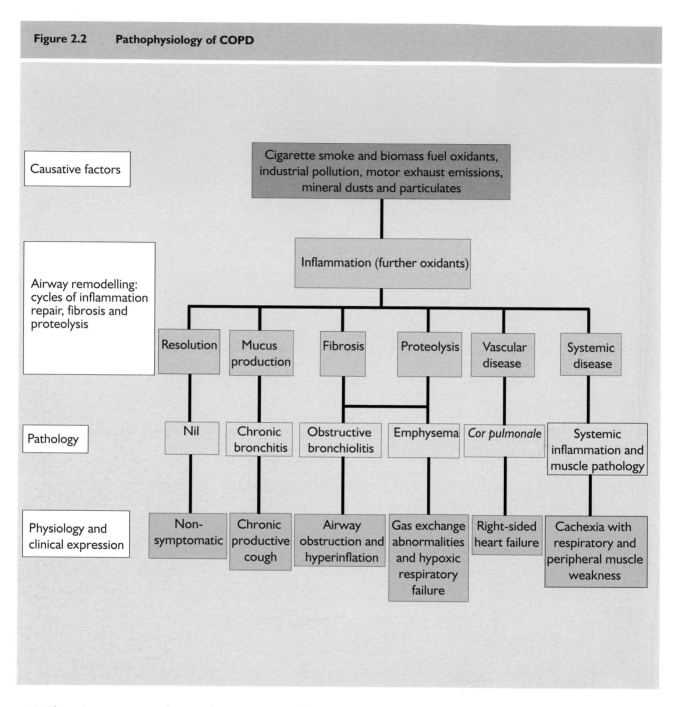

Oxidants in cigarette smoke are the major cause of COPD, but a variety of other factors contribute. An amplified inflammatory response is a feature of COPD, and is associated with cycles of resolution, mucus production, fibrosis and proteolysis. The pathology of COPD involves five sites: the large central airways (chronic bronchitis), the small peripheral airways (obstructive bronchiolitis), the lung parenchyma (emphysema), the cardiovascular system (*cor pulmonale*) and respiratory and peripheral muscles (systemic disease).

TOBACCO SMOKE

Cigarette smoke is a heterogeneous aerosol generated by incomplete burning of tobacco leaves. It is composed of gaseous, volatile and particulate components, with up to 95% of the weight of smoke in the gaseous phase. Each inhalation of cigarette smoke is said to contain of the order of 10^{17} reactive oxygen species (ROS) molecules. More than 400 substances are present in cigarette smoke, including oxidants, pharmacologically active compounds such as nicotine, mutagens and carcinogens, as well as antigenic and cytotoxic components. Nicotine is a toxic plant alkaloid that stimulates acetylcholine receptors at autonomic ganglia of both the sympathetic and parasympathetic systems. In addition, nicotine has stimulant activities at neuromuscular receptor sites and in the central nervous system.

Carbon monoxide interferes with oxygen transport and utilization due to formation of carboxyhemoglobin, while carcinogens include aromatic hydrocarbons, amines, and nitrosamines.

AMPLIFIED INFLAMMATION

Cigarette smoking and other inhaled irritants initiate an inflammatory response in the peripheral airways and lung parenchyma. Inflammation in normal smokers is very similar in terms of inflammatory cells, mediators and proteases to inflammation in patients with COPD, but is less pronounced. This suggests that the inflammation in lungs of patients with COPD represents an exaggeration of the normal inflammatory response to irritants such as cigarette smoke (Figure 2.3)[1]. The mechanisms for

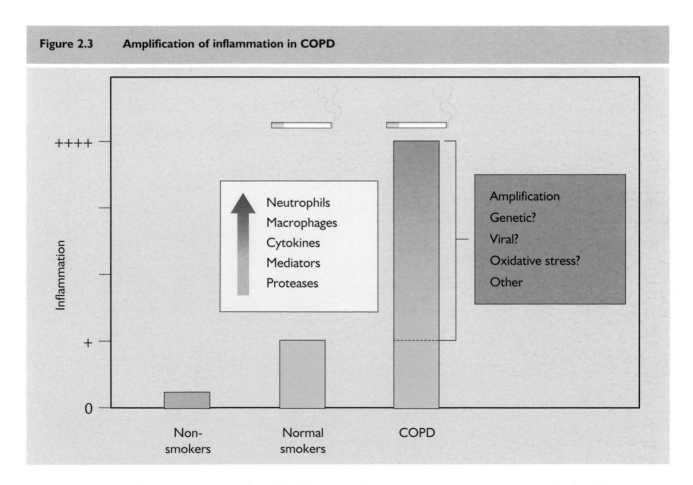

Figure 2.3   Amplification of inflammation in COPD

Heavy smokers without COPD ('normal smokers') have an inflammatory response to cigarette smoke, but this appears to be amplified in patients with COPD. This has become established from studies on sputum and bronchoalveolar lavage (BAL) in COPD, which have demonstrated elevation in numbers and activity of neutrophils and macrophages, cytokines, inflammatory mediators and proteins. The molecular mechanisms of this amplification are currently unknown but may result from genetic factors, viruses (adenovirus and respiratory infections during exacerbations) and increased levels of oxidative stress.

this amplification are not yet certain, but may be determined by genetic factors[2], latent viruses (such as adenovirus)[3,4] and impaired histone deacetylase activity. Histone acetylation causes the activation of nuclear core histones, resulting in the transcription of genes that cause inflammation. The reversal of this process by histone deacetylase is impaired in alveolar macrophages from patients with COPD[5,6].

CELLS AND THEIR ACTIONS

COPD causes a particular type of inflammation especially associated with mononuclear cells (macrophages and CD8+ T cells), as well as neutrophils. This inflammation may resolve or become associated with fibrosis, proteolysis and remodelling. The natures of the inflammatory infiltrate are broadly similar in large and small airways, as well as within the alveoli and pulmonary artery wall.

Macrophages

Macrophages are activated by cigarette smoke and other inhaled irritants, and are thought to play an important role in driving the inflammatory process in COPD (Figure 2.4). Macrophage numbers are

Figure 2.4	Macrophages in COPD

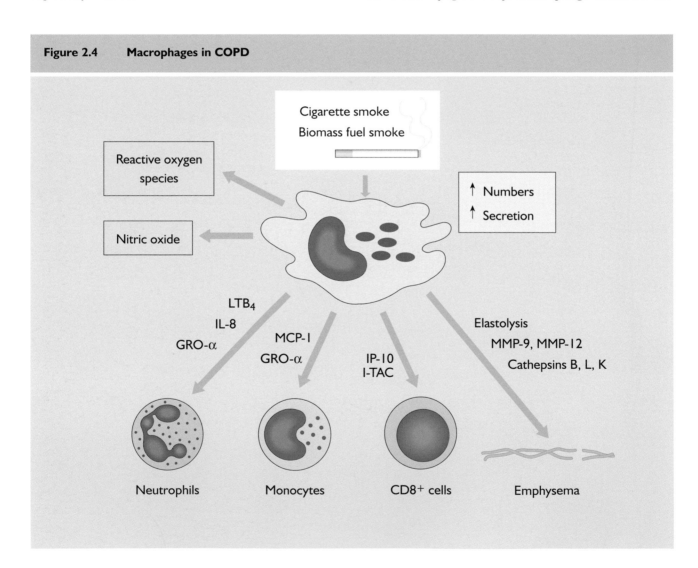

Increased numbers of macrophages are present in the airways and parenchyma of patients with COPD. These macrophages generate reactive oxygen species, nitric oxide and chemokines that attract neutrophils, monocytes and T cells into inflamed tissue. LTB$_4$, leukotriene B$_4$; IL-8, interleukin-8; MCP-1, monocyte chemotactic protein-1; GRO-α, growth-related oncogene-α; IP-10, interferon γ-inducible protein-10; MMP, matrix metalloproteinase, I-TAC, interferon-inducible T cell alpha chemoattractant

increased in bronchoalveolar lavage (BAL) fluid of patients with COPD[7], and are concentrated in the centriacinar zones where emphysema is most marked[3,8]. Furthermore, the number of macrophages in the alveolar wall correlates with the amount of parenchymal destruction in emphysema[8], and the number of macrophages in the airways correlates with the severity of airways obstruction[9]. Macrophages may be responsible for the continued proteolytic activity in the lungs of patients with emphysema, and they release increased amounts of inflammatory mediators and proteinases in COPD. Indeed, macrophages may be activated by cigarette smoke to release inflammatory mediators, including tumor necrosis factor-α (TNF-α), interleukin-8 (IL-8), leukotriene B$_4$ (LTB$_4$) and reactive oxygen species. Alveolar macrophages are long-lived cells,

and there is indirect evidence that they may have prolonged survival in COPD, since the anti-apoptotic protein Bcl-XL is increased[10]. Significant increases are reported in the numbers of subepithelial CD68+ macrophages in chronic bronchitis[11–13].

T cells

Significant increases are reported in the numbers of CD45 (total leukocytes), CD3 (T lymphocytes), CD25+ and VLA-1+ (very late antigen) cells in chronic bronchitis[11]. T lymphocytes increase in the surface epithelium and the subepithelium[12,13]. In COPD, the CD8+ (cytotoxic/suppressor) lymphocyte increases in number and proportion to become the predominant T cell subset (Figure 2.5). The increases of CD8+ cells are associated with a decline

Figure 2.5   Cytotoxic T cells and interferon-γ (IFN-γ) in COPD

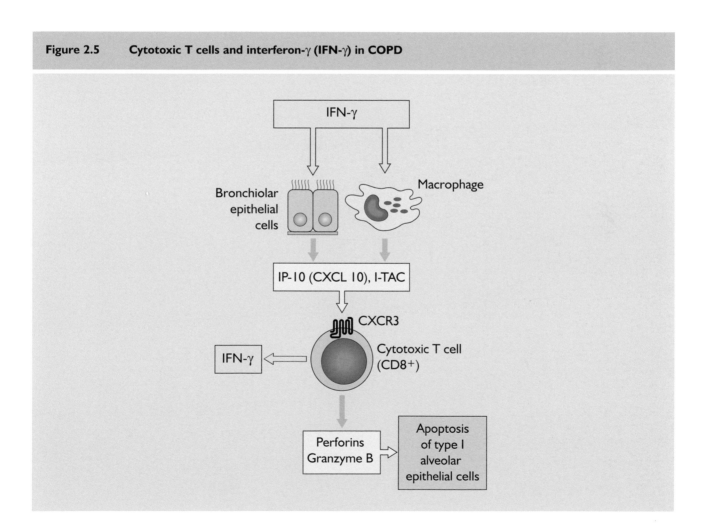

CD8+ T cells are a prominent population in the airways of patients with COPD, and these cells are attracted chemotactically via CXCR3 by interferon γ-inducible protein-10 (IP-10). CD8+ T cells produce interferon-γ, perforins, granzyme B and TNF-α; these induce apoptosis in type I alveolar cells, destruction of which could contribute to emphysema. I-TAC, interferon-inducible T cell alpha chemoattractant

in lung function[12]. The increases of the CD8 pheno-type and of the CD8/CD4 ratio occur in both the mucosa and submucosa, and are associated with mucus-secreting glands[12,14]. There are increased numbers of CD8+ T cells in the central and periph-eral airways as well as lung parenchyma in COPD[8,12,15,16]. These cells may contribute to patho-physiology via the release of granzymes, perforins and TNF-α, which induce apoptosis in type I alveo-lar cells[15,17,18]. It is not known whether the CD8+ T cells in COPD are predominantly Tc1 (interferon-γ-producing) or Tc2 (IL-4-producing)[19].

Neutrophils

The role of the neutrophil in COPD is controversial (Figure 2.6). It is not understood why the increased number of neutrophils found in BAL fluid and sputum from subjects with COPD[20–24] is not usually seen in the bronchial mucosa, at least in the subepithelial zone where the biopsy is generally quantified[8,12,22]. This may be due to rapid transit of neutrophils through the airways and parenchyma. Other studies demonstrate the close relationship of neutrophils with the surface epithelium and mucus-secreting

---

Figure 2.6   Neutrophils in COPD

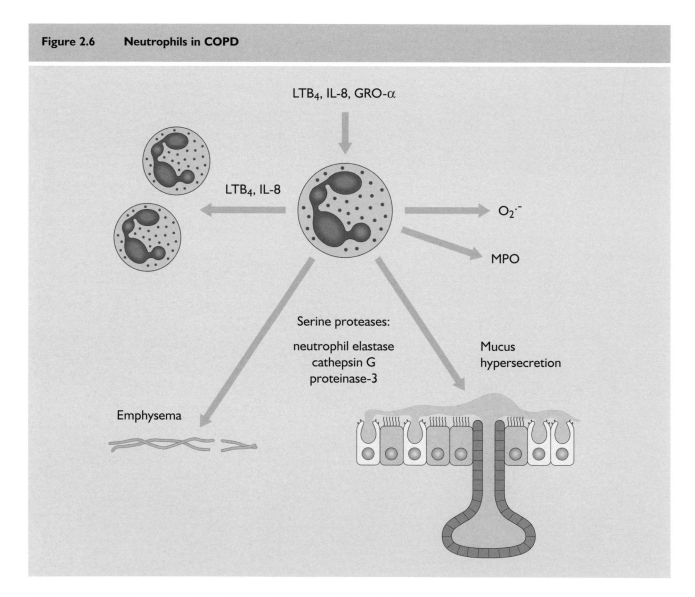

Neutrophils (polymorphonuclear leukocytes) are circulating leukocytes that are attracted into tissue sites by leukotriene B_4 (LTB$_4$), interleukin-8 (IL-8) and growth-related oncogene-α (GRO-α). Neutrophils themselves produce LTB$_4$ and IL-8, superoxide anion (O_2^-) and myeloperoxidase (MPO). Neutrophils contain potent serine proteases including neutrophil elastase, cathepsin-G and proteinase-3. These proteases may contribute to emphysema and the mucus hypersecretion of chronic bronchitis.

glands[14,25]. The reasons and consequences of the compartmentalization of distinct inflammatory cells in the airway mucosa will need to be considered in the future. Interestingly, rapid decline in FEV_1 in smokers is associated with increased levels of sputum neutrophils[26]. Mucosal biopsies and induced sputum from ex-smokers show similar inflammatory processes, suggesting that inflammation may persist in the airway once established[27,28].

Neutrophils secrete serine proteases, including neutrophil elastase, cathepsin G, and proteinase-3. These enzymes may contribute to alveolar destruction, and are also potent mucus stimulants. Neutrophil recruitment to the airways involves vascular adhesion, and E-selectin is upregulated on the bronchial endothelium in COPD[29]. It is likely that neutrophil chemotactic factors are released from activated macrophages and possibly from epithelial cells and CD8+ (cytotoxic) T lymphocytes; these include IL-8 and LTB$_4$. Neutrophilia is likely to be linked to mucus hypersecretion in chronic bronchitis, and neutrophil numbers in bronchial biopsies and sputum are correlated with disease severity[9,21]. However, a negative association has been reported between the number of neutrophils and the extent of alveolar destruction[8]. Although neutrophils have the capacity to cause elastolysis, this is not a prominent feature of cystic fibrosis and bronchiectasis, where chronic airway neutrophilia is more prominent.

Eosinophils

There are some reports of increased numbers of inactive eosinophils in the airways and BAL of patients with stable COPD, although others have not found these increases[30]. It has been noted that the presence of eosinophils predicts a response to corticosteroids, and may indicate coexisting asthma with COPD[31,32]. It is possible that eosinophils may have degranulated and no longer be recognizable in COPD, since eosinophil cationic protein and eosinophil peroxidase are elevated in sputum from COPD patients[23]. In support of this, neutrophil elastase causes degranulation of human eosinophils *in vitro*[33]. There is a small, but significantly increased, number of tissue eosinophils in COPD compared to that found in healthy control subjects, although it has been suggested that these eosinophils do not degranulate[22]. Airways resected from the lungs of heavy smokers demonstrate marked gene expression for both IL-4 and IL-5, and this eosinophilia is associated

with the bronchial glands of subjects with chronic bronchitis[34]. However, the most pronounced eosinophilia occurs when there is an exacerbation of COPD[29,35-37]. Sputum eosinophilia also occurs in cases of 'eosinophilic bronchitis', in patients without a history of asthma and without bronchial hyper-responsiveness[38].

Epithelial cells

Airway epithelial cells are likely to be an important source of mediators in COPD. Epithelial cells are activated by cigarette smoke to produce TNF-α and IL-8, while transforming growth factor (TGF)-β may induce local fibrosis[39]. Vascular endothelial growth factor (VEGF) may be necessary to maintain alveolar cell survival, and blockade of VEGF receptors (VEGFR2) in rats induces apoptosis of alveolar cells and an emphysema-like pathology[40].

Fibroblasts

Overactivity of fibroblasts results in excessive production of extracellular matrix proteins within the small airways. Small airway fibrosis is prominent in obstructive bronchiolitis.

INFLAMMATORY MEDIATORS

There are multiple cells and mediators involved in the pathology of COPD (Figure 2.7).

Leukotriene B$_4$

There are increased amounts of LTB$_4$, a potent chemoattractant of neutrophils, in the sputum of patients with COPD[41]. LTB$_4$ is probably derived from alveolar macrophages and the neutrophils themselves. Alveolar macrophages from patients with α_1-antitrypsin deficiency secrete greater amounts of LTB$_4$[42].

IL-8 and chemokines

IL-8, a chemoattractant for neutrophils, is present in high concentrations in induced sputum of patients with COPD[21,43], and is found in increased amounts in BAL fluid[7]. IL-8 may be secreted by macrophages, neutrophils and by airway epithelial cells[44]. IL-8 may be important in the neutrophilic inflammation found in induced sputum of patients with COPD and is

29

Figure 2.7   Multiple cells and mediators in COPD

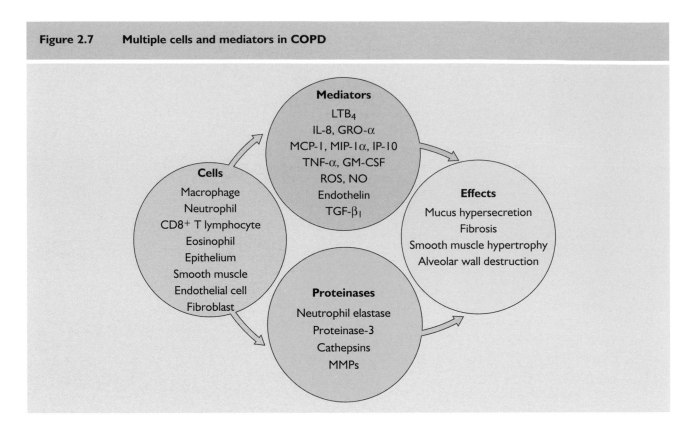

LTB$_4$, leukotriene B$_4$; IL-8, interleukin-8; GRO-α, growth-related oncogene-α; MCP-1, monocyte chemotactic protein-1; MIP-1α, monocyte inflammatory protein-1α; GM-CSF, granulocyte-macrophage colony stimulating factor; ROS, reactive oxygen species; NO, nitric oxide; MMP, matrix metalloproteinases.

Figure 2.8   CXC chemokine receptors

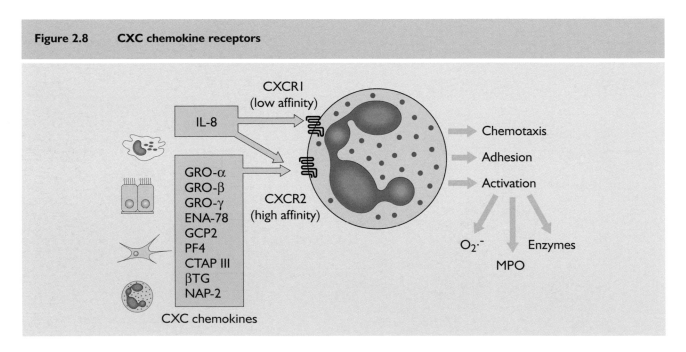

Interleukin-8 (IL-8) binds to both a low affinity CX chemokine receptor (CXCR1) as well as a high affinity CX chemokine receptor (CXCR2). Amongst the family of CXC chemokines are growth-related oncogene-α, -β, -γ (GRO-α, -β, -γ), epithelial-derived neutrophil-activating peptide (ENA-78), granulocyte chemotactic protein (GCP), platelet factor 4 (PF4), chemokine connective tissue-activating peptide III (CTAP III), β-thromboglobulin (βTG), neutrophil-activating peptide-2 (NAP-2). Neutrophils produce superoxide anion (O$_2$·$^-$) and myeloperoxidase (MPO).

correlated with the number of neutrophils, which in turn correlate with the degree of airflow obstruction.

IL-8 signals through two receptors (Figure 2.8): a low-affinity CXCR1 specific for IL-8 that is involved in neutrophil activation, and a high-affinity CXCR2 that is activated by a range of CXC chemokines, including IL-8, growth-related oncogene (GRO-α, -β, -γ), and epithelial-derived neutrophil activating peptide, ENA-78. CXCR2 is involved in the chemotaxis of neutrophils and monocytes. The CC chemokine, macrophage chemotactic peptide-1 (MCP-1), is increased in BAL of COPD patients[45]. MCP-1 is a potent chemoattractant for monocytes, and acts via CCR2. GRO-α is elevated in COPD[46] and is chemotactic for monocytes as well as neutrophils. It may therefore contribute to the increased numbers of macrophages that are derived from blood monocytes in COPD.

TNF-α

TNF-α is present in high concentration in the sputum of COPD patients[21], especially during exacerbations[47]. TNF-α may activate the transcription of NF-κB, which switches on the transcription of inflammatory genes, including chemokine (IL-8) genes and proteases, in macrophages and epithelial cells[48] (Figure 2.9). Serum concentrations of TNF-α and stimulated TNF-α production from peripheral blood monocytes are increased in weight-losing COPD patients[49], and TNF-α inhibits the expression of skeletal muscle proteins via activation of NF-κB[50]. Inhibitors of TNF-α may be useful to reduce both the inflammatory response and skeletal muscle wasting seen in COPD[51].

Figure 2.9   TNF-α and IL-8 in COPD

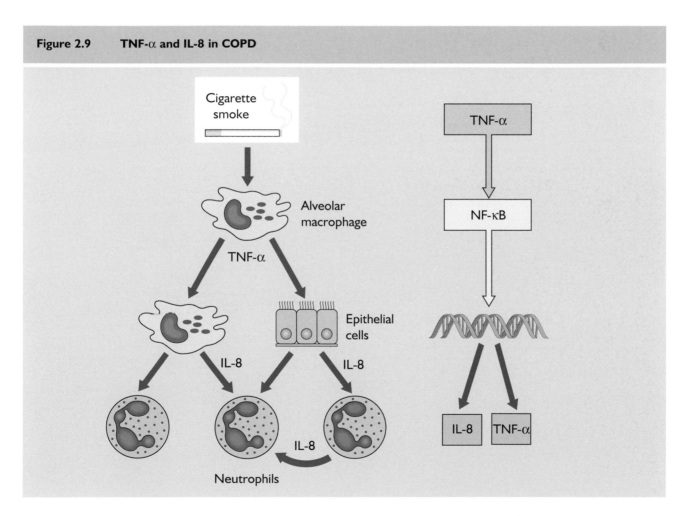

Cigarette smoke activates macrophages to release tumor necrosis factor-α (TNF-α) which releases interleukin-8 (IL-8) via activation of the transcription factor nuclear factor-κB (NF-κB). IL-8 attracts neutrophils, which themselves secrete IL-8 to perpetuate the response. There are increased levels of TNF-α and IL-8 in induced sputum of patients with COPD compared to normal subjects, cigarette smokers without airway obstruction and patients with asthma.

TGF-β_1

Transforming growth factor-β_1 shows increased expression in small airway and alveolar epithelial cells in COPD, and participates in the fibrotic processes that take place in the small airways[39,52].

IL-13

IL-13 and interferon-γ are overexpressed in a murine form of emphysema that is mediated by increased expression of MMPs and cathepsins[53,54].

Endothelin-1

Endothelin-1 (ET-1) levels are increased in the sputum of patients with COPD, particularly during exacerbations[55,56]. ET-1 may be important in pulmonary vascular remodelling in severe pulmonary hypertension[57].

OXIDATIVE STRESS

Reactive oxygen species

There is considerable evidence that oxidative stress is increased in patients with COPD and that reactive oxygen species (ROS) contribute to the pathophysiology of COPD[58-62]. Each puff of cigarette smoke contains of the order of 10^{17} ROS molecules, and ROS are also produced endogenously by activated inflammatory cells, including neutrophils and

---

Figure 2.10   Oxidative stress in COPD

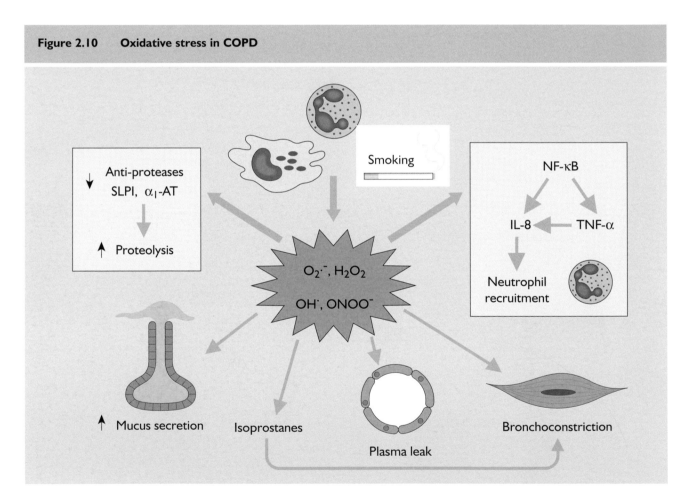

Reactive oxygen species (ROS) from cigarette smoke or from inflammatory cells result in several damaging effects in COPD, and are mediated by superoxide anion ($O_2^{\cdot-}$), hydrogen peroxide (H_2O_2), hydroxyl radicals ($OH^{\cdot}$) and peroxynitrite ($ONOO^-$). ROS cause decreased anti-protease defences, through inactivation of secretory leukoprotease inhibitor (SLPI) and α_1-antitrypsin (α_1-AT), and also mediate increased proteolysis. In addition, ROS cause activation of nuclear factor-κB (NF-κB), resulting in increased secretion of the cytokines interleukin-8 (IL-8) and tumor necrosis factor-α (TNF-α). For further details, see reference 62.

macrophages. A range of ROS cause a spectrum of effects in COPD (Figure 2.10):

- *Hydrogen peroxide* Increased levels of hydrogen peroxide (H_2O_2) are present in expired condensates from patients with COPD, particularly during exacerbations[63].

- *Ethane* There is an increase in concentrations of ethane in exhaled air, this being a product of lipid peroxidation[64].

- *Isoprostanes* Oxidative stress leads to the formation of isoprostanes by direct oxidation of arachidonic acid. 8-Isoprostane is found in exhaled breath condensate of COPD patients at elevated levels, which are related to disease severity[65,66]. Isoprostanes have several effects on airway function, including bronchoconstriction, increased plasma leakage and mucus hypersecretion.

- *Peroxynitrite* Superoxide anions ($O_2^{\cdot -}$) rapidly combine with nitric oxide ($NO\cdot$) to form the potent radical peroxynitrite ($ONOO^-$), which itself generates $OH^{\cdot}$. Peroxynitrite reacts with tyrosine residues within certain proteins to form 3-nitrotyrosines. These may be detected immunologically, with increased reactivity in

sputum macrophages from patients with COPD[60].

Impaired antioxidant defenses

There is evidence for a reduction in antioxidant defenses in patients with COPD, which may further enhance oxidative stress[58,61] (Figure 2.11). ROS are normally counteracted by endogenous (glutathione, uric acid, bilirubin) and exogenous (dietary vitamins C and E) antioxidants.

Mechanisms of oxidant damage

- *Proteases* Oxidants may contribute to the pathophysiology of COPD by induction of serum protease inhibitors, potentiation of elastase activity, direct activation of MMPs, and inactivation of antiproteases such as α_1-antitrypsin (α_1-AT) and secretory leukocyte protease inhibitor. Oxidants thus both directly increase proteolytic activity and decrease the antiprotease shield.

- *Mucus* Oxidants are potent mucus secretagogues

| Figure 2.11 | Oxidant–antioxidant imbalance in COPD |

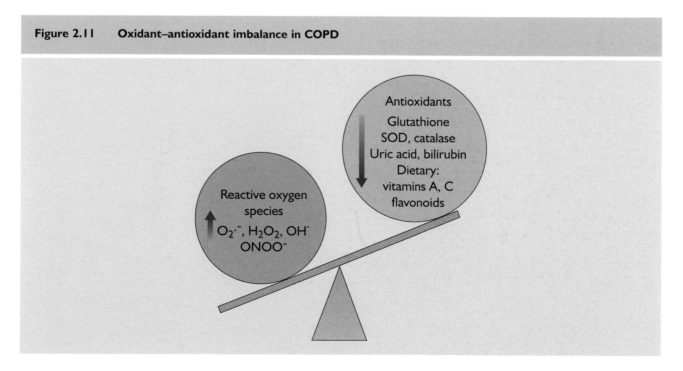

There is an excess of reactive oxygen species (ROS), including superoxide anion ($O_2^{\cdot -}$), hydrogen peroxide (H_2O_2), hydroxyl radicals ($OH^{\cdot}$) and peroxynitrite ($ONOO^-$). There is also a deficiency in antioxidants, including superoxide dismutase (SOD).

33

Figure 2.12   Protease–antiprotease imbalance in COPD

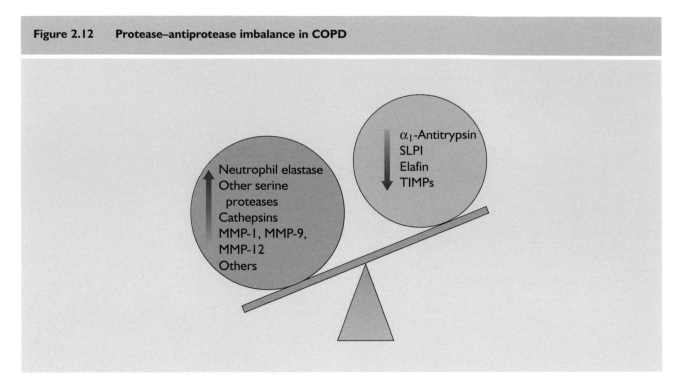

In COPD, the balance is tipped in favor of increased proteolysis. There is an increase in proteases, including neutrophil elastase, cathepsins and matrix metalloproteinases (MMP). There is also a deficiency in antiproteases, including α_1-antitrypsin, elafin, secretory leukoprotease inhibitor (SLPI) and tissue inhibitors of matrix metalloproteinases (TIMPs).

- *NF-κB* Oxidants activate the transcription factor, NF-κB, which orchestrates the transcription of many inflammatory genes, including IL-8, TNF-α, inducible NO synthase (iNOS) and inducible cyclooxygenase (COX-2).

- *Smooth muscle and vascular effects* Hydrogen peroxide directly constricts airway smooth muscle *in vitro*, while hydroxyl radicals (OH⁻) potently induce plasma exudation in airways.

PROTEASE–ANTIPROTEASE IMBALANCE

Emphysema is due to an imbalance between proteases (which digest elastin and other structural proteins in the alveolar wall) and antiproteases, that protect against this attack[67] (Figure 2.12).

Several proteases are likely to be involved in lung parenchymal destruction:

- *Neutrophil elastase*, a neutral serine protease, is a major constituent of lung elastolytic activity and also potently stimulates mucus secretion. In addition, neutrophil elastase induces IL-8 release from epithelial cells and therefore may perpetuate the inflammatory state. Although

neutrophil elastase is likely to be the major mechanism mediating elastolysis in patients with α_1-AT deficiency, it may well not be the major elastolytic enzyme in smoking-related COPD, and it is important to consider other enzymes as targets for inhibition.

- *Proteinase 3* is another neutral serine protease in neutrophils and may contribute to the elastolytic activity of these cells.

- *Cathepsin G* is another serine protease in neutrophils that has elastolytic activity. Cathepsins B, K, L and S are cysteine proteases that are released from macrophages and also have elastolytic activity.

- *Matrix metalloproteinases* (MMP) are a group of over 20 closely related endopeptidases that are capable of degrading all of the components of the extracellular matrix of lung parenchyma, including elastin, collagen, proteoglycans, laminin and fibronectin. They are produced by neutrophils, alveolar macrophages and airway epithelial cells[68] (Figure 2.13). Increased levels of collagenase (MMP-1) and gelatinase B (MMP-9) have been detected in BAL fluid of

Figure 2.13   Matrix metalloproteinases in COPD

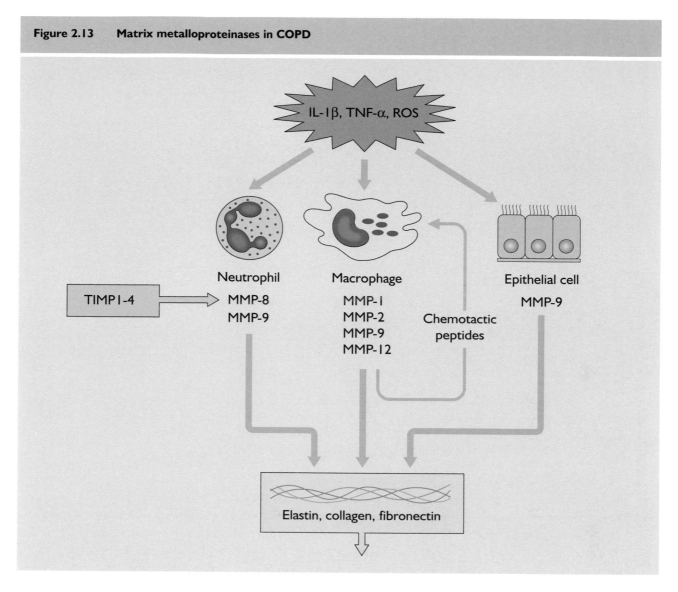

Interleukin-1β (IL-1β), tumor necrosis factor-α (TNF-α) and reactive oxygen species (ROS) cause activation of neutrophils, macrophages and epithelial cells. These cells release matrix metalloproteinases (MMPs), which are antagonized by tissue inhibitors of matrix metalloproteinases (TIMPs).

patients with emphysema[69]. BAL macrophages from patients with emphysema express more MMP-9 and MMP-1 than do cells from control subjects, suggesting that these cells, rather than neutrophils, may be the major cellular source[70,71]. Alveolar macrophages also express a unique MMP, macrophage metalloelastase (MMP-12). MMP-12 knock-out mice do not develop emphysema and do not show the expected increases in lung macrophages after long-term exposure to cigarette smoke[72]. MMP-12 does not appear to play a major role in humans, and MMP-9 is likely to be a major elastolytic enzyme in emphysema.

Counterbalancing these proteases are a range of antiproteases:

- α_1-AT, also known as α_1-protease inhibitor, is the major antiprotease in lung parenchyma. It is mainly derived from plasma and synthesized in the liver. Inheritance of homozygous α_1-AT deficiency may result in severe emphysema, particularly in cigarette smokers, but this genetic disease accounts for < 1% of cases of COPD. α_1-AT is not the only antiprotease.

- α_1-Antichymotrypsin is also present in the lungs, and heterozygous individuals who have lower than normal levels have an increased risk of COPD.

- *Secretory leukocyte protease inhibitor* (SLPI) is the most important protective mechanism in the airways. It is derived from airway epithelial cells and provides a local protective mechanism.

- *Tissue inhibitors of metalloproteinases* (TIMPs) counteract the effect of matrix metalloproteinases.

- *Cystatins* counteract the effect of cathepsins.

FIBROSIS

MMP-9 may play a role in the activation of TGF-β_1[73,74], as well as with the release of chemotactic peptides and activation of α_1-AT (Figure 2.14), this being involved closely with both proteolysis and fibrosis. Protease-activated receptor 2 (PAR-2) is a transmembrane receptor preferentially activated by trypsin and tryptase, and PARs play an important role in matrix remodelling, cell migration and proliferation, and inflammation. PAR-2 has increased expression on the smooth muscle of bronchial vessels in chronic bronchitis when compared to patients with COPD[75]. PAR-2 induces the proliferation of human airway smooth muscle cells[76] and human lung fibroblast proliferation[77], as well as MMP-9 release from airway epithelial cells[78]. Hence MMP-9, PAR-2 and TGF-β_1 may be interrelated in causing fibrosis in COPD.

Figure 2.14   Matrix metalloproteinase-9: role in elastolysis and fibrosis

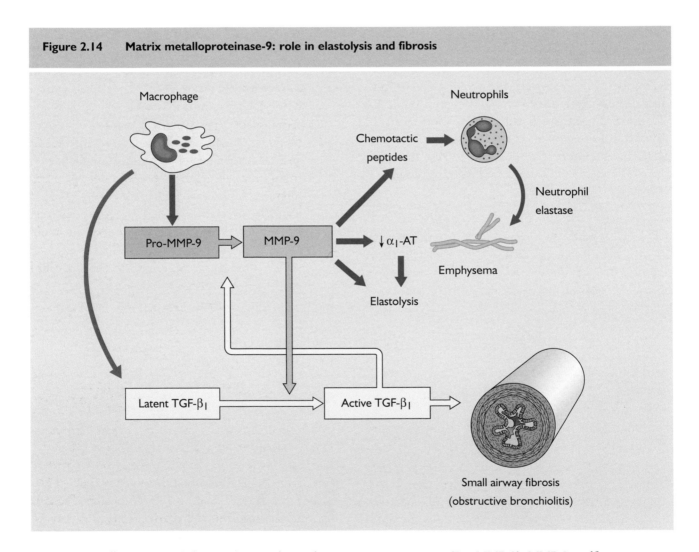

Matrix metalloproteinase-9 (MMP-9) is synthesized as an inactive precursor (Pro-MMP-9). MMP-9 itself causes activation of latent transforming growth factor-β_1 (TGF-β_1) to active TGF-β_1, which has potent fibrogenic activity. MMP-9 has proteolytic activity and causes release of chemotactic peptides, as well as inactivation of α_1-antitrypsin (α_1-AT) and reduced antiprotease defence. Active TGF-β_1 activates MMP-9.

THE PATHOLOGY OF COPD

The pathology of COPD has been the subject of a number of recent reviews[30,79–85], as well as being covered in textbooks of lung pathology[86]. We will discuss five types of pathology that may occur in COPD, although in advanced COPD all five features can be present in a single patient (Figure 2.1). In order to understand the histopathological features of COPD, it is important first to appreciate the structure and histology of the normal airways and lung parenchyma (Figures 2.15–2.18).

Chronic bronchitis

Normal bronchus

The epithelium of the normal bronchus is pseudo-stratified respiratory epithelium consisting largely of ciliated columnar cells, interspersed with occasional mucus cells (Figure 2.17). These mucus cells have prominent secretory vesicles containing mucus, and, due to their shape, are commonly called goblet cells. The normal bronchus has two incomplete bands of smooth muscle inside the submucosal bronchial gland layer (Figure 2.19). Outside this, there are plates of cartilage and the bronchial adventitia.

Macroscopic

At postmortem, the bronchi of a patient with chronic bronchitis contain an abundance of mucus that overlies a dusky red mucous membrane[86]. Chronic bronchitis affects mainly the intermediate-sized bronchi with an internal diameter of 2–4 mm.

Microscopic

Working from the lumen outwards into the bronchial wall, the following features are present (Figures 2.19–2.21):

- *Mucus*: increased mucus is present on the surface of the lumen.
- *Epithelial changes*: goblet cell hyperplasia occurs, with an increased proportion of goblet cells at the expense of ciliated epithelial cells. Epithelial atrophy[87], focal squamous metaplasia[88], and ciliary abnormalities are also present[89–92]. However, the altered epithelium is generally intact[93] and the thickness of the reticular basement membrane is within the normal range in the majority of studies[94].

- *Inflammation* occurs in the mucosa as well as in the smooth muscle and submucosal glands. Inflammation provides a better morphological indication of chronic bronchitis than mucous gland hypertrophy[95]. In bronchial mucosal biopsy specimens of subjects with stable COPD and exacerbations of bronchitis, there is convincing evidence of a mononuclear inflammatory cell infiltration by macrophages, CD8+ T cells and plasma cells[11,12,22,93,96], associated with up-regulation of cell-surface adhesion molecules[29,97].

- *Smooth muscle hypertrophy* may be present to a minor extent, but can be difficult to assess. Some bronchi do not have a complete band of smooth muscle; rather they have two interlocking longitudinal spirals.

- *Enlargement of the submucosal bronchial glands* is a major histological feature of chronic bronchitis[98,99]. There is a shift in the proportion of serous to mucous acini in the glands, with a reduction in serous cells containing the antibacterial agents lysozyme and lactoferrin. Mucus plugging of the airways can occur in COPD, and tenacious secretions may be difficult to expectorate[100]. The Reid index describes the relative thickness of the submucosal mucus gland layer relative to that of the airway wall from the base of the epithelium to the inner cartilage surface. The normal index is 0.3, the submucosal glands occupying about one-third of the airway wall thickness.

- *Degeneration of bronchial cartilage* is a late manifestation[101,102].

Physiology

Mucus hypersecretion may arise through activation of sensory nerve endings in the airways with reflex (local peptidergic and spinal cholinergic) increase in mucus secretion and direct stimulatory effects of enzymes, such as neutrophil elastase and chymase (*see* Figure 8.16). Recent studies suggest that epidermal growth factor (EGF) is a key mediator of mucus hyperplasia and mucus hypersecretion and may be the final common pathway that mediates the effects of many stimuli, including cigarette smoke, on mucus secretion[103]. With time, there is hyperplasia of submucosal glands and proliferation of goblet cells under the influence of growth factors such as EGF.

Figure 2.15   The normal airways

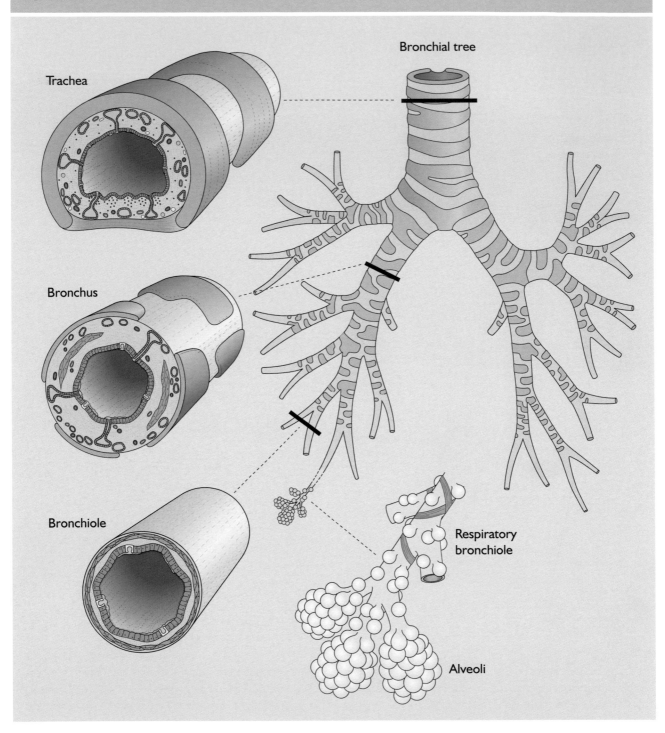

Diagrammatic representation of four sections at different points in the airways. According to the Weibel model of the bronchial tree, there is repeated branching (asymmetrical dichotomy) of the airways up to 23 times before the furthest alveoli are reached, although, near the hilum, alveoli can be reached in eight divisions.

Trachea The trachea is protected ventrally by 'C'-shaped cartilage (in blue) that can be palpated under the skin in the neck. Dorsally, there is a band of smooth muscle (in brown) that links the two horns of the cartilage. Longitudinal mucosal ridges are present on the posterior wall of the trachea, and correspond to thick longitudinal bundles of elastin in the subepithelial lamina propria. This elastin contributes to elastic recoil on expiration, and the elastin fibers could link up with those in the airways, including alveolar ducts and walls. *Continued on next page*

Figure 2.16   Histology of the normal airways and lung parenchyma

Location	Generation	Epithelium	Muscle	Cartilage
Trachea (T)	1	pseudostratified columnar epithelium with ciliated, mucus (goblet) and basal cells	trachealis muscle: single band between two dorsal cartilaginous horns	prominent 'C'-shaped rings
Bronchus (B)	2–8		two bands in form of opposing spirals	plates
Membranous bronchiole (MB)	9–15	simple cuboidal epithelium with ciliated, Clara and serous cells: becomes non-ciliated and free of mucus (goblet) cells	complete well-defined layer	nil
Terminal bronchiole (TB)	16		RB have thin spiral-forming knobs between mouths of alveoli on cross-section	
Respiratory bronchiole (RB)	17–19			
Alveolar ducts (AD)	20–23	type I alveolar epithelial cells: attenuated cytoplasm for gas exchange type II alveolar epithelial cells: vacuoles of surfactant	nil	nil
Alveolar sacs (AS)				

Figure 2.15   Continued . . .

Bronchi The right main bronchus is larger than the left, carrying 55% of each breath. The two main bronchi divide into five lobar bronchi, and these then progressively divide to form the 19 bronchopulmonary segments. Bronchi have interlocking spirals of smooth muscle bands, prominent submucosal mucus glands of mixed seromucinous type (yellow) and patches of cartilage (blue). Approximately eight generations of bronchi may be present, and the central conducting airways of internal diameter > 2 mm are the major site of resistance to airflow in the normal lung.

Membranous (conducting) bronchiole The transition from bronchus to bronchiole takes place in airways of about 1 mm diameter. There are around seven generations of membranous bronchioles (MB). The last order of MB is confusingly named the terminal bronchiole (TB), despite them leading into further generations of respiratory bronchioles. The membranous bronchiole has a continuous layer of smooth muscle (brown), but lacks submucosal glands and cartilage in the wall.

Respiratory bronchiole and alveoli Respiratory bronchioles (RB) have alveoli directly attaching to their wall, so are capable of gas transfer, and have thin bands of smooth muscle (brown) spiralling around their wall. There are generally about three generations of respiratory bronchioles, and four generations of alveolar ducts (AD), eventually terminating in the alveolar sacs (AS).

Figure 2.17   The normal bronchi

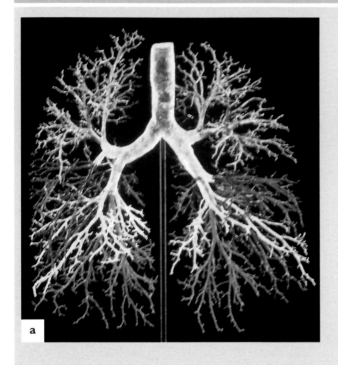

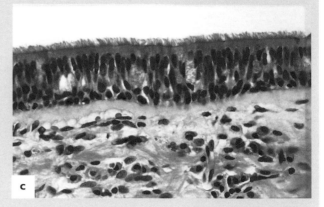

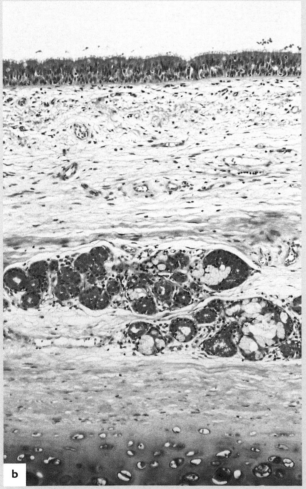

(a) *The central airways* A plastic cast of the proximal airways with individual segments distinguished by color.

(b) *Normal bronchial wall* The mucosa consists of surface epithelium resting on elastin-rich connective tissue, beneath which are the submucosal glands and cartilage. The glands are of a mixed seromucous type. The apparent absence of submucosal muscle at this point is attributable to its double-spiral arrangement.

(c) *Normal bronchial epithelium* Bronchial epithelium composed of pseudostratified columnar ciliated cells interspersed with occasional mucus-secreting (goblet) cells.

All photographs are reprinted by kind permission of Professor Bryan Corrin and Elsevier Science, from *Pathology of the Lungs* by B. Corrin, © 2000, ISBN 0 443 057133.

Figure 2.18   Respiratory epithelia

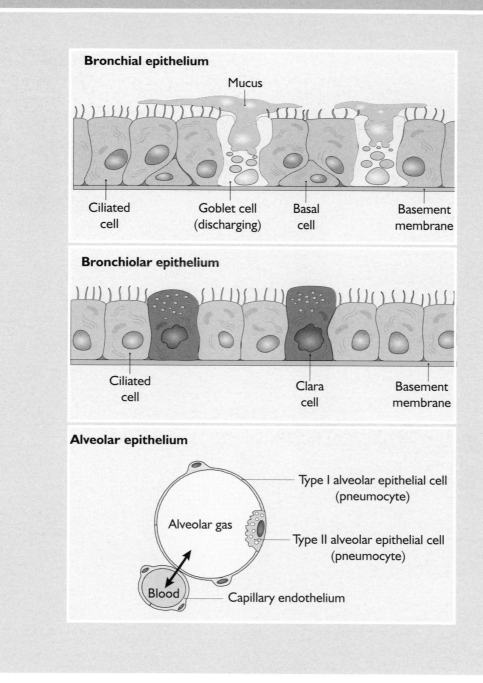

Bronchial epithelium The epithelium of the trachea and bronchi is pseudostratified, with all cells resting on the basement membrane, but not all reaching the lumen. The majority of cells are columnar ciliated epithelial cells, but there also goblet-shaped mucus cells, basal cells, brush cells and neuroendocrine cells. In addition, there are occasional fine nerve terminals and T cells, mast cells and eosinophils.

Bronchiolar epithelium The airway epithelium becomes cuboidal in the bronchioles, and the mucus cells decrease in number. In the small airways, Clara and serous cells become more prominent.

Alveoli The alveolar epithelium consists mainly of type I and type II alveolar epithelial cells. Type I alveolar epithelial cells have thin attenuated cytoplasm that extends large distances from the cell nucleus. They may cover up to 5000 µm of alveolar surface but only be 0.2 µm in thickness. Their function is to provide a complete but very thin covering, to aid gas exchange but hinder fluid loss. Type II alveolar epithelial cells are taller and more numerous than type I cells, but occupy < 10% of the alveolar surface. They have prominent secretory vacuoles containing pulmonary surfactant.

Figure 2.19   Normal bronchus and chronic bronchitis

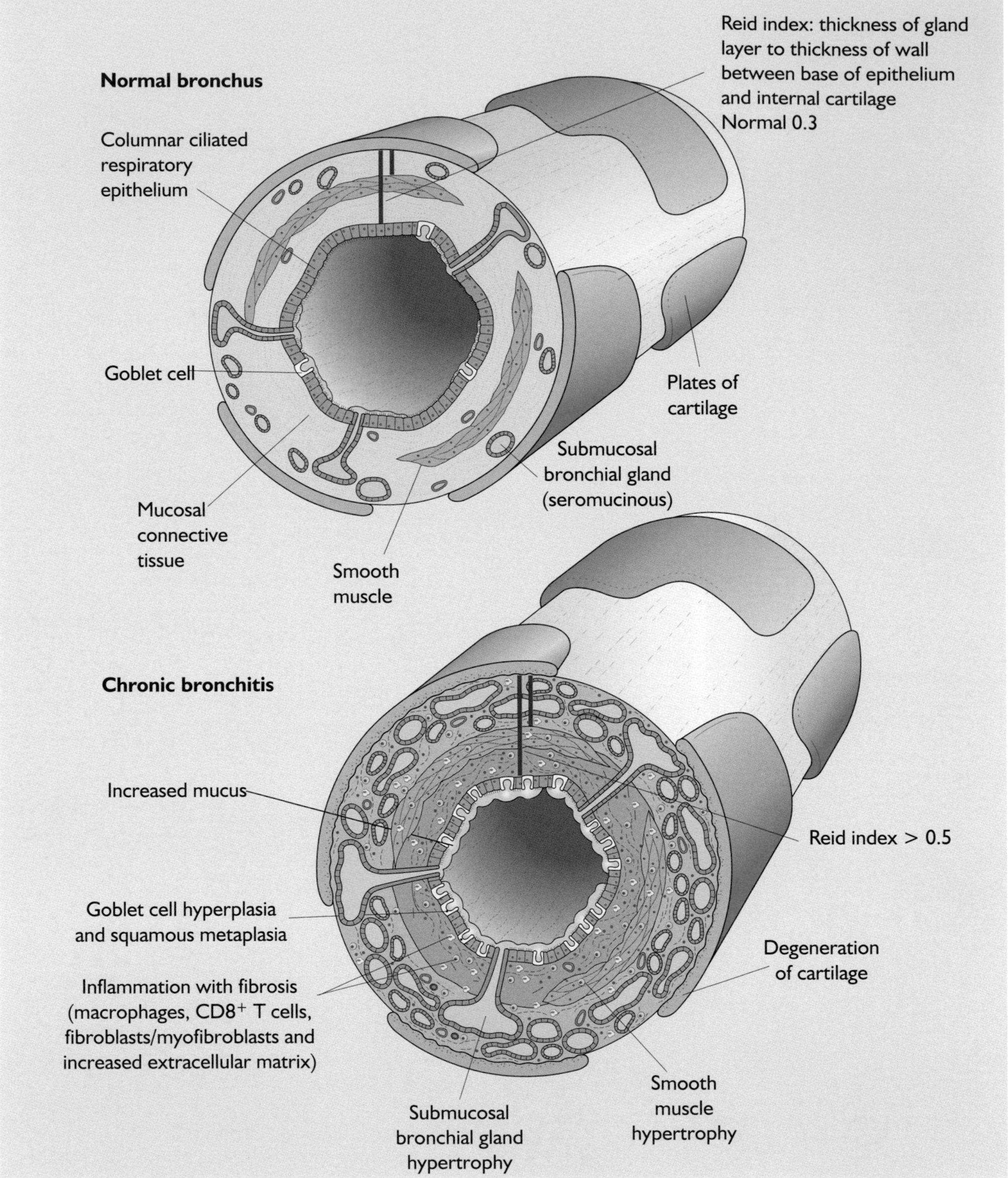

Reid index: thickness of gland layer to thickness of wall between base of epithelium and internal cartilage
Normal 0.3

Normal bronchus

Columnar ciliated respiratory epithelium

Goblet cell

Plates of cartilage

Mucosal connective tissue

Smooth muscle

Submucosal bronchial gland (seromucinous)

Chronic bronchitis

Increased mucus

Reid index > 0.5

Goblet cell hyperplasia and squamous metaplasia

Degeneration of cartilage

Inflammation with fibrosis (macrophages, CD8$^+$ T cells, fibroblasts/myofibroblasts and increased extracellular matrix)

Submucosal bronchial gland hypertrophy

Smooth muscle hypertrophy

The normal bronchus has a pseudostratified ciliated columnar epithelium containing scattered goblet cells. There are two interlocking spirals of smooth muscle band that do not form a complete layer. Bronchi have submucosal mucus glands of mixed seromucinous type (yellow) and patches of cartilage (blue).
In chronic bronchitis, changes are demonstrated when working from the lumen outwards into the bronchial wall; see text for details.

Figure 2.20   Histology of chronic bronchitis

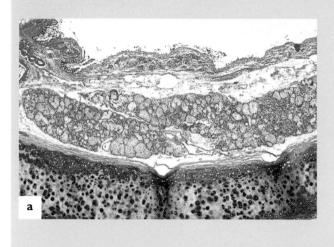

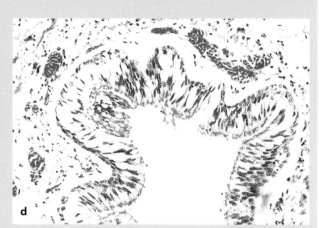

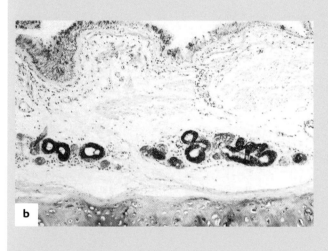

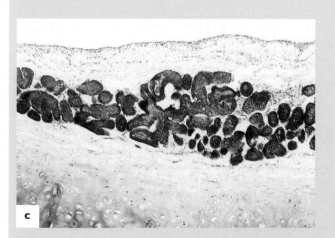

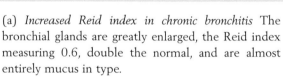

(a) *Increased Reid index in chronic bronchitis* The bronchial glands are greatly enlarged, the Reid index measuring 0.6, double the normal, and are almost entirely mucus in type.

(b) *Submucosal glands in normal bronchus.*

(c) *Submucosal glands in chronic bronchitis* As well as enlargement of the submucosal glands, chronic bronchitis is characterized by a shift in the nature of the glands from the normal mixed seromucus pattern to one that is almost entirely mucus, while, within the mucus acini, there is a shift from mixed neutral and acidic (red/blue) mucus to purely acidic (blue) mucus. A further shift within the acidic mucus, one from sialomucin to sulphomucin, is not apparent with this Alcian blue-periodic acid-Schiff stain.

(d) *Chronic bronchitis epithelium* In the surface epithelium, goblet cells are increased at the expense of the ciliated cells.

All figures are reprinted by kind permission of Professor Bryan Corrin and Elsevier Science, from *Pathology of the Lungs* by B. Corrin, © 2000, ISBN 0 443 057133.

Figure 2.21   Pathological changes of the central airways in COPD

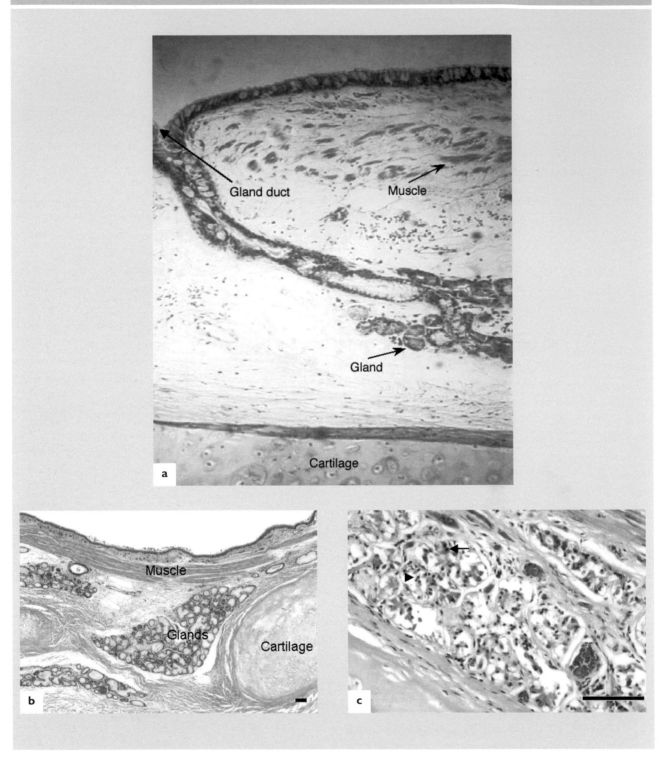

(a) A central bronchus from the lung of a cigarette smoker with normal lung function. Only small amounts of muscle are present and the epithelial glands are small. This contrasts sharply with a diseased bronchus (b), where the muscle appears as a thick bundle and the glands are enlarged. (c) These enlarged glands are shown at a higher magnification. There is evidence of a chronic inflammatory process involving polymorphonuclear (arrowhead) and mononuclear cells, including plasma cells (arrow).

Printed with permission of Dr James C. Hogg and Stuart Greene.

Chronic stimulation leads to up-regulation of mucin (MUC) genes. There are at least eight MUC genes now recognized in humans[104]; however, it is not yet certain which genes are overexpressed in chronic bronchitis. It was once thought that mucus hypersecretion played no role in airflow obstruction, but epidemiological data show that mucus hypersecretion is a risk factor for airflow obstruction and it is likely that viscous mucus may contribute to reduced airflow[105]. However, a 15-year study has found that GOLD Stage 0 with chronic bronchitis does not identify subsequent airways obstruction[106].

Obstructive bronchiolitis

Normal bronchiole histology

The structure of the normal bronchiole is illustrated in diagram form and from microscopy (Figures 2.22–2.24). Goblet cells are sparse in the normal bronchiole, submucosal glands are absent, and non-ciliated secretory and ciliated cells are the main cell types[107,108]. The Clara cell is the major secretory phenotype as well as the progenitor from which ciliated and newly formed mucus cells develop (Figure 2.18). There is a complete layer of smooth muscle in the membranous bronchiole that becomes an incomplete layer in the respiratory bronchioles (Figure 2.15), although cartilage is absent from the walls of bronchioles.

Pathology

Obstructive bronchiolitis involves the small or peripheral airways, and is an inflammatory condition of small airways (Figures 2.22–2.24).

Working from the lumen outwards through the wall of the bronchiole, the following histological features are present:

- *Collapsed lumen with increased mucus*, unlike in asthma where the lumen is maintained.

- *Epithelium with goblet cell (mucus) metaplasia* Clara cells are replaced by goblet cells[109], and mucus appears in peripheral airways by the process of goblet cell metaplasia[109–111]. The replacement of the normal surfactant lining by mucus leads to an abnormally high surface tension and small airway instability, and predisposes to early airway closure during expiration[112].

- *Inflammation* Bronchial biopsies have demonstrated an infiltration with mononuclear cells; macrophages and cytotoxic (CD8+) T lymphocytes, rather than neutrophils[1,81,113,114]. In studies that examined the peribronchiolar inflammation of smokers whose lungs had been resected for localized tumor, those with chronic bronchitis and COPD had increased numbers of CD8+ cells[115,116]. These inflammatory changes to small airways appear to be related to clinical airflow obstruction in COPD, and this association with loss in FEV$_1$ appears to be stronger than that seen in the bronchi[114,117–121]. Histologically, one of the most consistently observed early effects of cigarette smoke in patients with COPD is a marked increase in the number of macrophages in the bronchioli, and an associated respiratory bronchiolitis and alveolitis[121]. Increased numbers of macrophages can also be detected in BAL[111,123,124]. In stable COPD, macrophages predominate in mild to moderate disease, while neutrophils are more prominent in severe to very severe disease. In mild exacerbations of COPD, eosinophils are commonly prominent, while neutrophils predominate in more severe exacerbations.

- *Fibrosis* There are increased numbers of fibroblasts and myofibroblasts, and increased extracellular matrix. The injury and resolution process result in a structural remodelling of the airway wall, with increased collagen content and scar formation, which narrows the lumen and produces fixed airways obstruction[125]. The resultant stenotic narrowing of bronchioles has been convincingly demonstrated[126], and has been documented in terms of peripheral airway resistance[127]. Fibrosis in the small airways is characterized by the accumulation of mesenchymal cells (fibroblasts and myofibroblasts) and extracellular connective tissue matrix.

- *Smooth muscle hypertrophy* Key structural changes in obstructive bronchiolitis include smooth muscle hypertrophy, mural edema and an increased number of airways that are < 400 mm in diameter[111,123,128,129]. Smooth muscle hypertrophy is most striking in small bronchi and bronchioli[115,130].

- *Loss of alveolar attachments* In the small airways, the inflammation moves into the interstitium

Figure 2.22   Normal bronchiole and obstructive bronchiolitis

Normal bronchiole

Goblet
cell

Alveolar
attachments

Smooth
muscle

Obstructive bronchiolitis

Collapsed lumen

Increased mucus

Goblet cell metaplasia

Loss of
attachments

Smooth
muscle hypertrophy

Inflammation with fibrosis
(macrophages, CD8+ T cells,
fibroblasts/myofibroblasts and
increased extracellular matrix)

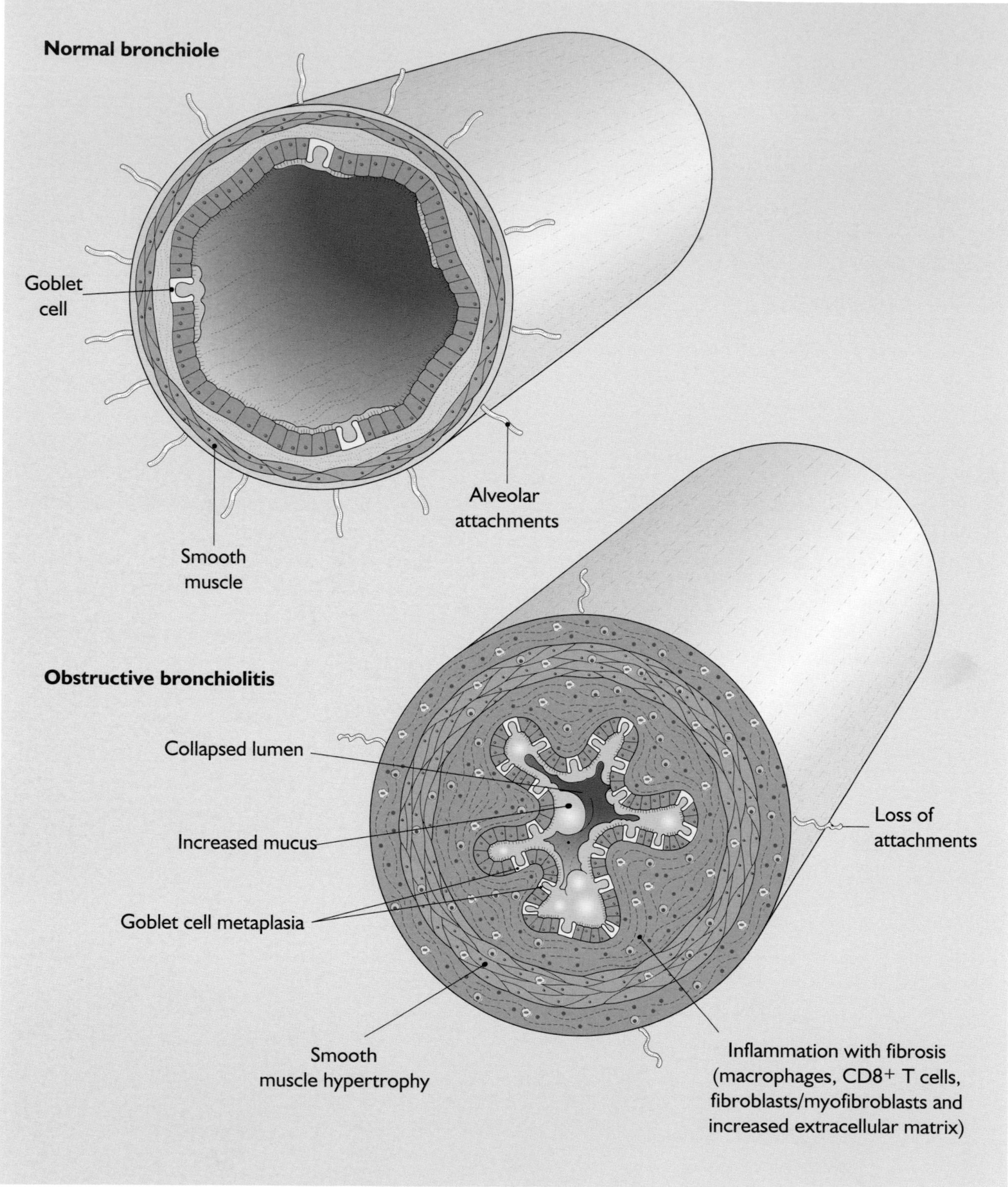

The normal bronchiole has a columnar ciliated respiratory epithelium. Goblet cells are sparse, and the Clara cell more prominent. There is a continuous layer of smooth muscle within the membranous bronchioles (MB), but only two spirals in the respiratory bronchioles (RB).

In obstructive bronchiolitis, collapse of the lumen and fibrosis of the inflamed wall are prominent. Changes are shown from the lumen outwards into the airway wall; see text for details.

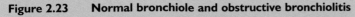

Figure 2.23   Normal bronchiole and obstructive bronchiolitis

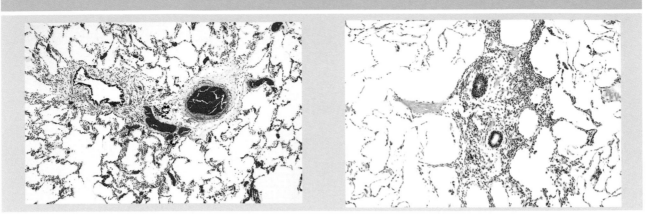

(a) Bronchioles and pulmonary arteries lie alongside each other in the centers of the lung acini, sharing a connective tissue sheath. (b) Peribronchiolitis and fibrosis in small airway disease. Reprinted by kind permission of Professor Bryan Corrin and Elsevier Science, from *Pathology of the Lungs* by B. Corrin, © 2000, ISBN 0 443 057133.

Figure 2.24   Pathological changes of the peripheral airways in COPD

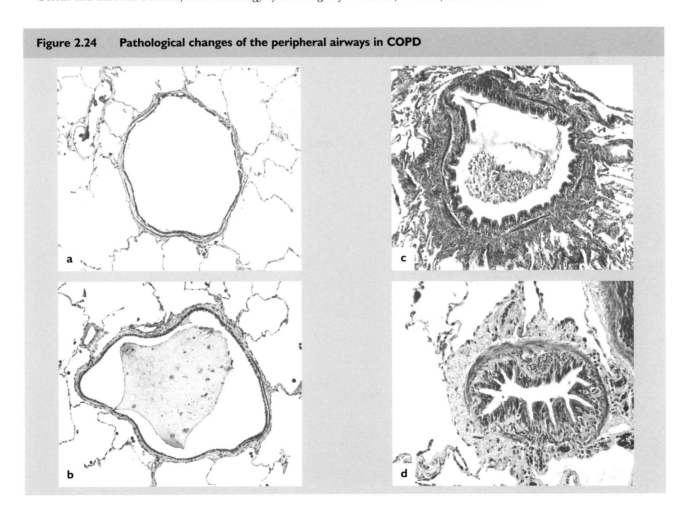

Histological sections of peripheral airways from patients who are cigarette smokers. (a) shows a nearly normal airway; (b) shows a plug of mucoid exudate in the lumen with little or no evidence of inflammation in the wall; (c) shows the presence of an inflammatory exudate in the wall and lumen of the airway; and (d) shows an airway with reduced lumen, structural reorganization of the airway wall, increased smooth muscle, and deposition of peribronchial connective tissue. Printed with permission of Dr James C. Hogg and Stuart Greene.

to destroy the alveolar attachments that provide parenchymal support to the bronchiole. A loss of alveolar attachments to the bronchiole perimeter contributes to the loss of elastic recoil and favors increased tortuosity and early closure of bronchioles during expiration in patients with COPD[131-134].

Physiology

There is debate about whether the airflow obstruction in COPD is primarily due to obstruction of the lumen of small airways as a result of bronchiolitis and fibrosis[135], or whether it is due to loss of elasticity and closure of small airways as a result of parenchymal destruction and loss of alveolar attachments. Loss of lung elasticity may occur in COPD, even in the absence of emphysema, and it is likely that this may be an important contributor to airway obstruction in all patients with COPD. It is probable that bronchiolitis and loss of the 'guy-rope' tractional effects of alveolar attachments both contribute to airway obstruction.

Figure 2.25   Alveoli and the lung parenchyma

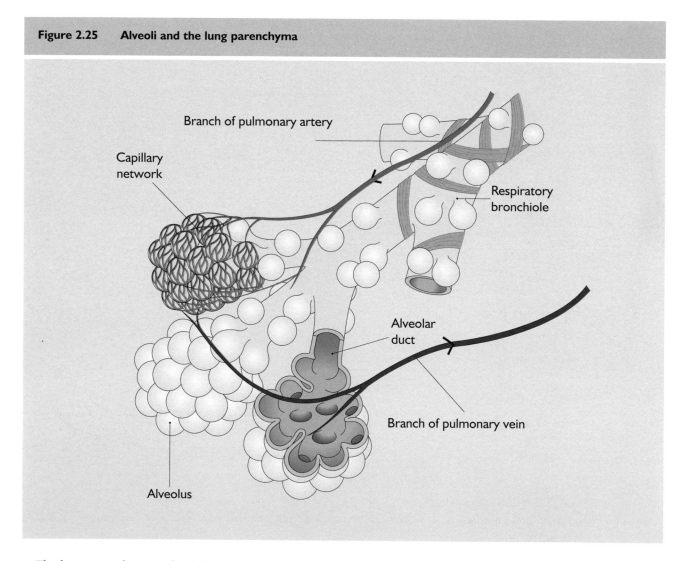

The lung parenchyma is divided into secondary lobules bounded by indistinct fibrous septa. Each secondary lobule contains three to ten acini, each being supplied by a terminal bronchiole. Bronchioles and pulmonary arteries lie alongside each other in the center of the acini. The vein, artery and terminal bronchiole are adjacent at entry into the lung lobule. The primary lobule is the portion of the respiratory tract distal to an alveolar duct. The branches of the pulmonary artery carry deoxygenated blood to the alveolar capillary network where gaseous exchange occurs. The capillaries drain into pulmonary veins that run in the interlobular fibrous septa before returning to the heart.

Emphysema

Normal lung parenchymal anatomy

The lung parenchyma contains the alveoli and their rich capillary bed that comprise the gas transfer area of the lung (Figure 2.25). This parenchyma is divided into secondary lobules bounded by indistinct fibrous septa, which are visible on the cut surface of the lungs (Figure 2.26). Each secondary lobule contains three to ten acini, each acinus being supplied by a terminal bronchiole, and measuring about 0.5–1 cm in length. The primary lobule is that portion of the respiratory tract distal to an alveolar duct. Each acinus comprises about 2000 alveoli, with both lungs containing 300 million alveoli, each measuring about 250 mm in diameter, with a resulting gas transfer area of about 70 m² (approximately the area of a tennis court) involved in handling approximately 10 000 liters of air each day.

Figure 2.26   The lung parenchyma

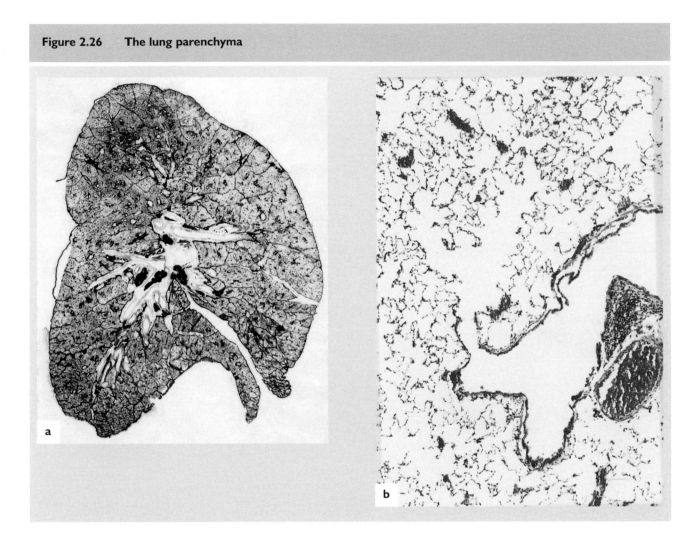

(a) *Secondary lung lobules* A Gough–Wentworth paper-mounted whole lung section of a city-dweller's lung in which the interlobular septa and centriacinar structures are particularly well seen because of dust in the lymphatics and lymphorecticular aggregates.

(b) *Normal lung parenchyma* A terminal bronchiole dividing into alveolated respiratory bronchioles, this represents the termination of the purely conductive membranous bronchioles, and the commencement of the transitional zone of the lung and the apex of a pulmonary acinus. A pulmonary artery is seen alongside the bronchiole. Artery and bronchiole are of roughly the same caliber. Between them is a lymphorecticular aggregate, this marking the point at which lymphatics commence.

Reprinted by kind permission of Professor Bryan Corrin and Elsevier Science, from *Pathology of the Lungs* by B. Corrin, © 2000, ISBN 0 443 057133.

Lambert's canals (30 μm) are communications between terminal and respiratory bronchioles and alveoli, while the interalveolar pores of Kohn have a diameter of 2–12 μm. Bronchioles and pulmonary arteries lie alongside each other in the center of the acini (Figure 2.26), while pulmonary veins run in the interlobular fibrous septa. The vein, artery and terminal bronchiole are adjacent at entry into the lung lobule.

Pathology

Emphysema is defined by permanent, destructive enlargement of the air spaces distal to the terminal bronchioli, affecting the respiratory bronchioles and, sometimes, the alveoli (Figure 2.27). The enlargement is best not called a dilatation, since this implies a reversible bronchodilation, as occurs in asthma. The mechanism of this process is poorly understood, but it is thought to be an inflammatory condition of the lung parenchyma mediated by T lymphocytes, neutrophils and alveolar macrophages. Inflammation is associated with the release of excessive amounts of proteolytic enzymes such as neutrophil elastase and matrix metalloproteinases. Inflammation and proteolysis are accompanied by destruction of lung parenchyma, fibrosis and remodelling.

Forms of emphysema

- *Centrilobular emphysema* This is the most common cause of cigarette smoking-induced emphysema in COPD. It involves the dilatation and destruction of the respiratory bronchioles (Figures 2.28 and 2.29)[136,137]. Centrilobular emphysema occurs more frequently in the upper lung fields in mild disease. In more advanced disease, lesions are more diffuse and also involve destruction of the capillary bed.

- *Panacinar emphysema* This comprises the characteristic lesion seen in α_1-antitrypsin deficiency[138]. It extends throughout the entire acinus, involving the dilatation and destruction of the alveolar ducts and sacs as well as the respiratory bronchioles (Figures 2.27 and 2.29). Since it usually affects all the acini in the secondary lobule, it is also referred to as panlobular emphysema. Panacinar emphysema tends to affect the lower more than the upper lung regions.

Macroscopic appearance

In postmortem necropsy material, holes are visible in lung sections in patients with severe emphysema.

Alveolar wall fenestrae

The early changes of emphysema may include subtle disruption to elastic fibers, with an accompanying loss of elastic recoil, bronchiolar and alveolar distortion. It has been postulated that fenestrae (pores of Kohn) may enlarge to develop microscopic emphysema[139,140].

Inflammation and proteolysis

Lymphocytes have been demonstrated to form a significant component of the alveolar wall inflammatory infiltrate in COPD[8,141]. The greater the number of T lymphocytes, the less alveolar tissue is present[16]. Neutrophil elastase is a powerful proteolytic enzyme, and neutrophils have also been implicated in lung damage. It has been recently demonstrated in a mouse model that alveolar wall apoptosis causes lung destruction and emphysematous changes[142,143].

Loss of bronchoalveolar attachments and lung parenchyma

Later changes involve the loss of the interacinar septa, as well as the airspace walls[144]. This may lead to progressively enlarging holes > 1 mm in diameter, which can be detected with the naked eye.

Alveolar wall fibrosis

The destructive process is accompanied by a net increase in the mass of collagen with alveolar wall fibrosis, even in emphysematous lungs[145].

Physiology

Emphysema is due to enzymatic destruction of the alveolar walls and destruction of alveolar attachments to the bronchioles. This results in the loss of driving pressure and airway narrowing, with a consequent reduction in FEV_1. The fundamental defect is ventilation/perfusion (Va/Q) imbalance which becomes reflected in abnormalities in gas transfer that eventually become manifest as respiratory failure.

Figure 2.27   Emphysema

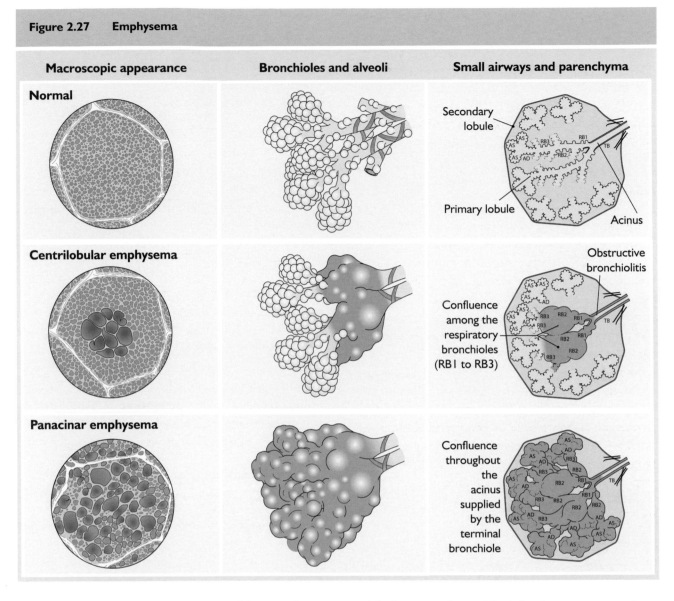

| Macroscopic appearance | Bronchioles and alveoli | Small airways and parenchyma |

Top row: *Diagrammatic representation of the normal appearance of the lung parenchyma.* The left column represents the macroscopic (naked eye) appearance of the secondary lung lobule, the middle column demonstrates the morphology of the respiratory bronchioles and alveoli, while the right column illustrates the morphology of the small airways and parenchyma within the secondary lobule. Secondary lung lobules are irregularly polyhedral in shape, 1–2 cm in diameter, and defined loosely by fibrous septa. The secondary lung lobule can frequently be visualized macroscopically on the cut surface of the lung and through the pleura, and is well visualized in health and disease with high-resolution CT scans. Each secondary lung lobule contains three to ten acini, an acinus being the lung parenchyma supplied by a terminal bronchiole (TB), comprising the respiratory bronchioles (RB1–3), the alveolar ducts (AD) and the alveolar sacs (AS). The primary lobule is the alveolar duct and its distal structures. The terminal bronchiole at the center of the secondary lobule is accompanied by a pulmonary artery, while the pulmonary vein and lymphatic branches are within the fibrous septa. For simplicity, only one order of alveolar ducts is drawn (not to scale).

Middle row: *Centrilobular emphysema.* This consists of destructive enlargement and confluence, especially of the third-order respiratory bronchioles (RB3), which spares the alveolar ducts (AD) and alveolar sacs (AS). Hence the destruction and apparent dilatation are central within the secondary lobule. Centrilobular emphysema predominantly affects the upper lobes and is associated with cigarette smoking. Spaces of diameter > 1 cm are termed bullae.

Bottom row: *Panacinar emphysema.* There is destructive confluence throughout the acinus supplied by the terminal bronchiole (TB), and the acinus is affected uniformly. This is the characteristic lesion seen in α_1-antitrypsin deficiency and involves the respiratory bronchioles (RB), alveolar ducts and alveolar sacs. It usually affects the lower lung regions, and is also termed panlobular emphysema because it affects all the acini in a secondary lobule.

Figure 2.28   Normal respiratory bronchioles and centrilobular emphysema

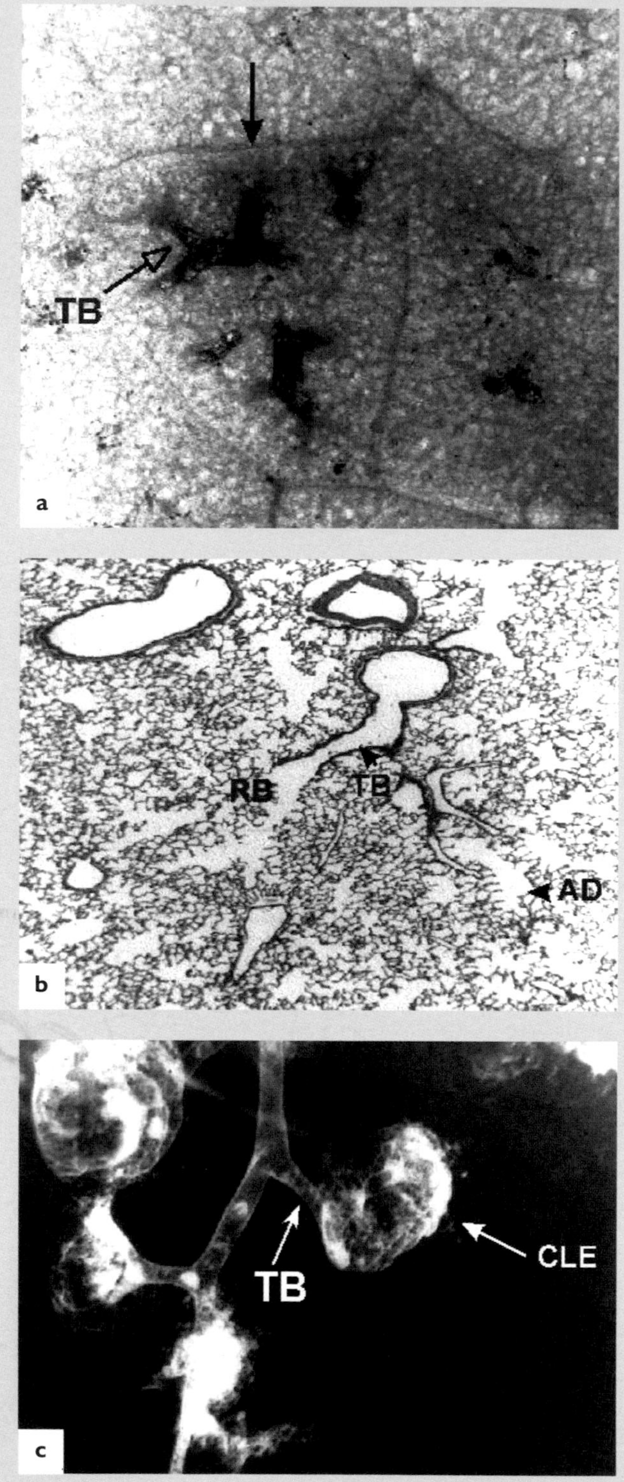

(a) A photomicrograph of the pleural surface of a normal lung, with a secondary lobule defined by a connective tissue septum (solid arrow) and several terminal bronchioles (TB) filled with opaque material. (b) A low–lower photomicrograph of a normal terminal bronchiole (TB) branching into a respiratory bronchiole (RB), which eventually ends in alveolar ducts (AD). (c) The bronchographic appearance of this lesion (CLE, centrilobular emphysema).
Printed with permission of Dr James C. Hogg and Stuart Greene.

Figure 2.29   Emphysema

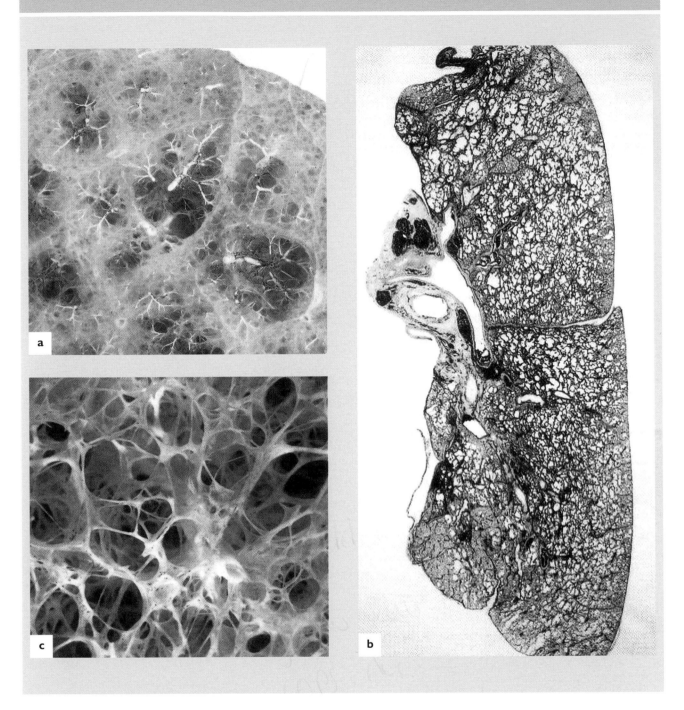

(a) *Centrilobular (centriacinar) emphysema* Destruction of lung parenchyma is demonstrated by inflation fixation and barium sulfate precipitation. Dust-pigmented deficiencies in the lung substance are confined to the centers of the acini. As well as using barium sulfate to emphasize the emphysema, the pulmonary arteries have been injected with a barium gelatine preparation for angiography.

Reproduced by permission of the late Professor B.E. Heard, Brompton, UK. Reprinted by kind permission of Professor Bryan Corrin and Elsevier Science, from *Pathology of the Lungs* by B. Corrin, © 2000, ISBN 0 443 057133.

(b) *Panacinar emphysema* The whole of the lung acinus is affected uniformly. Paper-mounted whole lung section; (c) barium sulfate precipitation.

Reproduced by permission of the late Professor B.E. Heard, Brompton, UK. Reprinted by kind permission of Professor Bryan Corrin and Elsevier Science, from *Pathology of the Lungs* by B. Corrin, © 2000, ISBN 0 443 057133.

Figure 2.30   Histology of a small arteriole and pulmonary vascular disease

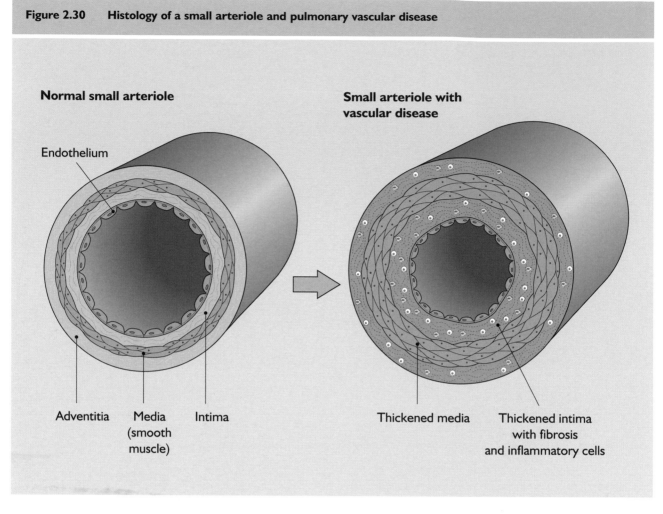

The pulmonary arteriole has an internal endothelial layer, bounded by the loose intima, then the smooth muscle media, and finally the connective tissue adventitia. The vascular changes in COPD include thickening of the intima, increase in the media, and infiltration of the vessel wall with inflammatory cells. There is progressive deposition of proteoglycan and collagen within the vessel wall, and there may be destruction of the capillary bed in advanced emphysema.

Pulmonary vascular disease

Normal pulmonary artery

The pulmonary arteriole has an internal endothelial layer, bounded by the loose intima, then the smooth muscle media, and finally the connective tissue adventitia (Figures 2.30 and 2.31).

Pathology

Pulmonary vascular changes in COPD begin early in the course of COPD as intimal thickening, followed by smooth muscle hypertrophy and inflammatory infiltration. This may be followed by pulmonary hypertension and destruction of the capillary bed.

Endothelial dysfunction of the pulmonary arteries may be caused directly by cigarette smoke products[146] or indirectly by inflammatory mediators[147]. Endothelial dysfunction may then initiate the sequence of events that results in structural changes[148–150], possibly mediated through endothelial derived relaxing factors.

Early in the natural history of COPD, thickening of the intima begins in the walls of the muscular pulmonary arteries. This intimal hyperplasia is believed to occur when lung function is reasonably well maintained, and when pulmonary vascular pressures are normal at rest[148].

An increase in vascular smooth muscle occurs, although only a moderate degree of muscular

Figure 2.31   Pathological changes of the pulmonary vasculature in COPD

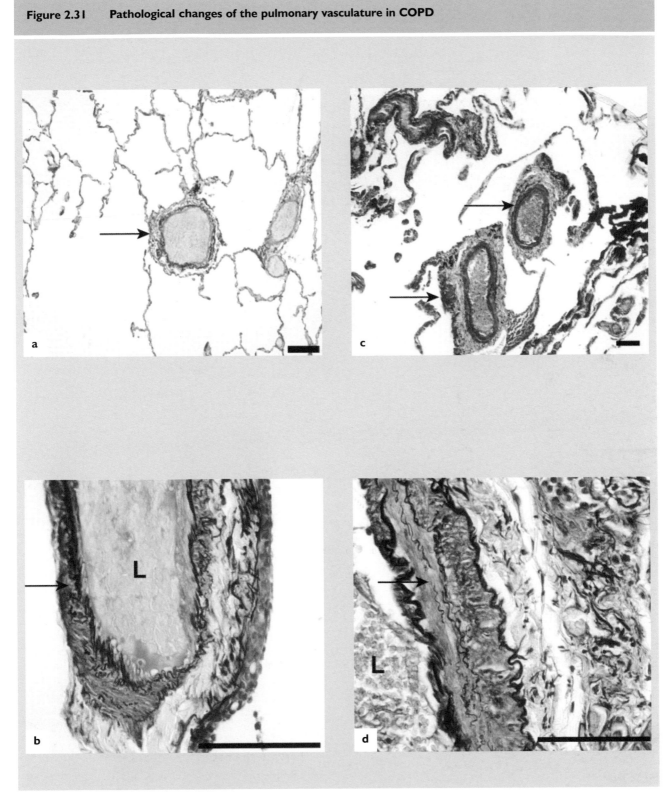

Photomicrographs of small (a) and large (b) vessels in the lung of a heavy smoker with normal lung function, and small (c) and large (d) vessels in the lung of a patient with severe emphysema. Note that the smaller vessel has thicker walls (compare arrows in (a) and (c)) and that the larger vessel has a thicker media (compare arrows in (b) and (d)) in the patient with severe emphysema. L, vessel lumen; magnification bars, 100 μm.
Printed with permission of Dr James C. Hogg and Stuart Greene.

hypertrophy has been reported[129], with extension of vascular smooth muscle to vessels that normally lack muscle. Infiltration of the vessel wall by inflammatory cells including macrophages and CD8+ T cells occurs[16,147]. Increasing amounts of smooth muscle, proteoglycans and collagen further thicken the vessel wall, and fibrosis may obliterate some vessels.

Hypoxic pulmonary vasoconstriction may contribute to pulmonary hypertension (Figure 2.32), while advanced COPD is associated with emphysematous destruction of the pulmonary capillary bed[149].

Endothelin

The mechanisms of vascular remodelling are not yet understood and it is likely that several growth factors, including vascular endothelial growth factor and fibroblast growth factor, may be involved. ET-1 is strongly expressed in pulmonary vascular endothelium of patients with pulmonary hypertension secondary to chronic hypoxia[57]; urinary ET-1 excretion is increased in patients with COPD[150] and sputum ET-1 levels are increased in exacerbations[56]. ET-1, acting mainly via ET$_A$ receptors, induces fibrosis and hyperplasia of pulmonary vascular smooth muscle, implying a role in the pulmonary hypertension secondary to COPD.

Physiology

Although pulmonary hypertension and *cor pulmonale* are common sequelae of COPD, the precise mechanisms of increased vascular resistance are unclear[149,151]. Structural changes in the pulmonary arteries are correlated with an increase in pulmonary vascular pressure (pulmonary hypertension) which develops first with exercise and then at rest.

- Chronic hypoxia results in widespread pulmonary vasoconstriction;

Figure 2.32   Vascular pathology in COPD

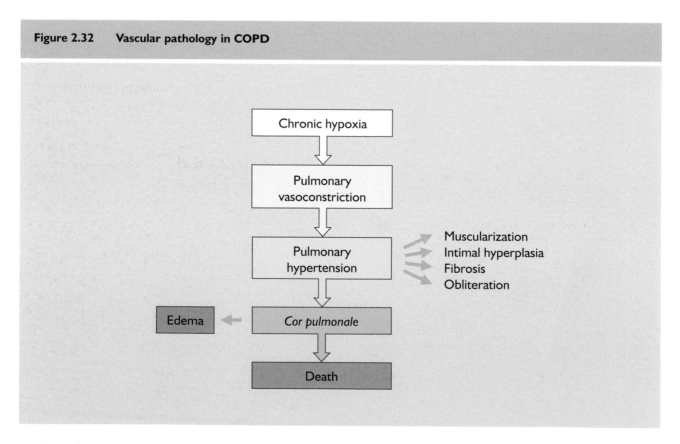

Chronic hypoxia results in hypoxic pulmonary vasoconstriction and, over time, leads to structural changes, resulting in secondary pulmonary hypertension. Eventually, this may lead to right heart failure (*cor pulmonale*), which may be manifest as limb edema, an enlarged pulsatile liver, and a raised jugular venous pressure. *Cor pulmonale* has a poor prognosis.

- Remodelling of the pulmonary circulation with pulmonary hypertension;
- Right heart failure (*cor pulmonale*) in some patients.

Systemic extrapulmonary effects

Systemic features of COPD include disturbances in metabolism with cachexia, as well as increased respiratory and skeletal muscle fatigue with wasting[152]. Particularly patients with predominant emphysema may develop profound weight loss, and this is a predictor of increased mortality that is independent of poor lung function[153]. Weight loss in COPD has been associated with increased levels of TNF-α and soluble TNF-α receptors[49,154–156]. The skeletal muscle weakness may exacerbate dyspnea, and skeletal and respiratory muscle training is an important aspect of pulmonary rehabilitation. Improved nutrition and a short course of anabolic steroids have been shown to improve lung function in patients with COPD[157].

Figure 2.33   Overlap between COPD and asthma

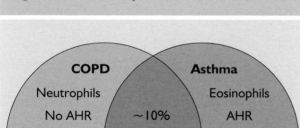

Venn diagram to show that COPD and asthma are common but distinct diseases and frequently co-exist in 10% of cases. The underlying inflammation of asthma is mainly eosinophilic and driven by CD4+ T lymphocytes, while in COPD there are more neutrophils and macrophages and involvement of CD8+ T cells. AHR, airway hyperreactivity.

ASTHMA COMPARED WITH COPD

Asthma differs markedly from COPD in that there is a greater reversibility of lung function spontaneously and on treatment with bronchodilators or steroids[80,83,113,158]. Some patients with asthma have progressive irreversible airflow obstruction and therefore have a form of COPD, and some patients may have coexistent asthma and COPD (Figure 2.33). It is unlikely that atopy predisposes to the development of COPD in cigarette smokers (the 'Dutch hypothesis'). Asthma should be regarded as a separate condition from COPD, with different causes, different cellular mechanisms and different responses to treatments. Approximately 10% of patients with COPD may have features of asthma, and this is probably due to the coincidence of these common diseases in some patients.

In general, there are striking differences in inflammation between asthma and COPD, with differences in inflammatory cells, mediators, inflammatory effects and location of the inflammatory process (Figures 2.34 and 2.35). The distinctions between COPD and asthma at the tissue level are by no means always clear[22,80,159,160]. In the bronchial wall of patients with asthma, there is frequently a prominent eosinophil infiltrate, while, in conditions such as asthma death, the airway lumen is normally maintained, although it may be plugged with mucus (Figure 2.36). In contrast, in COPD, the bronchiole wall is considerably thickened with extensive fibrosis and a mononuclear inflammatory infiltrate, and the lumen may be collapsed with decreased alveolar attachments (Figure 2.36). Oral prednisolone administration uncovers a subgroup of patients with COPD who show a degree of airway reversibility associated with histological features of asthma[161], and there are patients with sputum eosinophilia who do not show the characteristic clinical features of asthma. Smokers with the combined structural and inflammatory features of both COPD and asthma are likely to be more frequent than appreciated from the currently reported studies that compare highly selected groups of smokers with mild COPD and non-smokers with asthma. In severe stable asthma, there may be an increase in neutrophils[162], whereas, in exacerbations of COPD, there may be an increase in eosinophils[35].

Figure 2.34   Comparison of inflammation in COPD and asthma

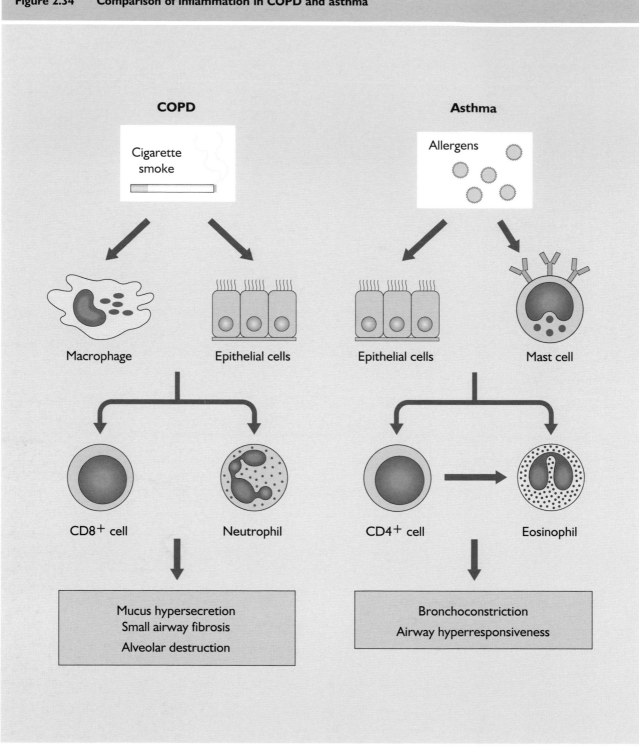

COPD involves an amplified inflammatory response to oxidants in cigarette smoke, which activates airway and alveolar macrophages and epithelial cells, resulting in the recruitment of CD8+ T cells and neutrophils. In response to increased levels of proteases and disturbance in inflammatory mediators and cytokines, mucus hypersecretion, small airway fibrosis and alveolar destruction occur.

In contrast, asthma may be triggered by allergens that cause the degranulation of mast cells, the activation of epithelial cells, and the recruitment of CD4+ T cells and eosinophils. Characteristic features of asthma are intermittent and reversible bronchoconstriction, associated with airway hyperresponsiveness.

Figure 2.35   Comparison of the pathophysiology of COPD and asthma

	COPD	Asthma
Lung function: airflow obstruction	Fixed, irreversible and progressive	Variable and reversible in mild and moderate asthma. Can become fixed and irreversible in severe asthma with extensive airway remodelling
Bronchodilator response (FEV$_1$) Steroid response (FEV$_1$) Peak flow reversibility	< 15%	> 15%
Postmortem: macroscopic	Excessive mucus Small airway disease Emphysema: holes	Hyperinflation and airway plugging in asthma death
Sputum	Neutrophils and macrophages 2 : 1 ratio (normal 1 : 2)	Eosinophilia Creola bodies Charcot–Leyden crystals Curschmann's spirals
Bronchial epithelium	Bronchial goblet cell hyperplasia and squamous metaplasia	Fragile with stripping and denudation
Reticular subepithelial basement membrane	No change	Thickened and hyaline
Congestion/edema	Present	Present
Remodelling	Fibrosis in bronchioles Destruction of alveoli	Smooth muscle hypertrophy and fibrosis in advanced disease
Bronchial smooth muscle	Enlarged mass (small airways)	Enlarged mass (large airways)
Bronchial glands	Prominent enlargement and increased acid glycoprotein in chronic bronchitis	Moderate enlargement
Cellular infiltrate	CD8$^+$ T cells neutrophils macrophages	CD4$^+$ T cells eosinophils mast cells

Figure 2.36   Comparative histology of the bronchiole in asthma and COPD

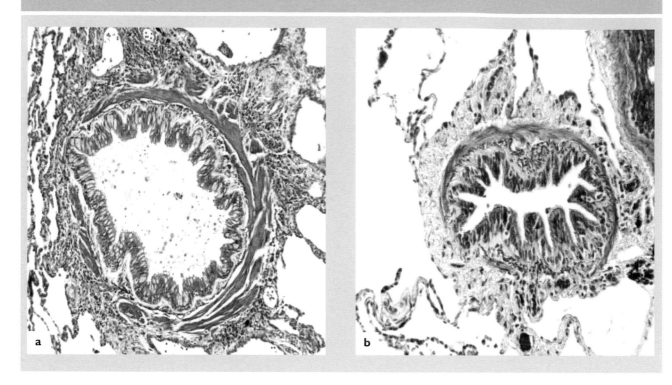

(a) Peripheral conducting airway from a patient who died of asthma. The airway lumen is filled with an inflammatory exudate that contains plasma proteins, inflammatory cells, sloughed epithelial cells, and mucus. There are metaplastic changes in the epithelium, with increased numbers of goblet cells. There is also an increase in muscle and connective tissue, but the caliber of the airway lumen is not reduced. Increased numbers of mast cells and eosinophils are present in the airway wall.

(b) Airway from a patient with COPD, where the caliber of the airways is reduced by airway collapse, with the wall thickness increased by peribronchiolar inflammatory process with connective tissue deposition in the adventitia, and loss of alveolar attachments.

Reproduced with permission of Dr James C. Hogg and the publishers, from *Asthma and COPD: Basic Mechanisms and Clinical Management*, edited by P.J. Barnes *et al.*, Academic Press, 2002.

REFERENCES

1.   Barnes PJ. Chronic obstructive pulmonary disease. *N Engl J Med* 2000;343:269–80

2.   Barnes PJ. Molecular genetics of chronic obstructive pulmonary disease. *Thorax* 1999;54:245–52

3.   Meshi B, Vitalis TZ, Ionescu D, Elliott WM, Liu C, Wang XD, *et al*. Emphysematous lung destruction by cigarette smoke. The effects of latent adenoviral infection on the lung inflammatory response. *Am J Respir Cell Mol Biol* 2002;26:52–7

4.   Gilmour PS, Rahman I, Hayashi S, Hogg JC, Donaldson K, MacNee W. Adenoviral E1A primes alveolar epithelial cells to PM(10)-induced transcription of interleukin-8. *Am J Physiol Lung Cell Mol Physiol* 2001;281:L598–606

5.   Ito K, Barnes PJ, Adcock IM. Glucocorticoid receptor recruitment of histone deacetylase 2 inhibits interleukin-1b-induced histone H4 acetylation on lysines 8 and 12. *Mol Cell Biol* 2000;20:6891–903

6.   Ito K, Lim S, Caramori G, Chung KF, Barnes PJ, Adcock IM. Cigarette smoking reduces histone deacetylase 2 expression, enhances cytokine expression and inhibits glucocorticoid actions in alveolar macrophages. *FASEB J* 2001;15:1100–2

7.   Pesci A, Balbi B, Majori M, Cacciani G, Bertacco S, Alciato P, *et al*. Inflammatory cells and mediators in bronchial lavage of patients with chronic obstructive pulmonary disease. *Eur Respir J* 1998;12:380–6

8.   Finkelstein R, Fraser RS, Ghezzo H, Cosio MG. Alveolar inflammation and its relation to emphy-

sema in smokers. *Am J Resp Crit Care Med* 1995;152:1666–72

9. Di Stefano A, Capelli A, Lusuardi M, Balbo P, Vecchio C, Maestrelli P, *et al.* Severity of airflow limitation is associated with severity of airway inflammation in smokers. *Am J Respir Crit Care Med* 1998;158:1277–85

10. Tomita K, Caramori G, Lim S, Ito K, Hanazawa T, Oates T, *et al.* Increased p21(CIP1/WAF1) and B cell lymphoma leukemia-x(L) expression and reduced apoptosis in alveolar macrophages from smokers. *Am J Respir Crit Care Med* 2002;166:724–31

11. Saetta M, Di Stefano A, Maestrelli P, Ferraresso A, Drigo R, Potena A, *et al.* Activated T-lymphocytes and macrophages in bronchial mucosa of subjects with chronic bronchitis. *Am Rev Respir Dis* 1993;147:301–6

12. O'Shaughnessy TC, Ansari TW, Barnes NC, Jeffery PK. Inflammation in bronchial biopsies of subjects with chronic bronchitis: inverse relationship of CD8+ T lymphocytes with FEV1. *Am J Respir Crit Care Med* 1997;155:852–7

13. Fournier M, Lebargy F, Le Roy LF, Lenormand E, Pariente R. Intraepithelial T-lymphocyte subsets in the airways of normal subjects and of patients with chronic bronchitis. *Am Rev Respir Dis* 1989;140:737–42

14. Saetta M, Turato G, Facchini FM, Corbino L, Lucchini RE, Casoni G, *et al.* Inflammatory cells in the bronchial glands of smokers with chronic bronchitis. *Am J Respir Crit Care Med* 1997;156:1633–9

15. Majo J, Ghezzo H, Cosio MG. Lymphocyte population and apoptosis in the lungs of smokers and their relation to emphysema. *Eur Respir J* 2001;17:946–53

16. Saetta M, Baraldo S, Corbino L, Turato G, Braccioni F, Rea F, *et al.* CD8+ve cells in the lungs of smokers with chronic obstructive pulmonary disease. *Am J Respir Crit Care Med* 1999;160:711–17

17. Liu AN, Mohammed AZ, Rice WR, Fiedeldey DT, Liebermann JS, Whitsett JA, *et al.* Perforin-independent CD8(+) T-cell-mediated cytotoxicity of alveolar epithelial cells is preferentially mediated by tumor necrosis factor- alpha: relative insensitivity to Fas ligand. *Am J Respir Cell Mol Biol* 1999;20:849–58

18. Hashimoto S, Kobayashi A, Kooguchi K, Kitamura Y, Onodera H, Nakajima H. Upregulation of two death pathways of perforin/granzyme and FasL/Fas in septic acute respiratory distress syndrome. *Am J Respir Crit Care Med* 2000;161:237–43

19. Vukmanovic-Stejic M, Vyas B, Gorak-Stolinska P, Noble A, Kemeny DM. Human Tc1 and Tc2/Tc0 CD8 T-cell clones display distinct cell surface and functional phenotypes. *Blood* 2000;95:231–40

20. Thompson AB, Daughton D, Robbins RA, Ghafouri MA, Oehlerking M, Rennard SI. Intraluminal airway inflammation in chronic bronchitis. Characterization and correlation with clinical parameters. *Am Rev Respir Dis* 1989;140:1527–37

21. Keatings VM, Collins PD, Scott DM, Barnes PJ. Differences in interleukin-8 and tumour necrosis factor-alpha in induced sputum from patients with chronic obstructive pulmonary disease or asthma. *Am J Respir Crit Care Med* 1996;153:530–4

22. Lacoste JY, Bousquet J, Chanez P, Van Vyve T, Simony-Lafontaine J, Lequeu N, *et al.* Eosinophilic and neutrophilic inflammation in asthma, chronic bronchitis, and chronic obstructive pulmonary disease. *J Allergy Clin Immunol* 1993;92:537–48

23. Keatings VM, Barnes PJ. Granulocyte activation markers in induced sputum: comparison between chronic obstructive pulmonary disease, asthma, and normal subjects. *Am J Respir Crit Care Med* 1997;155:449–53

24. Peleman RA, Rytila PH, Kips JC, Joos GF, Pauwels RA. The cellular composition of induced sputum in chronic obstructive pulmonary disease. *Eur Respir J* 1999;13:839–43

25. O'Shaughnessy TC, Ansari TW, Barnes NC. Inflammatory cells in the airway surface epithelium of smokers with and without bronchitic airflow obstruction. *Eur Respir J* 1996;9(Suppl 23):14s

26. Stanescu D, Sanna A, Veriter C, Kostianev S, Calcagni PG, Fabbri IM, *et al.* Airways obstruction, chronic expectoration, and rapid decline of FEV1 in smokers are associated with increased levels of sputum neutrophils. *Thorax* 1996;51:267–71

27. Turato G, Di Stefano A, Maestrelli P, Mapp CE, Ruggieri MP, Roggeri A, *et al.* Effect of smoking cessation on airway inflammation in chronic bronchitis. *Am J Respir Crit Care Med* 1995;152:1262–7

28. Rutgers SR, Postma DS, ten Hacken NH, Kauffman HF, Der Mark TW, ter GH, *et al.* Ongoing airway inflammation in patients with COPD who do not currently smoke. *Thorax* 2000;55:12–18

29. Di Stefano A, Maestrelli P, Roggeri A, Turato G, Calabro S, Potena A, *et al.* Upregulation of adhesion molecules in the bronchial mucosa of subjects with chronic obstructive bronchitis. *Am J Respir Crit Care Med* 1994;149:803–10

61

30. Turato G, Zuin R, Saetta M. Pathogenesis and pathology of COPD. *Respiration* 2001;68:4–19

31. Brightling CE, Monteiro W, Ward R, Parker D, Morgan MD, Wardlaw AJ, *et al.* Sputum eosinophilia and short-term response to prednisolone in chronic obstructive pulmonary disease: a randomised controlled trial. *Lancet* 2000;356:1480–5

32. Papi A, Romagnoli M, Baraldo S, Braccioni F, Guzzinati I, Saetta M, *et al.* Partial reversibility of airflow limitation and increased exhaled NO and sputum eosinophilia in chronic obstructive pulmonary disease. *Am J Respir Crit Care Med* 2000;162:1773–7

33. Liu H, Lazarus SC, Caughey GH, Fahy JV. Neutrophil elastase and elastase-rich cystic fibrosis sputum degranulate human eosinophils *in vitro*. *Am J Physiol* 1999;276:L28–34

34. Zhu J, Majumdar S, Qui Y, Ansari T, Oliva A, Kips JC, *et al.* Interleukin-4 and interleukin-5 gene expression and inflammation in the mucus-secretion glands and subepithelial tissue of smokers with chronic bronchitis. *Am J Respir Crit Care Med* 2001;164:2220–8

35. Saetta M, Di Stefano A, Maestrelli P, Turato G, Ruggieri MP, Roggeri A, *et al.* Airway eosinophilia in chronic bronchitis during exacerbations. *Am J Respir Crit Care Med* 1994;150:1646–52

36. Saetta M, Di Stefano A, Maestrelli P, Turato G, Mapp CE, Pieno M, *et al.* Airway eosinophilia and expression of interleukin-5 protein in asthma and in exacerbations of chronic bronchitis. *Clin Exp Allergy* 1996;26:766–74

37. Zhu J, Qiu YS, Majumdar S, Gamble E, Matin D, Turato G, *et al.* Exacerbations of bronchitis: bronchial eosinophilia and gene expression for interleukin-4, interleukin-5, and eosinophil chemoattractants. *Am J Respir Crit Care Med* 2001;164:109–16

38. Gibson PG, Hargreaves FE, Girgis-Gabardo A. Chronic cough with eosinophilic bronchitis and examination for variable airflow obstruction and response to corticosteroid. *Allergy* 1995;25:127–32

39. Takizawa H, Tanaka M, Takami K, Ohtoshi T, Ito K, Satoh M, *et al.* Increased expression of transforming growth factor-beta1 in small airway epithelium from tobacco smokers and patients with chronic obstructive pulmonary disease (COPD). *Am J Respir Crit Care Med* 2001;163:1476–83

40. Kasahara Y, Tuder RM, Taraseviciene-Stewart L, Le Cras TD, Abman S, Hirth PK, *et al.* Inhibition of VEGF receptors causes lung cell apoptosis and emphysema. *J Clin Invest* 2000;106:1311–19

41. Hill AT, Bayley DL, Stockley RA. The interrelationship of sputum inflammatory markers in patients with chronic bronchitis. *Am J Respir Crit Care Med* 1999;160:893–8

42. Hubbard RC, Fells G, Gadek J, Pacholok S, Humes J, Crystal RG. Neutrophil accumulation in the lung in alpha 1-antitrypsin deficiency. Spontaneous release of leukotriene B4 by alveolar macrophages. *J Clin Invest* 1991;88:891–7

43. Yamamoto C, Yoneda T, Yoshikawa M, Fu A, Tokuyama T, Tsukaguchi K, *et al.* Airway inflammation in COPD assessed by sputum levels of interleukin-8. *Chest* 1997;112:505–10

44. Kwon OJ, Au BT, Collins PD, Adcock IM, Mak JC, Robbins RR, *et al.* Tumor necrosis factor-induced interleukin-8 expression in cultured human airway epithelial cells. *Am J Physiol* 1994;267:L398–405

45. Capelli A, Stefano ADi, Gnemmi I, Balbo P, Cerutti CG, Balbi B, *et al.* Increased MCP-1 and MIP-1beta in bronchoalveolar lavage fluid of chronic bronchitics. *Eur Respir J* 1999;14:160–5

46. Traves SL, Culpitt SV, Russell RE, Barnes PJ, Donnelly LE. Increased levels of the chemokines GROalpha and MCP-1 in sputum samples from patients with COPD. *Thorax* 2002;57:590–5

47. Aaron SD, Angel JB, Lunau M, Wright K, Fex C, Le Saux N, *et al.* Granulocyte inflammatory markers and airway infection during acute exacerbation of chronic obstructive pulmonary disease. *Am J Respir Crit Care Med* 2001;163:349–55

48. Barnes PJ, Karin M. Nuclear factor-kb-A pivotal transcription factor in chronic inflammatory diseases. *N Engl J Med* 1997;336:1066–71

49. de Godoy I, Donahoe M, Calhoun WJ, Mancino J, Rogers RM. Elevated TNF-alpha production by peripheral blood monocytes of weight-losing COPD patients. *Am J Respir Crit Care Med* 1996;153:633–7

50. Langen RC, Schols AM, Kelders MC, Wouters EF, Janssen-Heininger YM. Inflammatory cytokines inhibit myogenic differentiation through activation of nuclear factor-kappaB. *FASEB J* 2001;15:1169–80

51. Barnes PJ. Cytokine modulators as novel therapies for airway disease. *Eur Respir J* 2001;18:67S–77S

52. de Boer WI, van Schadewijk A, Sont JK, Sharma HS, Stolk J, Hiemstra PS, *et al.* Transforming growth factor beta1 and recruitment of macrophages and mast cells in airways in chronic obstructive pulmonary disease. *Am J Respir Crit Care Med* 1998;158:1951–7

53. Zheng T, Zhu Z, Wang Z, Homer RJ, Ma B, Riese RJ Jr, et al. Inducible targeting of IL-13 to the adult lung causes matrix metalloproteinase- and cathepsin-dependent emphysema. J Clin Invest 2000; 106:1081–93

54. Wang Z, Zheng T, Zhu Z, Homer RJ, Riese RJ, Chapman HA Jr, et al. Interferon gamma induction of pulmonary emphysema in the adult murine lung. J Exp Med 2000;192:1587–600

55. Chalmers GW, Macleod KJ, Sriram S, Thomson LJ, McSharry C, Stack BH, et al. Sputum endothelin-1 is increased in cystic fibrosis and chronic obstructive pulmonary disease. Eur Respir J 1999;13:1288–92

56. Roland M, Bhowmik A, Sapsford RJ, Seemungal TA, Jeffries DJ, Warner TD, et al. Sputum and plasma endothelin-1 levels in exacerbations of chronic obstructive pulmonary disease. Thorax 2001;56:30–5

57. Giaid A, Yanagisawa M, Langleben D, Michel RP, Levy R, Shennib H, et al. Expression of endothelin-1 in the lungs of patients with pulmonary hypertension. N Engl J Med 1993;328:1732–9

58. Repine JE, Bast A, Lankhorst I. Oxidative stress in chronic obstructive pulmonary disease. Oxidative Stress Study Group. Am J Respir Crit Care Med 1997;156:341–57

59. MacNee W. Oxidants/antioxidants and COPD. Chest 2000;117(5 Suppl 1):303S–17S

60. Ichinose M, Sugiura H, Yamagata S, Koarai A, Shirato K. Increase in reactive nitrogen species production in chronic obstructive pulmonary disease airways. Am J Respir Crit Care Med 2000;162:701–6

61. MacNee W. Oxidative stress and lung inflammation in airways disease. Eur J Pharmacol 2001;429: 195–207

62. Seventeenth Transatlantic Airway Conference Supplement: Oxidants and antioxidants. Am J Respir Crit Care Med 2002;166:S1–66

63. Dekhuijzen PN, Aben KK, Dekker I, Aarts LP, Wielders PL, van Herwaarden CL, et al. Increased exhalation of hydrogen peroxide in patients with stable and unstable chronic obstructive pulmonary disease. Am J Respir Crit Care Med 1996;154: 813–16

64. Paredi P, Kharitonov SA, Leak D, Ward S, Cramer D, Barnes PJ. Exhaled ethane, a marker of lipid peroxidation, is elevated in chronic obstructive pulmonary disease. Am J Respir Crit Care Med 2000;162: 369–73

65. Montuschi P, Collins JV, Ciabattoni G, Lazzeri N, Corradi M, Kharitonov SA, et al. Exhaled 8-isoprostane as an in vivo biomarker of lung oxidative stress in patients with COPD and healthy smokers. Am J Respir Crit Care Med 2000;162:1175–7

66. Pratico D, Basili S, Vieri M, Cordova C, Violi F, Fitzgerald GA. Chronic obstructive pulmonary disease is associated with an increase in urinary levels of isoprostane F2alpha-III, an index of oxidant stress. Am J Respir Crit Care Med 1998;158:1709–14

67. Stockley RA. The role of proteinases in the pathogenesis of chronic bronchitis. Am J Respir Crit Care Med 1994;150:S109–13

68. Shapiro SD. Elastolytic metalloproteinases produced by human mononuclear phagocytes. Potential roles in destructive lung disease. Am J Respir Crit Care Med 1994;150:S160–4

69. Finlay GA, Russell KJ, McMahon KJ, D'arcy EM, Masterson JB, FitzGerald MX, et al. Elevated levels of matrix metalloproteinases in bronchoalveolar lavage fluid of emphysematous patients. Thorax 1997;52:502–6

70. Finlay GA, O'Driscoll LR, Russell KJ, D'arcy EM, Masterson JB, FitzGerald MX, et al. Matrix metalloproteinase expression and production by alveolar macrophages in emphysema. Am J Respir Crit Care Med 1997;156:240–7

71. Shapiro SD, Kobayashi DK, Ley TJ. Cloning and characterization of a unique elastolytic metalloproteinase produced by human alveolar macrophages. J Biol Chem 1993;268:23824–9

72. Hautamaki RD, Kobayashi DK, Senior RM, Shapiro SD. Requirement for macrophage metalloelastase for cigarette smoke-induced emphysema in mice. Science 1997;277:2002–4

73. Dallas SL, Rosser JL, Mundy GR, Bonewald LF. Proteolysis of latent transforming growth factor-beta (TGF-beta)-binding protein-1 by osteoclasts. A cellular mechanism for release of TGF-beta from bone matrix. J Biol Chem 2002;277:21352–60

74. Kranenburg AR, de Boer WI, van Krieken JH, Mooi WJ, Walters JE, Saxena PR, et al. Enhanced expression of fibroblast growth factors and receptor FGFR-1 during vascular remodeling in chronic obstructive pulmonary disease. Am J Respir Cell Mol Biol 2002;27:517–25

75. Miotto D, Hollenberg MD, Bunnett NW, Papi A, Braccioni F, Boschetto P, et al. Expression of protease activated receptor-2 (PAR-2) in central airways of smokers and non-smokers. Thorax 2002;57:146–51

76. Berger P, Perng DW, Thabrew H, Compton SJ, Cairns JA, McEuen AR, et al. Tryptase and agonists of PAR-

2 induce the proliferation of human airway smooth muscle cells. *J Appl Physiol* 2001;91:1372–9

77. Akers IA, Parsons M, Hill MR, Hollenberg MD, Sanjar S, Laurent GJ, *et al*. Mast cell tryptase stimulates human lung fibroblast proliferation via protease-activated receptor-2. *Am J Physiol Lung Cell Mol Physiol* 2000;278:L193–201

78. Vligoftis H, Schwingshackl A, Milne CD, Duszyk M, Hollenberg MD, Wallace JL, *et al*. Proteinase-activated receptor-2-mediated matrix metalloproteinase-9 release from airway epithelial cells. *J Allergy Clin Immunol* 2000;106:537–45

79. Saetta M, Turato G, Maestrelli P, Mapp CE, Fabbri LM. Cellular and structural bases of chronic obstructive pulmonary disease. *Am J Respir Crit Care Med* 2001;163:1304–9

80. Jeffery PK. Comparison of the structural and inflammatory features of COPD and asthma. Giles F. Filley Lecture. *Chest* 2000;117(Suppl 1):251S–60S

81. Calhoun WJ, Retamales I, Elliott WM, Meshi B, Coxson HO, Havashi S, *et al*. More inflammation than lung in emphysema. *Am J Respir Crit Care Med* 2002;165:730B–1

82. Hogg JC. Chronic obstructive pulmonary disease: an overview of pathology and pathogenesis. *Novartis Found Symp* 2001;234:4–19

83. Jeffery PK. Remodeling in asthma and chronic obstructive lung disease. *Am J Respir Crit Care Med* 2001;164:S28–38

84. Jeffery PK. Lymphocytes, chronic bronchitis and chronic obstructive pulmonary disease. *Novartis Found Symp* 2001;234:149–61

85. Jeffery PK, Laitinen A, Venge P. Biopsy markers of airway inflammation and remodelling. *Respir Med* 2000;94(Suppl F):S9–15

86. Corrin B. *Pathology of the Lungs*. London: Churchill Livingstone, 2000

87. Wright RR, Stuart CM. Chronic bronchitis with emphysema: a pathological study of the bronchi. *Medicina Thoracalis* 1965;22:210–18

88. Klienerman J, Boren HG. Morphologic basis of chronic obstructive lung disease. In Baum GL, ed. *Textbook of Pulmonary Disease*. Boston, MA: Little Brown 1974:571

89. Ailsby RL, Ghadially FN. Atypical cilia in human bronchial mucosa. *J Pathol* 1973;109:75–8

90. Chang SC. Microscopic properties of whole mounts and sections of human bronchial epithelium of smokers and nonsmokers. *Cancer* 1957;10:1246–62

91. Wanner A. Clinical aspects of mucociliary transport. *Am Rev Respir Dis* 1977;116:73–125

92. Miskovits G, Appel J, Szule P. Ultrastructural changes of ciliated columnar epithelium and goblet cells in chronic bronchitis biopsy material. *Acta Morphol Acad Sci Hung* 1974;22:91–103

93. Ollerenshaw SL, Woolcock AJ. Characteristics of the inflammation in biopsies from large airways of subjects with asthma and subjects with chronic airflow limitation. *Am Rev Respir Dis* 1992;145:922–7

94. O'Shaughnessy TC, Ansari TW, Barnes NC. Reticular basement membarne thickness in moderately severe asthma and smokers' chronic bronchitis with and without airflow obstruction. *Am J Respir Crit Care Med* 1996;153:A879

95. Mullen JB, Wright JL, Wiggs BR, Pare PD, Hogg JC. Reassessment of inflammation of airways in chronic bronchitis. *Br Med J (Clin Res Ed)* 1985;291:1235–9

96. Grashoff WF, Sont JK, Sterk PJ, Hiemstra PS, de Boer WI, Stolk J, *et al*. Chronic obstructive pulmonary disease: role of bronchiolar mast cells and macrophages. *Am J Pathol* 1997;151:1785–90

97. Vignola AM, Campbell AM, Chanez P, Bousquet J, Paul-Lacoste P, Michel FB, *et al*. HLA-DR and ICAM-1 expression on bronchial epithelial cells in asthma and chronic bronchitis. *Am Rev Respir Dis* 1993;148:689–94

98. Reid L. Pathology of chronic bronchitis. *Lancet* 1954;1:275–9

99. Reid L. Measurement of the bronchial mucous gland layer: a diagnostic yardstick in chronic bronchitis. *Thorax* 1960;6:132–41

100. Dunnill MS, Massarella GR, Anderson JA. A comparison of the quantitative anatomy of the bronchi in normal subjects, in status asthmaticus, in chronic bronchitis, and in emphysema. *Thorax* 1969;24:176–9

101. Haraguchi M, Shimura S, Shirato K. Morphometric analysis of bronchial cartilage in chronic obstructive pulmonary disease and bronchial asthma. *Am J Respir Crit Care Med* 1999;159:1005–13

102. Thurlbeck WM, Pun R, Toth J, Frazer RG. Bronchial cartilage in chronic obstructive lung disease. *Am Rev Respir Dis* 1974;109:73–80

103. Takeyama K, Dabbagh K, Lee HM, Agusti C, Lausier JA, Ueki IF, *et al*. Epidermal growth factor system regulates mucin production in airways. *Proc Natl Acad Sci USA* 1999;96:3081–6

104. Reid CJ, Gould S, Harris A. Developmental expression of mucin genes in the human respiratory tract. *Am J Respir Cell Mol Biol* 1997;17:592–8

105. Vestbo J, Prescott E, Lange P. Association of chronic mucus hypersecretion with FEV1 decline and chronic obstructive pulmonary disease morbidity. *Am J Respir Crit Care Med* 1996;153:1530–5

106. Vestbo J, Lange P. Can GOLD Stage 0 provide information of prognostic value in chronic obstructive pulmonary disease? *Am J Respir Crit Care Med* 2002;166:329–32

107. Jeffery PK, Reid L. New observations of rat airway epithelium: a quantitative and electron microscopic study. *J Anat* 1975;120:295–320

108. Jeffery PK. Structural, immunologic, and neural elements of the normal human airway wall. In Busse WWHS, ed. *Asthma and Rhinitis.* Oxford, UK: Blackwell Scientific Publications, 1995:80–106

109. Ebert RV, Terracio MJ. The bronchiolar epithelium in cigarette smokers. Observations with the scanning electron microscope. *Am Rev Respir Dis* 1975;111:4–11

110. Ebert RV, Hanks PB. Mucus secretion by the epithelium of the bronchioles of cigarette smokers. *Br J Dis Chest* 1981;75:277–82

111. Cosio MG, Hale KA, Niewoehner DE. Morphologic and morphometric effects of prolonged cigarette smoking on the small airways. *Am Rev Respir Dis* 1980;122:265–21

112. Macklem PT, Proctor DF, Hogg JC. The stability of peripheral airways. *Respir Physiol* 1970;8:191–203

113. Jeffery PK. Structural and inflammatory changes in COPD: a comparison with asthma. *Thorax* 1998;53:129–36

114. Saetta M, Turato G, Baraldo S, Zanin A, Braccioni F, Mapp CE, *et al.* Goblet cell hyperplasia and epithelial inflammation in peripheral airways of smokers with both symptoms of chronic bronchitis and chronic airflow limitation. *Am J Respir Crit Care Med* 2000;161:1016–21

115. Saetta M, Di Stefano A, Turato G, Facchini FM, Corbino L, Mapp CE, *et al.* CD8+ T-lymphocytes in peripheral airways of smokers with chronic obstructive pulmonary disease. *Am J Respir Crit Care Med* 1998;157:822–6

116. Lams BEA, Sousa AR, Rees PJ, Lee TH. Immunopathology of the small-airway submucosa in smokers with and without chronic obstructive pulmonary disease. *Am J Respir Crit Care Med* 1998;158:1518–23

117. Elliot WM, Retamales I, Meshi B. Inflammatory cell recruitment in emphysema. *Am J Respir Crit Care Med* 1999;159:A810

118. Snider GL. Chronic obstructive pulmonary disease – a continuing challenge. *Am Rev Respir Dis* 1986;133:942–4

119. Thurlbeck WM. Chronic airflow obstruction: correlation of structure and function. In Petty TL, ed. *COPD, 2nd edn.* New York: Markel Dekker, 1985:129–203

120. Wright JL, Lawson LM, Pare PD, Wiggs BJ, Kennedy S, Hogg JC. Morphology of peripheral airways in current smokers and ex-smokers. *Am Rev Respir Dis* 1983;127:474–7

121. Verbeken EK, Cauberghs M, Mertens I, Lauweryns JM, Van de Woestijne KP. Tissue and airway impedance of excised normal, senile, and emphysematous lungs. *J Appl Physiol* 1992;72:2343–53

122. Wright JL, Hobson JE, Wiggs B, Pare PD, Hogg JC. Airway inflammation and peribronchiolar attachments in the lungs of nonsmokers, current and ex-smokers. *Lung* 1988;166:277–86

123. Niewoehner DE, Kleinerman J, Rice DB. Pathologic changes in the peripheral airways of young cigarette smokers. *N Engl J Med* 1974;291:755–8

124. Reynolds HY. Bronchoalveolar lavage. *Am Rev Respir Dis* 1987;135:250–63

125. Matsuba K, Thurlbeck WM. The number and dimensions of small airways in emphysematous lungs. *Am J Pathol* 1972;67:265–75

126. Bignon J, Khoury F, Even P, Andre J, Brouet G. Morphometric study in chronic obstructive bronchopulmonary disease. Pathologic, clinical, and physiologic correlations. *Am Rev Respir Dis* 1969;99:669–95

127. Hogg JC, Macklem PT, Thurlbeck WM. Site and nature of airway obstruction in chronic obstructive lung disease. *N Engl J Med* 1968;278:1355–60

128. Mitchell RS, Stanford RE, Johnson JM, Silvers GW, Dart G, George MS. The morphologic features of the bronchi, bronchioles, and alveoli in chronic airway obstruction: a clinicopathologic study. *Am Rev Respir Dis* 1976;114:137–45

129. Hale KA, Ewing SL, Gosnell BA, Niewoehner DE. Lung disease in long-term cigarette smokers with and without chronic air-flow obstruction. *Am Rev Respir Dis* 1984;130:716–21

130. Jamal K, Cooney TP, Fleetham JA, Thurlbeck WM. Chronic bronchitis. Correlation of morphologic find-

ings to sputum production and flow rates. *Am Rev Respir Dis* 1984;129:719-22

131. Saetta M, Ghezzo H, Kim WD, King M, Angus GE, Wang NS, *et al.* Loss of alveolar attachments in smokers. A morphometric correlate of lung function impairment. *Am Rev Respir Dis* 1985;132:894–900

132. Finkelstein R, Ma HD, Ghezzo H, Whittaker K, Fraser RS, Cosio MG. Morphometry of small airways in smokers and its relationship to emphysema type and hyperresponsiveness. *Am J Respir Crit Care Med* 1995;152:267–76

133. Linhartova A, Anderson AEJ, Foraker AG. Further observations on luminal deformity and stenosis of nonrespiratory bronchioles in pulmonary emphysema. *Thorax* 1977;32:50–3

134. Anderson AEJ, Foraker AG. Relative dimensions of bronchioles and parenchymal spaces in lungs from normal subjects and emphysematous patients. *Am J Med* 1962;32:218–26

135. Gelb AF, Hogg JC, Muller NL, Schein MJ, Kuei J, Tashkin DP, *et al.* Contribution of emphysema and small airways in COPD. *Chest* 1996;109:353–9

136. Leopold JG, Gough J. Centrilobular form of hypertrophic emphysema and its relation to chronic bronchitis. *Thorax* 1957;12:219–35

137. Cosio MG, Cosio Piqueras MG. Pathology of emphysema in chronic obstructive pulmonary disease. *Monaldi Arch Chest Dis* 2000;55:124–9

138. Kim WD, Eidelman DH, Izquierdo JL, Ghezzo H, Saetta MP, Cosio MG. Centrilobular and panlobular emphysema in smokers. Two distinct morphologic and functional entities. *Am Rev Respir Dis* 1991;144:1385–90

139. Gillooly M, Lamb D. Microscopic emphysema in relation to age and smoking habit. *Thorax* 1993;48:491–5

140. Lamb D, McLean A, Gillooly M, Warren PM, Gould GA, MacNee W. Relation between distal airspace size, bronchiolar attachments, and lung function. *Thorax* 1993;48:1012–17

141. Eidelman D, Saetta MP, Ghezzo H, Wang NS, Hoidal JR, King M, *et al.* Cellularity of the alveolar walls in smokers and its relation to alveolar destruction. Functional implications. *Am Rev Respir Dis* 1990;141:1547–52

142. Aoshiba K, Yokohori N, Nagai A. Alveolar wall apoptosis causes lung destruction and emphysematous changes. *Am J Respir Cell Mol Biol* 2003;28:555–62

143. Tuder RM, Petrache I, Elias JA, Voelkel NF, Henson PM. Apoptosis and emphysema: the missing link. *Am J Respir Cell Mol Biol* 2003;28:551–4

144. Vlahovic G, Russell ML, Mercer RR, Crapo JD. Cellular and connective tissue changes in alveolar septal walls in emphysema. *Am J Resp Crit Care Med* 1999;160:2086–92

145. Lang MR, Fiaux GW, Gillooly M, Stewart JA, Hulmes DJ, Lamb D. Collagen content of alveolar wall tissue in emphysematous and non-emphysematous lungs. *Thorax* 1994;49:319–26

146. Sekhon HS, Wright JL, Churg A. Cigarette smoke causes rapid cell proliferation in small airways and associated pulmonary arteries. *Am J Physiol* 1994;267:L557–63

147. Peinado VI, Barbera JA, Abate P, Ramirez J, Roca J, Santos S, *et al.* Inflammatory reaction in pulmonary muscular arteries of patients with mild chronic obstructive pulmonary disease. *Am J Respir Crit Care Med* 1999;159:1605–11

148. Peinado VI, Barbera JA, Ramirez J, Gomez FP, Roca J, Jover L, *et al.* Endothelial dysfunction in pulmonary arteries of patients with mild COPD. *Am J Physiol* 1998;274:L908–13

149. Barbera JA, Peinado VI, Santos S. Pulmonary hypertension in COPD: old and new concepts. *Monaldi Arch Chest Dis* 2000;55:445–9

150. Sofia M, Mormile M, Faraone S, Carratu P, Alifano M, Di Benedetto G, *et al.* Increased 24-hour endothelin-1 urinary excretion in patients with chronic obstructive pulmonary disease. *Respiration* 1994;61:263–8

151. Barbera JA, Riverola A, Roca J, Ramirez J, Wagner PD, Ros D, *et al.* Pulmonary vascular abnormalities and ventilation-perfusion relationships in mild chronic obstructive pulmonary disease. *Am J Respir Crit Care Med* 1994;149:423–9

152. Bernard S, LeBlanc P, Whittom F, Carrier G, Jobin J, Belleau R, *et al.* Peripheral muscle weakness in patients with chronic obstructive pulmonary disease. *Am J Respir Crit Care Med* 1998;158:629–34

153. Schols AM, Slangen J, Volovics L, Wouters EF. Weight loss is a reversible factor in the prognosis of chronic obstructive pulmonary disease. *Am J Respir Crit Care Med* 1998;157:1791–7

154. Schols AM, Buurman WA, Staal van den Brekel AJ, Dentener MA, Wouters EF. Evidence for a relation between metabolic derangements and increased levels of inflammatory mediators in a subgroup of

patients with chronic obstructive pulmonary disease. *Thorax* 1996;51:819–24

155. Schols AM, Creutzberg EC, Buurman WA, Campfield LA, Saris WH, Wouters EF. Plasma leptin is related to proinflammatory status and dietary intake in patients with chronic obstructive pulmonary disease. *Am J Respir Crit Care Med* 1999;160:1220–6

156. Eid AA, Ionescu AA, Nixon LS, Lewis-Jenkins V, Matthews SB, Griffiths TL, *et al*. Inflammatory response and body composition in chronic obstructive pulmonary disease. *Am J Respir Crit Care Med* 2001;164:1414–18

157. Schols AM, Soeters PB, Mostert R, Pluymers RJ, Wouters EF. Physiologic effects of nutritional support and anabolic steroids in patients with chronic obstructive pulmonary disease. A placebo-controlled randomized trial. *Am J Respir Crit Care Med* 1995;152:1268–74

158. Barnes PJ. Mechanisms in COPD: differences from asthma. *Chest* 2000;117(2 Suppl):10–14S

159. Fabbri L, Beghe B, Caramori G, Papi A, Saetta M. Similarities and discrepancies between exacerbations of asthma and chronic obstructive pulmonary disease. *Thorax* 1998;53:803–8

160. Jeffery PK. Differences and similarities between chronic obstructive pulmonary disease and asthma. *Clin Exp Allergy* 1999;29(Suppl 2):14–26

161. Chanez P, Vignola AM, O'Shaugnessy T, Enander I, Li D, Jeffery PK, *et al*. Corticosteroid reversibility in COPD is related to features of asthma. *Am J Respir Crit Care Med* 1997;155:1529–34

162. Jatakanon A, Uasuf C, Maziak W, Lim S, Chung KF, Barnes PJ. Neutrophilic inflammation in severe persistent asthma. *Am J Respir Crit Care Med* 1999;160:1532–9

3

Clinical aspects of COPD

CONTENTS

Clinical history: symptoms
Productive cough
Exertional dyspnea
Miscellaneous symptoms
Atypical symptoms
Exposure to risk factors

Physical examination: signs
Pink puffers and blue bloaters
Types of breathing
Breath sounds
Heart sounds
Chronic respiratory failure
Acute respiratory failure
Cor pulmonale
Pulmonary artery hypertension
Thromboembolic disease
Cachexia with nutritional depletion and
  muscle weakness/wasting
Sleep disorders

Differential diagnosis of COPD
Cigarette smoke-induced COPD
α_1-Antitrypsin deficiency
Primary ciliary dyskinesia
Asthma
Congestive heart failure

Ischemic heart disease
Bronchiectasis
Tuberculosis
Obliterative bronchiolitis
Diffuse panbronchiolitis
Need for referral

Investigations
Lung function
Blood, breath and sputum
Imaging
Electrocardiography
Echocardiography and esophageal
  cardiography
Miscellaneous

**Natural history, stages of
severity, monitoring, prognosis
and death**
Natural history
Stages of COPD severity
Decline in lung function
Horse-race effect
Smoking cessation
Prognosis
Death

SUMMARY

Chronic obstructive pulmonary disease (COPD) generally follows decades of heavy cigarette smoking, although other risk factors may be present, especially the burning of biomass fuels in developing countries (Figure 3.1).

COPD is a fixed obstructive airways disease distinct from other chronic obstructive lung conditions such as asthma, obliterative bronchiolitis, bronchiectasis and tuberculous lung disease.

Patients with COPD have variable pathology, including chronic bronchitis, obstructive bronchiolitis, emphysema and pulmonary vascular disease. More than one lung disease may be present at the same time, for example COPD and carcinoma of the lung commonly coexist in a heavy smoker, and some patients may have COPD and asthma.

Patients who have a chronic productive cough and insidious onset of dyspnea should have spirometry performed (Figure 3.1). Airflow limitation is confirmed by an FEV_1/FVC of $< 70\%$ and a pre-bronchodilator non-reversible FEV_1 of $< 80\%$ of that predicted for an individual of that height and weight. It is very important for every patient with COPD to stop smoking and to receive optimal bronchodilator therapy.

The natural history of COPD varies, and the two extremes are the 'pink puffer' and the 'blue bloater', although most patients have a mixed pattern. Patients with an FEV_1 of $< 40\%$ predicted, or with signs of respiratory failure such as central cyanosis, should have radial arterial blood gas tensions measured. Patients with more severe COPD may develop right heart failure (*cor pulmonale*) as well as nutritional depletion and cachexia.

High-resolution computerized tomography is proving useful in the assessment of COPD and is able to discern bronchial wall thickening (chronic bronchitis), ground-glass appearance (macrophage infiltrate of parenchyma), fluffy micronodules (bronchiolitis), areas of decreased attenuation (emphysema and bullae), as well as fibrosis and malignant lesions.

Monitoring of patients with COPD needs to involve lung function, as well as assessment for respiratory and cardiac failure, and nutritional depletion. The prognosis for patients with COPD remains bleak, although smoking cessation, optimal use of bronchodilators, and use of oxygen therapy and non-invasive ventilation are important therapeutic options.

Figure 3.1   The typical clinical picture of COPD

Symptoms

- Cough
- Sputum

Dyspnea =
abnormal awareness
of the act of breathing

Exposure to risk factors

- Tobacco smoke
- Occupation: coal mining
- Indoor/outdoor pollution
- Wood/biomass fuels
- Reduced lung growth
- Childhood pneumonia

Spirometry

- Reduced forced expiratory ratio (FEV_1/FVC) < 70%
- Reduced FEV_1% predicted post-bronchodilator
- Fixed, non-variable, slowly progressive obstruction
- Poorly reversible (< 12% with bronchodilator)

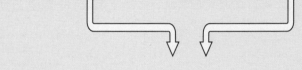

CLINICAL HISTORY: SYMPTOMS

Productive cough

A daily productive cough for at least 3 months of 2 consecutive years is part of the original clinical definition of chronic bronchitis (Figure 3.2). The cough is generally prominent in the morning on waking, and some patients claim that expectoration is assisted by having a cigarette. The sputum is mucinous but becomes purulent and increased in volume during exacerbations. A chronic productive cough can occur in isolation without development of airway obstruction.

Exertional dyspnea

Dyspnea is an abnormal awareness of the act of breathing, and dyspnea on exertion is usually the presenting symptom that causes the patient to consult their physician. As COPD progresses, dyspnea occurs with less and less effort, this exertional dyspnea being related to changes in end-expiratory volume during exercise[1,2]. Patients have usually lost a considerable amount of lung function by the time they present to a doctor, with FEV_1 values of < 50% predicted. During the early stages, most patients do not experience dyspnea except with significant exertion, and, by avoiding exertion, such individuals are able to avoid symptoms. Measurement of dyspnea using sensitive measures such as the Medical Research Council (MRC) dyspnea scale correlates weakly with FEV_1 and can be used to follow these patients objectively[3] (Figure 3.3). Patients generally present to the physician only after 50% of lung function is lost and when dyspnea is precipitated by relatively mild exertion[4–6]. Dyspnea is not closely correlated to arterial blood gases, as the typical 'blue bloater' with peripheral edema, hypoxemia and hypercapnia generally has less dyspnea, in contrast to the 'pink puffer' who generally does not have these blood gas abnormalities. Simple breathlessness (dyspnea) scores may be useful and may predict patients suitable for pulmonary rehabilitation and lung volume reduction surgery[3].

Miscellaneous symptoms

- Chest pains are common and may be due to concomitant ischemic heart disease or strain on intercostal muscles.

- Ankle swelling may be an important sign of right-sided heart failure when there is *cor pulmonale* (cardiac disease caused by lung disease).

- Anorexia and weight loss[7], as well as skeletal muscle wasting, are increasingly recognized[8,9].

- Muscle weakness and wasting: weight loss frequently occurs in advanced disease, and may be due to the increased work of breathing or increased production of TNF-α[10].

- The hallmarks of an exacerbation of COPD include increased cough, greater volumes of purulent sputum, increased dyspnea, and sometimes perceptible wheezing (see Chapter 6).

- Depression and malaise[11].

Atypical symptoms

The clinical features of COPD are usually characteristic, but care should be taken to carefully evaluate those symptoms and signs which are not typical. Some symptoms are not typical of COPD and should arouse suspicion that other pathology is present.

- Hemoptysis, rapid weight loss, recent onset of pneumonia or chest symptoms can occur due just to COPD, but their appearance in such a patient suggests the possibility of malignancy which must be carefully investigated. Hemoptysis complicating chronic bronchitis may occur with an infective episode.

- Seasonal exacerbations in spring or summer are more likely in asthma. Episodic and variable symptoms are more typical of asthma. Wheezing may occur during exacerbations of COPD and during periods of breathlessness, but is more typical of asthma. Excellent response to bronchodilators or steroids with definite symptom-free intervals is suggestive of asthma, not COPD.

- Continuous expectoration of purulent sputum is more typical of bronchiectasis than COPD.

- Breathlessness without productive cough or wheezing is more typical of cardiac disease or of other lung diseases such as interstitial pulmonary fibrosis.

Figure 3.2 Symptoms of COPD[1]

Cough
- Often discounted by the patient as an expected consequence of smoking
- Morning productive cough, often present on waking, but not disturbing sleep
- Often worse in winter months, after chest infection
- Initially intermittent, later present every day, often throughout the day
- May be unproductive, despite airflow limitation
- Cough syncope may occur after prolonged bouts of coughing

Sputum production
- Initially mucoid and not excessive (< 1 eggcupful/day)
- Purulent with exacerbation of COPD
- Continuous expectoration of purulent sputum suggests bronchiectasis
- Daily sputum production for 3 or more months in 2 consecutive years is the epidemiological definition of 'chronic bronchitis'
- May be difficult to evaluate due to swallowing rather than expectoration

Dyspnea: 'Abnormal awareness of the act of breathing'
- Sense of increased effort to breathe, heaviness, air hunger or gasping
- Hallmark symptom of COPD
- Commonly the reason why patients seek medical attention
- Major source of disability and anxiety associated with COPD
- Presents insidiously on exertion, becomes progressive and persistent
- Worse during exacerbations

Wheezing and chest tightness
- More characteristic of asthma or Stage III: severe COPD
- Audible wheeze may arise at a laryngeal level
- Widespread inspiratory or expiratory wheezes can be present
- Chest tightness often follows exertion
- May arise from isometric contraction of intercostal muscles

Other symptoms
- Chest pains may be due to ischemic heart disease or strain on intercostal muscles
- Swollen ankles may reflect *cor pulmonale* and right-sided heart failure
- Hemoptysis can occur during respiratory infection[2]
- Weight loss and anorexia often occur in advanced disease[2]
- Muscle weakness and wasting[2]

[1] Following long-term cigarette smoking, symptoms of COPD are slowly progressive over many years, in contrast to the variable and episodic symptoms of asthma.
[2] Assess for underlying carcinoma or tuberculosis.

Figure 3.3   MRC modified dyspnea scale

Grade 0	No breathlessness
Grade 1	Breathlessness with strenuous exercise
Grade 2	Short of breath when hurrying on the level *or* walking up a slight hill
Grade 3	Walks slower than people of same age on the level *or* stops for breath while walking at own pace on the level
Grade 4	Stops for breath after walking 100 yards
Grade 5	Too breathless to leave house *or* breathless when dressing or undressing

Exposure to risk factors

Certain aspects of the history of patients with COPD are important (Figure 3.4), especially exposure to risk factors for COPD.

- A detailed history of tobacco usage is required. Patients with COPD have generally been heavy cigarette smokers for decades, often having smoked for more than 20 pack-years, a pack-year representing 20 cigarettes daily for 1 year. A history of cigarette smoking should be taken in terms of cigarettes (tobacco and cannabis), pipe and cigars, and a calculation should be made of cigarette smoking in pack-years. The circumstances of smoking should be determined: in the home, workplace, and social smoking. Every effort should be made to encourage the patient to stop smoking, and appropriate support offered.

- The occupational history should include details of exposure to occupational smoke, chemicals and dust; hence a history of mining, chemical industry, construction and building work is relevant. For females from developing countries, consider exposure to biomass fuel smoke from cooking on open fires.

PHYSICAL EXAMINATION: SIGNS

The typical patient with established COPD may show some or all of the features listed in Figure 3.5, but, in mild-to-moderate COPD (Stages I and II, $FEV_1 > 50\%$ predicted), there may be no abnormal signs. Figure 3.5 initially considers the signs relating to respiratory failure, hypoxia (central cyanosis) and hypercapnia. Examination of the fingers may reveal tar-staining of the nails, with cyanosis (a bluish hue) of the nail bed. Clubbing is not a feature of COPD and suggests malignancy, bronchiectasis or some other lung disease. Tachypnea with rapid shallow breathing, and especially a prolonged expiration phase, is an important clinical sign of obstructive airway disease. Use of accessory muscles of respiration with the possible presence of pulmonary hyperinflation may be prominent. It is important to carefully examine the breath and heart sounds, and to look for signs of *cor pulmonale* with right-sided heart failure. Nutritional depletion with cachexia and muscle wasting is increasingly recognized as a feature of more severe COPD.

Pink puffers and blue bloaters

The classification of COPD patients into 'pink puffers' and 'blue bloaters' was an early attempt to

Figure 3.4   Aspects of the history of COPD   75

Risk factors

History of exposure to risk factors:

- tobacco smoke, cannabis
- occupational dusts and chemicals
- smoke from open fires
- cooking and heating fuels

Smoking history

- number of cigarettes /day, assess in pack-years
- types of cigarettes, filter-tipped or hand-rolled
- cannabis usage
- cigars, pipe
- attempts at cessation
- will to stop smoking

Past medical history

- asthma/allergy/sinusitis/nasal polyps
- premature baby, respiratory infections in childhood
- other respiratory diseases: tuberculosis, pneumonia
- cardiovascular diseases: hypertension, heart failure, ischemic heart disease, arrhythmias, peripheral vascular disease, rheumatic fever

Drug history

- appropriateness of current medical treatments for COPD
  short and long-acting β_2-agonists
  anticholinergics – ipratropium and tiotropium bromide
  oral theophylline slow-release (SR)
  inhaled corticosteroids
  oral corticosteroids are not generally given in stable COPD
- hypnotics, diuretics
- β-blockers are best avoided in COPD
- vaccination status: influenza and *Streptococcus pneumoniae*
  drug allergy or incompatibility – especially antibiotics

Social history   *NB: Also consider quality-of-life assessment*

- occupational history: mining and chemical industries
- impact of disease on patient's life: walking distance, stairs, exercise, hobbies
- social and family support, home conditions
- diet and alcohol consumption

Family history

- smoking
- COPD, asthma, lung cancer
- cardiovascular disease

Figure 3.5   Physical examination and clinical signs in COPD

Hypoxia: blue bloater
- central cyanosis – bluish lips, tongue and finger tips
- obese
- examine content of sputum pot

Hypercapnia:
CO_2 retention
- hand flap (asterixis)
- rapid bounding pulse
- peripheral vasodilation
- reduced consciousness

Normal blood gases: pink puffer

Fingers
- cyanosis
- tar-stained but *not* nicotine-stained
- clubbing is *not* a feature

Posture and use of accessory muscles of respiration
- Three-point posture (tripoding)
- fixing of shoulder girdle
- use of scalene, trapezius and sternocleidomastoid muscles

Nature of breathing
- tachypnea – respiration > 20 breaths/min
- shallow breathing
- prolonged expiration
- pursed lip breathing
- paradoxical breathing
- costal margin retraction

Pulmonary hyperinflation
- barrel-shaped chest – observe laterally
- reduced cardiac sounds
- wide xiphisternal angle
- depressed liver

Breath sounds
- quiet breath sounds
- crepitations early on inspiration
- rhonchi (wheeze) may be present
- prolonged expiratory time (> 6 s)

Heart sounds
- quiet heart sounds – listen over lower sternum (xiphoid area)

Pulmonary hypertension
- prominent systolic impulse along the lower left sternal border
- accentuation of the pulmonic component of the second heart sound (P2)
- murmurs of pulmonic or tricuspid insufficiency
- right ventricular gallop

Right heart failure
- raised jugular venous pressure
- orthopnea (breathless on lying flat)
- cardiomegaly
- loud pulmonic second heart sound (P2)
- large pulsatile tender liver
- ankle edema

Cachexia
- muscle weakness and wasting

base COPD classification on differences in ventilatory responses[12], although most patients with COPD have a mixed picture (Figure 3.6). These two characteristic body phenotypes may reflect distinct respiratory drive, lung pathology and systemic responses. Most patients with COPD have a mixed picture rather than the extremes of a pink puffer or blue bloater.

The pink puffer has good respiratory drive, utilizing rapid ventilation to maintain normal blood gases, thus having considerable dyspnea. Cough and sputum production are not generally prominent. Clinical examination reveals a thin, sometimes cachectic, often elderly individual. He/she has a pink complexion, with absence of cardiac and respiratory failure. The patient is alert, employing expiratory

---

Figure 3.6   Clinical syndromes in severe COPD

Type A: 'Pink puffer'

- Good respiratory drive

- Intense dyspnea with pursed-lip breathing
- Alert
- Leaning forward using accessory muscles of respiration
- Hyperinflation with increased total lung capacity
- Small sputum volume
- Severe airway obstruction on spirometry
- Emphysema on CT scan

- Thin body build – cachexia and muscle wasting

- Late onset of respiratory and heart failure
- Well-perfused with near-normal blood gases

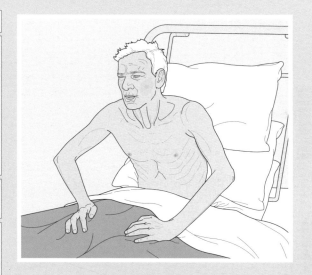

Type B: 'Blue bloater'

- Poor respiratory drive

- Relatively mild dyspnea
- Drowsy
- Central cyanosis at rest or on mild exertion – bluish lips, oral mucosa and finger tips
- Large sputum volume
- Moderate airway obstruction on spirometry
- Emphysema not detected on CT scan

- Often obese

- *Cor pulmonale* with right-sided heart failure – ankle edema, raised jugular venous pressure, hepatomegaly
- Respiratory failure: hypoxia and hypercapnia
- Nocturnal hypoxia during sleep
- Polycythemia

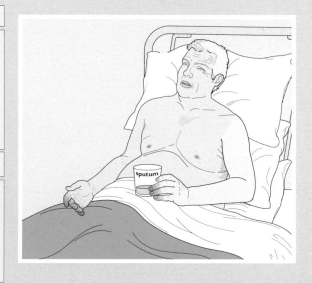

NB Most patients with COPD have a mixed pattern. Patients of the 'blue bloater' type should be treated with oxygen therapy.

Figure 3.7   Breathing patterns in COPD

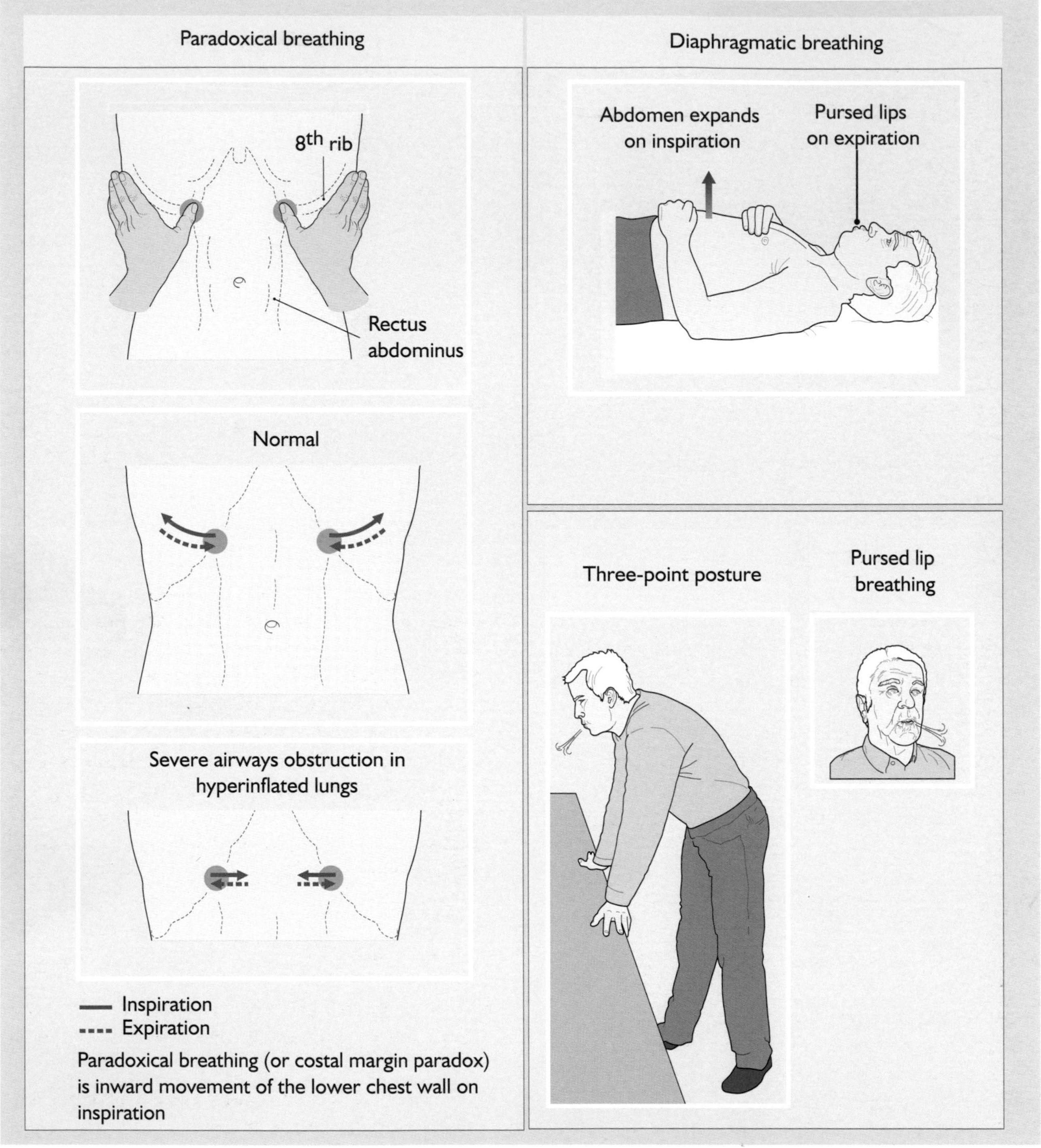

Paradoxical breathing

8th rib

Rectus abdominus

Normal

Severe airways obstruction in hyperinflated lungs

— Inspiration

---- Expiration

Paradoxical breathing (or costal margin paradox) is inward movement of the lower chest wall on inspiration

Diaphragmatic breathing

Abdomen expands on inspiration   Pursed lips on expiration

Three-point posture   Pursed lip breathing

pursed lip breathing that maintains the patency of the small airways (Figure 3.7), and using accessory muscles of respiration. He/she may be leaning onto a support to assist breathing, or leaning on their elbows or supporting their extended arms in a three-point position known as 'tripoding' (Figure 3.7). On examination, the patient may have lung hyper-inflation with a barrel chest (Figure 3.8). Spirometry demonstrates severe airflow limitation; plethysmo-graphy demonstrates pulmonary hyperinflation, and there is often decreased diffusion capacity of transfer factor for carbon monoxide. Blood tests may be normal, but there is radiological and pathological evidence of emphysema.

Figure 3.8   (a) Barrel chest; (b) cachexia in COPD

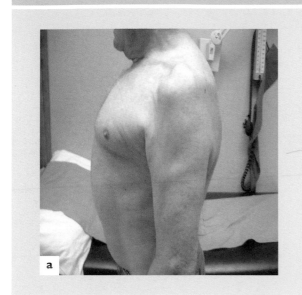
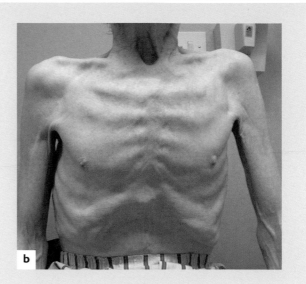

Photographs courtesy of Dr Onn Min Kon, St. Mary's Hospital, London.

The blue bloater has poor respiratory drive and early chronic respiratory and cardiac failure. The patient may be obese, sitting in bed slumped onto a pillow. This patient has prominent chronic bronchitis; their cough is productive, causing the patient to have large daily sputum volumes. Typically, the patient has no shortness of breath at rest, but relatively mild dyspnea on exertion. On clinical examination, the blue bloater has respiratory failure, with abnormal blood gases (hypoxia and perhaps hypercapnia), and central cyanosis manifesting as a bluish hue of the lips and fingers at rest. An important sign of cardiac failure is edema of the ankles, and there may be a loud second heart sound (P2) in the pulmonary area, although this may be difficult to hear due to hyperinflation. Lung function is relatively well preserved, although polycythemia and abnormal arterial blood gases may be present. There may be radiological evidence of cardiac failure/cardiomegaly, and mild emphysema may possibly be detected on high-resolution computerized tomography (CT)

Types of breathing

Paradoxical breathing or costal margin paradox (Figure 3.7) is an important sign in patients with severe airways obstruction and high inspiratory impedance in hyperinflated lungs. Expansion of the lower rib cage is assessed by spreading the hands with the fingers directed along the ribs and the thumbs near to the mid-line. In normal quiet breathing on inspiration, the thumbs move apart and, on expiration, they move back together. With paradoxical breathing on inspiration, there is movement of the thumbs together, and movement apart on expiration. Diaphragmatic breathing may be taught to patients to shift the breathing drive from the chest wall and musculature to the diaphragm; this involves the abdomen expanding outwards as the patient inspires.

Breath sounds

In many patients with COPD, physical examination reveals little abnormality especially during quiet breathing.

- Diminished breath sounds are associated with decreased heart sounds.

- Crepitations (coarse crackles) occurring early in inspiration have been associated with obstructive lung disease, although other adventitious sounds may be present.

- Rhonchi (musical wheezes) are more prevalent in patients complaining of dyspnea and are usually present both during inspiration and expiration. Wheezing is not a consistent finding and does not relate to the severity of obstruction.

- A prolonged expiratory time is the most consistent finding in patients with symptomatic COPD. This is best determined by listening over the larynx during a forced expiratory maneuver. Prolongation of the expiratory phase longer than the normal 4 s is indicative of significant obstruction.

Heart sounds

Quiet heart sounds may occur because the over-inflated lungs are interposed between the heart and the sternum. Physical findings of pulmonary hypertension include a prominent systolic impulse along the lower left sternal border, with accentuation of the pulmonic component of the second heart sound. There may be murmurs of pulmonic or tricuspid insufficiency, and a right ventricular gallop.

Chronic respiratory failure

Respiratory failure (hypoxia with or without hypercapnia) often develops insidiously and may be undetected in some patients with COPD. Hypoxia may be manifest as central cyanosis (Figure 3.5).

CO_2 retention with elevated arterial P_{CO_2} ($PaCO_2$) causes hypercapnic respiratory failure, and metabolic compensation may occur with elevated plasma bicarbonate and relatively normal pH.

Hypoxia may be disproportionate to elevated $PaCO_2$ because of concomitant ventilation/perfusion mismatching in the lungs. Hypoxia may become worse during sleep, and may be associated with mental confusion if severe. Chronic hypoxia often leads to *cor pulmonale*. When giving oxygen to correct hypoxia, patients may underventilate because ventilation is largely driven by hypoxia; therefore arterial blood gases should be regularly monitored, especially at the onset of treatment.

Acute respiratory failure

Acute respiratory failure may develop on the basis of chronic respiratory failure due to infection during an exacerbation, or because of some other complication such as pulmonary embolism or pulmonary artery thrombosis. The patient becomes more hypoxic with cyanosis, and underventilation may cause rising $PaCO_2$ and falling pH that may be best treated with non-invasive positive pressure ventilation (NIPPV).

Clinically, the patient becomes confused, drowsy and tired and ventilation deteriorates further, an important feature being that consciousness may be lost before respiratory arrest ensues. Arterial blood gas analyses are urgently required to monitor respiratory failure and oxygen therapy and to assess the need for non-invasive ventilation.

Cor pulmonale

Cor pulmonale is heart disease due to the effects of chronic hypoxia on the pulmonary vasculature. Chronic *cor pulmonale* is defined as enlargement of the right ventricle (hypertrophy or dilatation) due to increased right ventricular afterload from diseases of the lungs or pulmonary circulation.

Pulmonary artery hypertension

Resting mean pulmonary arterial pressures may rise to 30–40 mmHg in patients with advanced COPD, as opposed to the normal value of 10–18 mmHg. With exercise, mean pressures may rise as high as 50–60 mmHg or greater. There are several causes of the pulmonary hypertension in COPD[13,14]. Blood volume may be increased in patients with *cor pulmonale*, in part from impaired sodium and water excretion[15]. Increases in cardiac output occurring in response to hypoxemia may contribute to higher mean pulmonary arterial pressure in the presence of a restricted pulmonary vascular bed. Although left ventricular dysfunction is relatively uncommon in patients with *cor pulmonale* due to COPD, when such dysfunction is present, the occurrence of left ventricular failure and raised pulmonary venous pressure may also contribute to pulmonary hypertension.

The following are characteristic clinical features of pulmonary artery hypertension and *cor pulmonale* (right-sided heart failure):

- Edema of ankles

- Elevated jugular venous pressure

- Prominent pulmonary second heart sound on auscultation (difficult to hear because of over-inflation)

- Cardiomegaly on chest radiograph

- ECG showing P-pulmonale in lead 2 and right ventricular hypertrophy

- Echocardiography showing enlargement of right ventricle, pulmonary hypertension and reduced right ventricular ejection fraction

Thromboembolic disease

COPD patients are prone to develop chronic pulmonary thromboembolic disease, and this diagnosis should always be considered when the magnitude of pulmonary hypertension is out of proportion to a patient's underlying lung disease and arterial hypoxemia. Production of pro-inflammatory cytokines, such as interleukin 6 in the lung, may contribute directly to a prothrombotic state by increasing liver production of coagulation factors[16], as may polycythemia consequent to hypoxemia.

Cachexia with nutritional depletion and muscle weakness/wasting

It is becoming increasingly recognized that systemic effects are common in COPD and the assessment and treatment of nutritional depletion are important in management (see Chapter 7).

- Weight loss is now recognized as a poor prognostic feature in COPD[17] (Figure 3.8), and underweight individuals have considerably increased mortality. Studies have carefully described subjects with weight loss and nutritional depletion in patients with COPD[10,18–20]. Several mechanisms may contribute to weight loss in COPD, including the increased work of breathing, decreased appetite, difficulty in eating due to dyspnea, and circulating catabolic cytokines such as TNF-α.

- Skeletal muscle weakness is a better correlate of poor exercise performance in COPD than is dyspnea or impaired lung function[21]. Some of the weakness in COPD may be due to poor conditioning. A primary skeletal muscle defect, perhaps due to the effect of circulating cytokines, may also play a role.

Sleep disorders

The major cause of sleep-induced hypoxemia in COPD patients is thought to be hypoventilation during rapid eye movement (REM) sleep, related to rapid shallow breathing (see Chapter 7). An additional factor is reduction in functional residual capacity, accompanied by increased ventilation–

perfusion mismatch[22]. The blood gas abnormalities are greater during REM sleep than non-REM sleep[23]. The severity of decrease in arterial P_{O_2} tends to become greater as the night wears on, perhaps as a result of suppression of the cough reflex and retained secretions. Even patients with awake arterial P_{O_2} values of 60 mmHg or greater may experience periods of major nocturnal desaturation, which are of uncertain clinical significance[24].

Although patients with COPD may have long episodes of hypopnea during sleep, true sleep apnea is no more common than in the general population[25]. However, when sleep apnea does complicate COPD, nocturnal hypoxemia tends to be more severe than in the general population because of baseline hypoxemia.

DIFFERENTIAL DIAGNOSIS OF COPD

The differential diagnosis of COPD involves a great number of conditions (Figure 3.9).

Cigarette smoke-induced COPD

Most patients with COPD present with symptoms in their forties to sixties, following extensive cigarette smoking. They present insidiously with a smoker's productive cough and progressively worsening dyspnea on exertion. Spirometry is fundamental to establishing the diagnosis.

α_1-Antitrypsin deficiency

This is due to a severe reduction in hepatic production of the major anti-protease in lung parenchyma as a result of a genetic defect[26,27]. This renders the lung susceptible to the destructive effects of neutrophil elastase and other endogenous proteases, and results in severe basal panacinar emphysema, especially in smokers. This type of COPD appears at a much younger age (in the third to fourth decade) and may even appear in childhood. The condition is rare, accounting for < 1% of patients with COPD, and only occurs in homozygous carriers of the defective genes. Heterozygotes are usually healthy.

Primary ciliary dyskinesia

This is due to a defect in the ultrastructure of cilia throughout the body, that commonly results in chronic sinusitis, chronic otitis and COPD[28]. Males are sterile as their spermatozoa are immotile. In one

Figure 3.9   Differential diagnosis of COPD

COPD	Onset in mid-life Symptoms slowly progressive Commonly long smoking history Rarely α_1-antitrypsin deficiency Rarely primary ciliary dyskinesia	Dyspnea during exercise Largely irreversible airflow limitation
Asthma	Onset early in life (often childhood) Symptoms vary from day to day Symptoms at night/early morning	Allergy, rhinitis, or eczema also present Family history of asthma Responds to β_2-agonists: reversible airflow limitation
Congestive heart failure	Fine basilar crackles on auscultation Chest X-ray shows dilated heart, pulmonary edema	Pulmonary function tests include volume reduction, not airflow limitation – no obstructive pattern
Bronchiectasis	Bronchial dilation and suppuration Large volumes of purulent sputum Commonly associated with bacterial infection	Coarse crackles on auscultation Chest X-ray/CT shows bronchial dilation, bronchial wall thickening
Tuberculosis	Onset at all ages Chest X-ray shows lung infiltrate or nodular lesions	Microbiological confirmation High local prevalence of tuberculosis
Obliterative bronchiolitis	Onset in younger age, non-smokers May have history of rheumatoid arthritis or fume exposure	CT on expiration shows hypodense areas
Diffuse panbronchiolitis	Most patients are male and non-smokers Almost all have chronic sinusitis	Chest X-ray and high-resolution CT show diffuse small centrilobular nodular opacities and hyperinflation

form of the disease, there may be dextrocardia and bronchiectasis (Kartagener's syndrome), but most patients have a relatively mild type of COPD.

Asthma

Patients with asthma frequently have early onset of episodic airway obstruction, manifested as shortness of breath with wheeze. Asthma is commonly associated with allergy, is independent of smoking status, and airway obstruction measured by spirometry responds to bronchodilators and/or corticosteroids. Chronic severe asthma can have a fixed airways obstruction.

Congestive heart failure

There may be a history of orthopnea or paroxysmal nocturnal dyspnea, and the patient may describe malaise, anorexia and ankle swelling. On examination, signs include fine basal lung crepitations, ankle edema, and hepatomegaly. There is a characteristic chest X-ray with cardiomegaly (left or right ventricular hypertrophy), upper lobe blood diversion, and pulmonary edema. Spirometry does not generally show airway obstruction. Echocardiography and exercise stress testing assist the diagnosis.

Ischemic heart disease

This may also cause shortness of breath on exertion, but is usually associated with chest tightness and pain. ECG is generally helpful.

Bronchiectasis

Patients have generally had repeated episodes of pneumonia with copious purulent sputum. The diagnosis may be aided by computerized tomography to show the dilated bronchi.

Tuberculosis

Tuberculosis remains an important lung disease on a world-wide scale. There is onset at any age especially in high-risk subjects, since there is high prevalence in certain developing countries. Tuberculosis can cause obstructive lung disease with weight loss, thus mimicking systemic COPD. Chest X-rays show features such as lung infiltration, nodular lesions, fibrosis and cavitation. Sputum microscopy and culture as well as tuberculin testing may assist the diagnosis.

Obliterative bronchiolitis

This affects younger patients who are often non-smokers, and who may have rheumatoid arthritis, a history of exposure to toxic fumes, or who have undergone lung transplantation. CT on expiration shows characteristic hypodense (black) areas.

Diffuse panbronchiolitis

Most patients are Japanese non-smoking males, with a combination of obstructive airway disease and chronic sinusitis[29]. There is a characteristic chest X-ray and CT scan with diffuse small centrilobular nodular opacities and hyperinflation. Diffuse panbronchiolitis responds to treatment with macrolide antibiotics, such as erythromycin.

Need for referral

Referral to a respiratory physician of patients with productive cough and dyspnea may be useful to establish the diagnosis of COPD by spirometry and to differentiate it from asthma, and may also exclude other pathology, including a malignancy. In addition, the physician can reinforce the need to stop smoking and optimize therapy.

Referral is indicated in particular patients:

- Where there is early onset of disease
- Those with a family history of α_1-antitrypsin deficiency
- Those showing signs of *cor pulmonale*
- Those requiring assessment of need for long-term oxygen therapy or non-invasive ventilation or nebulizer therapy
- Those with a rapid decline in lung function (> 100 ml/year)
- Those with frequent infections who may have bronchiectasis
- Those showing any features suggestive of tuberculosis or lung cancer

Regular follow-up is important in order to:

- Assess disease progression with measurement of FEV_1
- Supervise smoking cessation
- Assess the benefits of drug treatment
- Assess clinical status in severe COPD to detect signs of *cor pulmonale* or respiratory failure

INVESTIGATIONS

Lung function

Investigations are essential to confirm the diagnosis of COPD (Figure 3.10). Any patient presenting with a history of cough, sputum production and breathlessness requires certain basic investigations which may, in turn, suggest the need for further investigations. Lung function tests are used for diagnosis, assessment of severity and following the course of the disease. Objective lung function tests are essential, as symptoms and physical signs cannot predict disease severity. The hallmark of COPD is chronic airflow obstruction which is largely irreversible. The obstruction is particularly marked in the smaller airways due to the pathological changes of chronic obstructive bronchitis and the loss of support for their walls due to emphysema. These small airways close off during expiration, trapping gas and increasing resting lung volume (functional residual capacity) and residual volume. Emphysema may also result in an increase in total lung capacity and loss of

Figure 3.10	Investigations in COPD

Abnormal results
• Spirometry: $\downarrow$FEV$_1$, FEV$_1$/FVC%
• Limited reversibility: bronchodilator response < 12%
• Inhaled steroid trial negative (excludes asthma)
• Hyperinflation: $\uparrow$total lung capacity, residual volume
• Impaired gas diffusion: $\downarrow$T$_{LCO}$, K$_{CO}$
• Chest X-ray: hyperinflation
• CT scan: emphysema
• Arterial blood gases: $\downarrow$ PaO$_2$, PaCO$_2$
• Exercise tests: impaired performance
• Health-related quality of life: impaired

Indications	
Routine	• FEV$_1$, FEV$_1$/FVC • Bronchodilator response • Chest X-ray • T$_{LCO}$/K$_{CO}$
Moderate/severe COPD	• Lung volumes • SaO$_2$ and/or blood gases • ECG • Hemoglobin
Persistent purulent sputum	• Sputum culture/sensitivity
Emphysema in young	• α_1-antitrypsin, genotype if low
Assessment of bullae	• CT scan
Disproportionate breathlessness	• Exercise test
Suspected asthma	• Trial of steroids • Peak expiratory flow monitoring • Airway responsiveness
Suspected sleep apnea	• Nocturnal sleep study

the alveolar surface area available for gas exchange. There are various tests which are useful in evaluating lung function in COPD (Figure 3.11).

Spirometry (Figures 3.12–3.14)

Forced expiratory volume in 1 second (FEV$_1$) FEV$_1$ measured by spirometry is the physiologic assessment that is necessary to establish the diagnosis of COPD, and then follow the course of the disease and assess prognosis. Lung function declines gradually over decades in patients with COPD[30], but recognition of early stages of COPD is possible with prompt use of lung function testing, particularly spirometry. Spirometry (including bronchodilator response) should ideally be measured at every clinic visit, and at least twice a year. The forced expiratory spirogram is the most useful test of airflow dynamics. Yearly measurement for at least 3 years is required to assess the rate of decline in FEV$_1$, and rates > 50 ml/year suggest accelerated decline.

FEV$_1$ has long been established as the main outcome measure in the monitoring of patients with COPD. Pre-bronchodilator FEV$_1$ is the mainstay of classification of severity of COPD (Figure 3.15) and it is strongly predictive of subsequent mortality from COPD[31–34]. Note that, in July 2003, the new GOLD clinical classification of severity for COPD was introduced. There are, however, limitations in the use of this measurement, since changes in FEV$_1$ over time are small in relation to repeatability of the measurement. Thus, it can take serial measurements over several years to demonstrate a declining trend in FEV$_1$ in one individual. In addition, the earliest changes in smokers' lungs occur in the peripheral airways[35], and may already be present whilst the FEV$_1$ remains normal. At present, pre- and post-bronchodilator FEV$_1$ remains the 'gold standard' to monitor progression of COPD, and to monitor the outcome of therapeutic interventions such as smoking cessation.

Figure 3.11   Lung function abnormalities in COPD

Lung function test	Parameter	Abbreviation (units)	Abnormality
Spirometry	Forced expiratory volume in 1 s	FEV_1 (l)	↓
	Forced vital capacity	FVC (l)	↓ airflow obstruction
	Forced expiratory ratio	FER = FEV_1/FVC (%)	↓
	Peak expiratory flow	PEF (l.s^{-1})	↓
Plethysmography	Total lung capacity	TLC (l)	↑
	Functional residual capacity	FRC (l)	↑ hyperinflation
	Residual volume	RV (l)	↑
	Specific airways conductance	sGaw (s^{-1}.kPa^{-1})	↓ airflow obstruction
Diffusion capacity (USA) or Transfer factor (Europe)	Diffusion capacity for lung carbon monoxide, CO = Transfer factor for lung CO	D_{LCO} T_{LCO} (mmol.min^{-1}.kPa^{-1})	↓
	Alveolar volume	V_A(l)	↓ impaired gas transfer
	Diffusion coefficient for CO = Transfer coefficient for CO	K_{CO} = D_{LCO}/V_A K_{CO} = T_{LCO}/V_A (mmol.min^{-1}.kPa^{-1}.l^{-1})	↓

FEV$_1$/FVC ratio The FEV$_1$/FVC ratio is diminished in patients with obstructive lung disease, but is maintained or increased in those with restrictive lung disease. In COPD, the FEV$_1$ and the FEV$_1$/FVC ratio fall progressively. The new GOLD guidelines define mild COPD as an FEV$_1$/FVC of < 70%, but a pre-bronchodilator FEV$_1$ of > 80% predicted[7].

Portable pneumotachograph-based spirometers are now available and may be used to monitor FEV$_1$, FVC and PEFR. During an exacerbation, the PEFR and FEV$_1$ may not be accurately determined by portable equipment and such values cannot be used interchangeably with those obtained by a volume displacement spirometer[36,37].

Peak expiratory flow The peak expiratory flow (PEF) is heavily effort-dependent and only a crude measure of lung function. The peak expiratory flow can be measured with relatively inexpensive peak flow meters, which patients can be taught to use them-selves. However, the peak expiratory flow is not as useful as FEV$_1$ in COPD, and should not be used for diagnosis. A peak flow pattern/diary may provide some useful information, and a normal peak expiratory flow does not exclude COPD.

Bronchodilator reversibility

The recent GOLD guidelines give specific advice on testing for reversibility to a bronchodilator[7]. The bronchodilator should be given by metered dose inhaler through a spacer device or by nebulizer (Figure 3.16). A suitable dose by metered dose inhaler would be salbutamol or albuterol at 400 μg. After 30–45 min, an increase in FEV$_1$ that is both greater than 200 ml and 12% above the pre-bronchodilator FEV$_1$ is considered significantly reversible. Many patients with COPD may have limited improvement in airflow in response to a bronchodilator, although airflow does not normalize.

Figure 3.12   A range of spirometers

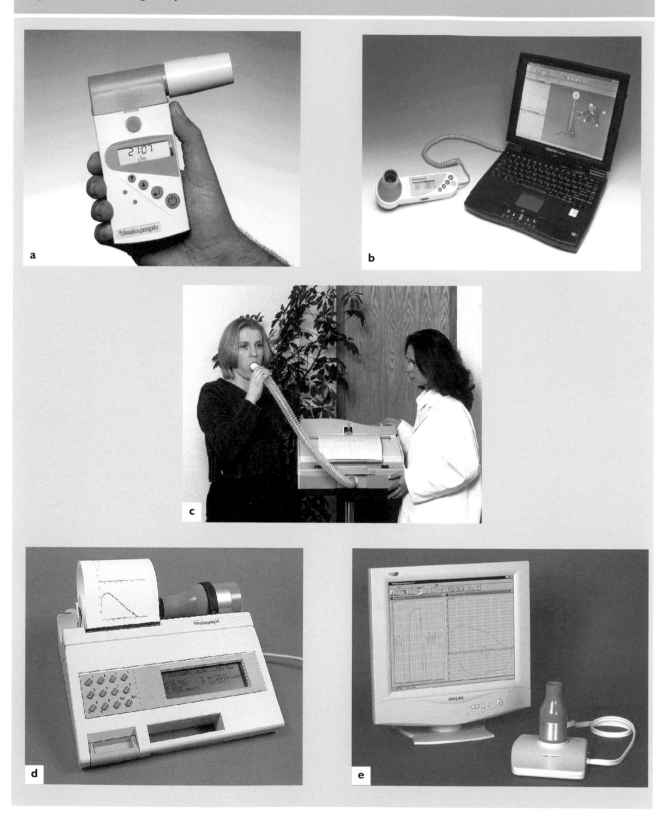

(a) Electronic PEF/FEV$_1$ diary; (b) 2120 handheld or PC based spirometer; (c) volume displacement spirometer; (d) Alpha III desktop spirometer with printer and screen; (e) Pneumotrac PC-based spirometry system. Pictures courtesy of Vitalograph Ltd.

Figure 3.13   Spirometry

Gold standard for diagnosis and monitoring
Spirometry is the gold standard for diagnosing COPD and monitoring its progression.

Airflow limitation
Spirometry is the simplest and best measurement of airways obstruction. It is standardized, reproducible, and the most objective measurement of airflow limitation available.

Early diagnosis
Spirometry should be undertaken for any patient who may have COPD, and can help identify patients early in the course of COPD. It should be performed in any patients with chronic cough and sputum production, even if they do not have dyspnea.

Access
Health-care workers who care for patients with COPD should have access to spirometry for diagnosis and monitoring of COPD.

Spirometry equipment
Spirometers need calibration on a regular basis.

Spirometers should produce hard copy to permit detection of technical errors.

Trained staff
The supervisor of spirometry needs training in its effective performance.

Maximal patient effort
The patient needs to be aware of how to perform the test and that maximal effort is required.

Techniques
These should meet published standards.

Spirometry should measure the maximum volume of air forcibly exhaled from the point of maximal inspiration (forced vital capacity, FVC) and the volume of air exhaled during the first second of this maneuver (forced expiratory volume in 1 second, FEV_1), and the ratio of these two measurements (FEV_1/FVC %) should be calculated.

Quality of trace
The expiratory volume/time trace should be smooth and free from irregularities.

The recording should go on long enough for a volume plateau to be reached, which may take > 12 s in severe disease.

Three recordings
Both FVC and FEV_1 recordings should each be the largest value from three technically satisfactory curves.

Variability
The FVC and FEV_1 values in the three curves should vary by no more than 6% or 100 ml, whichever is greater.

Reference values
Spirometry measurements are evaluated by comparison with reference values based on age, height, sex and race.

FEV_1/FVC, FEV_1 and reversibility testing
An early and sensitive measure of airflow limitation is when the FEV_1/FVC is < 70%, although, in mild COPD, FEV_1 may be > 80%.

The additional presence of FEV_1 < 80% is further evidence towards moderate COPD.

The hallmark of COPD is chronic airflow limitation which is largely irreversible: FEV_1/FVC < 70%, FEV_1 (% predicted) low, reversibility < 12% [100 x (post – pre)/pre]

However, it is important to recognize that some patients with COPD do have reversibility of > 12% following previous long-term cigarette smoking. These subjects have a clinical history typical of COPD, do not have clinical features of asthma, and lack allergy and eosinophilia. Hence, lack of reversibility is not an absolute diagnostic factor for COPD.

Figure 3.14   Spirometry in COPD

Spirograms in COPD of varying severity

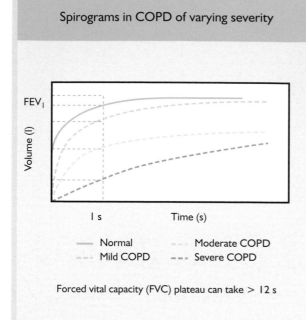

Normal — Mild COPD ---- Moderate COPD ---- Severe COPD ----

Forced vital capacity (FVC) plateau can take > 12 s

Flow volume loop: single breath forced maneuver

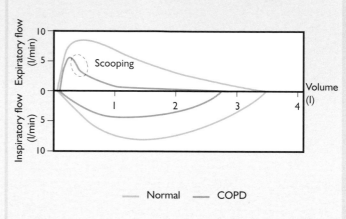

Normal — COPD —

Pneumotachograph: 'scooping' caused by expiratory airway collapse

Lung volumes

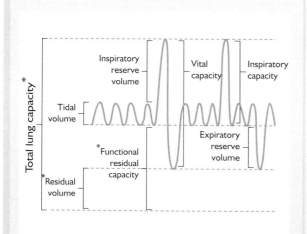

* Total lung capacity, residual volume and functional residual capacity are measured by plethysmography

Natural history: decline in FEV₁ with age

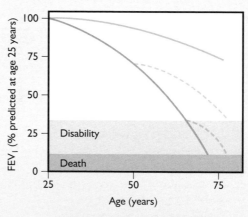

Non-smoker or non-susceptible smoker
Susceptible smoker (10–20%)
Stopped smoking aged 50 years
Stopped smoking aged 60 years

Fletcher C, Peto R. *Br Med J* 1977;1:1645–8

Figure 3.15   Classification of severity of COPD

| Stage | | Symptoms | FEV$_1$ (% predicted) | FEV$_1$/FVC (%) |
GOLD, 2003	GOLD, 2001			
0: At risk	0	chronic symptoms	normal	normal
I: Mild	I	+/- symptoms +/- cough/sputum	> 80	< 70
II: Moderate	IIA	+/- symptoms +/- cough/sputum/dyspnea	50–80	< 70
III: Severe	IIB		30–50	
IV: Very severe	III	cough/sputum/dyspnea +/- respiratory failure +/- right heart failure	< 30 or respiratory failure or right heart failure	< 70

Figure 3.16   Bronchodilator reversibility testing

Aims
Diagnosis: performed as part of the diagnosis of COPD – also rules out a diagnosis of asthma
Monitoring: establishes the post-bronchodilator best attainable lung function at that point in time
Prognosis: the post-bronchodilator FEV$_1$ is a more reliable prognostic marker than pre-bronchodilator FEV$_1$
The degree of bronchodilator reversibility is inversely related to the rate of FEV$_1$ decline in COPD patients
Potential treatment response: patients with a greater degree of reversibility are more likely to benefit from treatment with bronchodilators and glucocorticosteroids

Patient preparation
Stable COPD: tests should be performed when patients are clinically stable and free from respiratory infection
Withdraw therapy: patients should not have taken inhaled short-acting bronchodilators in the previous 6 h, long-acting β_2-agonists in the previous 12 h, tiotropium for 48 h, or sustained-release theophyllines in the previous 24 h

Method
Pre or baseline FEV$_1$: FEV$_1$ should be measured before a bronchodilator is given
Administration: the bronchodilator should be given by metered dose inhaler through a spacer device or by nebulizer to ensure it has been inhaled
Dose: the bronchodilator dose should be selected to be high on the dose/response curve:
- 400 μg β_2-agonist: salbutamol
- 80 μg anticholinergic: ipratropium bromide
- or salbutamol and ipratropium combined

Magnitude of reversibility [100 x (post – pre)/pre]
An acute change that exceeds both 200 ml and 12% of the baseline FEV$_1$ is evidence of reversibility. This is unlikely to have arisen by chance because between-day reproducibility of spirometry in the same individual is approximately 178 ml

Glucocorticosteroid (steroid) reversibility

The use of a therapeutic trial of inhaled cortico-steroids in order to predict long-term efficacy is controversial, although prescription of inhaled corticosteroids in COPD has been proposed in patients with repeated exacerbations or a significant FEV_1 response to steroids. A trial can be given with inhaled steroids for between 6 and 14 weeks (Figure 3.17). Oral prednisolone trials, while previously recommended, should be avoided. Morning peak expiratory flow should be measured daily and post-bronchodilator FEV_1 measured before and after steroid therapy. A post-bronchodilator FEV_1 increase of > 200 ml and > 12% above baseline is considered to be reversible.

Plethysmography for lung volumes: hyperinflation

The total lung capacity is increased in emphysema because the loss of elastic recoil permits the inspira-tory muscles to stretch the lungs to a greater maximal volume (Figures 3.11, 3.13 and 3.18). The residual volume is increased because of airway closure at a higher lung volume, which is due to a combination of loss of elastic recoil and premature airway closure. The functional residual capacity is increased because of loss of elastic recoil. Finally, the vital capacity is decreased because of the increase in residual volume.

Hyperinflation and dynamic hyperinflation

As airflow limitation develops, the rate of lung emptying is slowed and the interval between expiratory efforts does not allow expiration of the relaxation volume, leading to pulmonary hyperinflation[38]. Dynamic hyperinflation describes how pulmonary hyperinflation worsens with increasing respiratory rate, due to progressive air trapping, being a major cause of dyspnea on exertion (Figure 3.19). Dynamic

Figure 3.17   Trial of inhaled corticosteroids

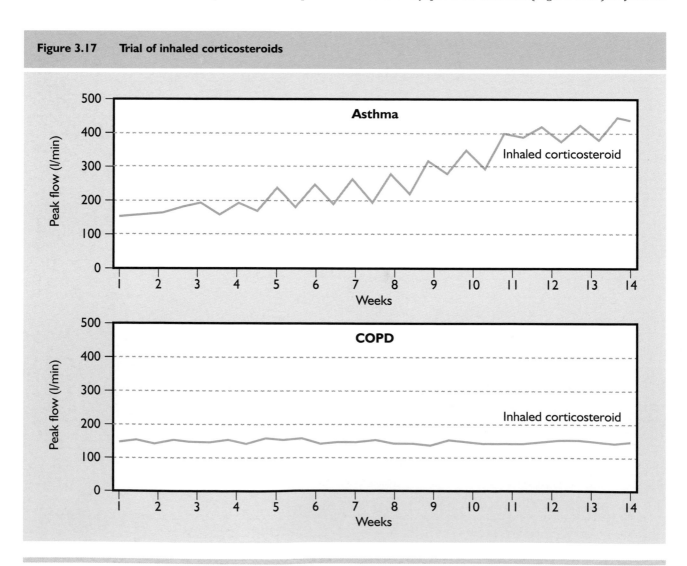

Figure 3.18   Lung function testing in COPD

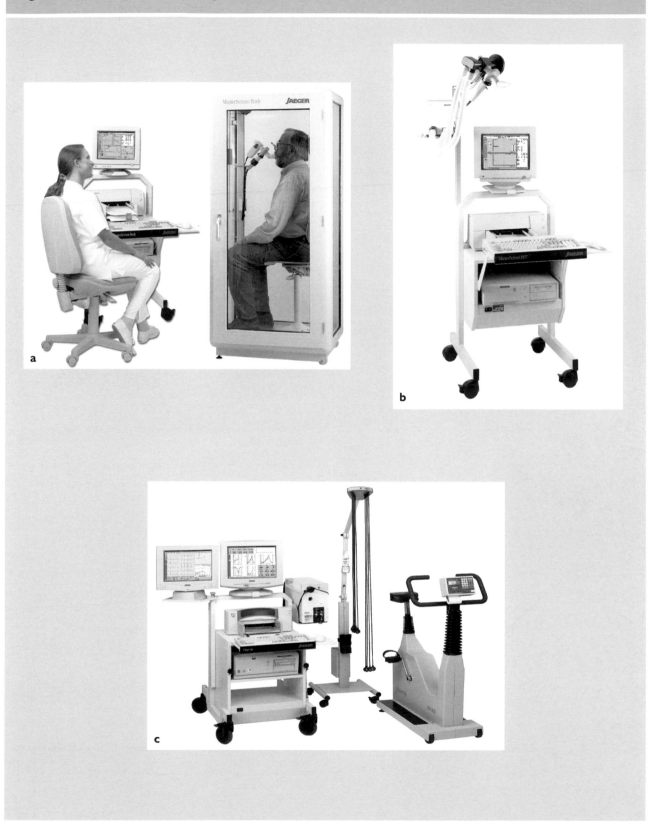

(a) Whole body plethysmography to measure lung volumes; (b) measurement of diffusion capacity, T_{LCO} or D_{LCO}; (c) cardiopulmonary exercise testing using bicycle ergometry. Pictures courtesy of Viasys/Jaeger Ltd.

Figure 3.19   Dynamic hyperventilation: operational lung volumes on exercise

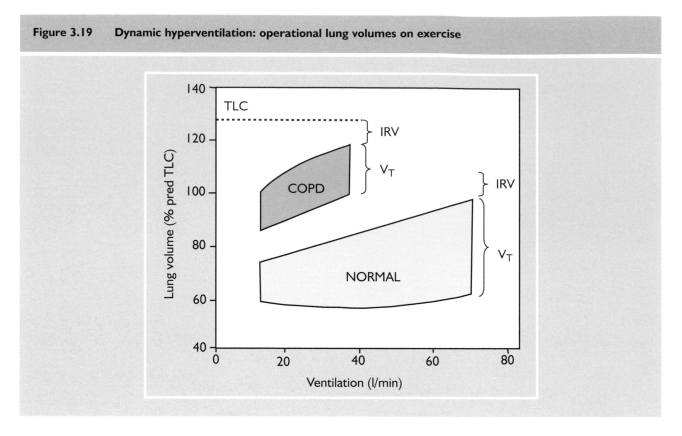

TLC, total lung capacity; IRV, inspiratory reserve volume; V$_T$, tidal volume. Adapted from O'Donnell DE. *Chest* 2000;117:42–7S.

lung hyperinflation is the response of the lung in terms of volumes after exercise[1,2,39], and has been shown to improve after bronchodilator therapy in COPD[40–42].

Diffusing capacity for carbon monoxide

The single-breath diffusing capacity is decreased in proportion to the severity of emphysema because of the destruction of the alveoli and the loss of alveolar capillary bed[43]. However, the measurement is not sensitive to low grades of emphysema[44] (Figures 3.11, 3.18 and 3.20). The diffusing capacity for carbon monoxide (D$_{LCO}$) is interchangeable with and usually called the transfer factor for carbon monoxide (T$_{LCO}$) in Europe[45]. The term conveys the ease of transfer of CO molecules from alveolar gas to pulmonary capillary hemoglobin. Thus, it involves the two processes of diffusion across the alveolar and capillary membranes and chemical combination with hemoglobin. D$_{LCO}$ values are lower in smokers than in non-smokers, even in young smokers who are not likely to have much emphysema[46].

Airway responsiveness

There is an increase in responsiveness to histamine and methacholine. This is much less than seen in asthma and is related to baseline lung function. Responses to indirect stimuli, such as adenosine monophosphate, sodium metabisulphite and exercise, are normal, however. Bronchial challenge tests are not useful in clinical practice and should not be conducted when FEV$_1$ is < 70% predicted normal.

Respiratory muscle function

A joint American Thoracic Society/European Respiratory Society statement on respiratory muscle testing has recently been published[47]. Maximum expiratory mouth pressure is usually normal until COPD is well advanced, but maximum inspiratory pressures are reduced due to hyperinflation. Function of skeletal muscles, such as quadriceps and deltoid, may be reduced in cachectic patients[48–50].

Figure 3.20   Pulmonary gas transfer

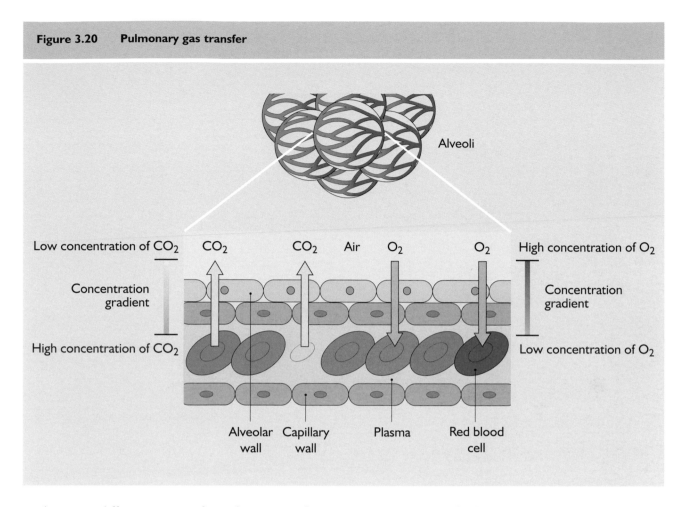

The terms 'diffusing capacity for carbon monoxide' (D_{LCO}, USA), and 'transfer factor' (T_{LCO}, Europe) are interchangeable. CO has high physical affinity for hemoglobin, binding 200 times more strongly than oxygen. CO transfer is diffusion-limited only.

Blood, breath and sputum

Serum α_1-antitrypsin levels

ZZ allele deficiency of α_1-antitrypsin (α_1-AT) or α_1-protease inhibitor (α_1-PI) is the best documented genetic factor for COPD[51–53] (Figure 3.21). The deficiency is a recessive trait seen in North Europeans in which severe deficiency of this major circulating inhibitor of serine proteases is often associated with early onset of emphysema in non-smokers. In smokers, α_1-PI deficiency is associated with the accelerated development of emphysema and mortality.

Intermediate levels are present in heterozygotes and persons with mixed phenotype, and these subjects may be at increased risk of developing COPD[54,55].

Polymorphisms in untranslated regions of the α_1-PI gene have been associated with an increased prevalence of COPD in some studies[56,57], although this has not been confirmed in another population[58].

Full blood count: erythrocytosis

In healthy individuals living at different altitudes, the development of erythrocytosis is proportional to arterial P_{O_2} values. In COPD, the literature is controversial, with various studies reporting that the response to P_{O_2} is normal, diminished, or even excessive[59]. Intermittent hypoxemia is a potent stimulus for erythropoietin production and both sleep and exercise can produce episodic desaturation in COPD. A relationship between arterial oxygen saturation of less than 80% in sleep and development of erythrocytosis has been shown[60]. Persistently

| Figure 3.21 | Blood tests in COPD |

α_1-antitrypsin

Estimation of serum α_1-antitrypsin levels is mandatory in the initial evaluation of patients with COPD presenting at < 45 years with prominent emphysema

Full blood count: polycythemia or anemia of chronic disease

Polycythemia (hematocrit > 47% in women or > 52% in men) is an indication of chronic hypoxia, and is most common in the 'blue bloater' type of COPD

Electrolytes

Electrolyte imbalance may occur in *cor pulmonale*, especially in those treated with diuretics, in whom hypokalemia may be a problem

Arterial blood gases

Take blood from radial artery if:
- FEV_1 is < 60% predicted
- exacerbation of COPD
- hypoxia
- oxygen therapy

Pulse oximetry for oxygen saturation (SaO_2)

---

elevated levels of blood carboxyhemoglobin contribute to the development of polycythemia in smokers[61]. Given the many factors that influence oxygen delivery to the tissues, a varying relationship between blood oxygen level and red blood cell mass should be expected in patients with COPD[59]. Other patients with COPD may have an anemia of chronic disease and this may be a systemic manifestation of COPD.

Pulse oximetry

Pulse oximetry measures oxygen saturation (SaO_2), but is not a good guide for diagnostic purposes, since it only indicates oxygenation and does not indicate changes in PCO_2. It may be useful for following the development of hypoxia as the disease advances, or in monitoring oxygen therapy. If SaO_2 is < 92%, blood gas tensions should be measured.

Arterial blood gases

More severe COPD is invariably accompanied by some degree of ventilation/perfusion mismatching, which results in arterial hypoxia in the patient breathing room air. In some patients, there is also a degree of respiratory failure, resulting in an increase in arterial $PaCO_2$ as FEV_1 falls below 1.5 l. In COPD patients with chronic respiratory failure, there should be metabolic compensation with an elevated base excess (or bicarbonate) and relatively normal pH (7.4).

Arterial blood gases taken from the radial artery with the patient breathing room air reveal mild or moderate hypoxemia without hypercapnia in the early stages of COPD. In the later stages of the disease, hypoxemia tends to become more severe and may be accompanied by hypercapnia with increased serum bicarbonate levels[43]. Blood gas abnormalities worsen during acute exacerbations and may also worsen during exercise[62] and sleep[63]. The relationship between impaired spirometric values and blood gas abnormalities is weak; hypercapnia is observed with increasing frequency with values of the FEV_1 of less than 1 liter.

- Arterial blood gases should be measured in patients with COPD in a stable state when breathing room air.

- Arterial blood gases should be measured during acute exacerbations of COPD to assess the degree of ventilatory failure. Because the pH is usually normal in stable COPD, a fall in pH is an indication of the severity of the exacerbation. It is important to assess $PaCO_2$ to decide on the need for non-invasive positive pressure ventilation.

Exhaled breath

A range of substances have been analyzed in exhaled breath and breath condensate from adults and children with lung disease. This includes nitric oxide (NO), ethane, isoprostanes, leukotrienes, prostaglandins, cytokines, products of lipid peroxidation, and nitrogenous derivatives. In addition, exhaled breath temperature may serve as a simple and inexpensive method for home monitoring of patients with asthma and COPD, and for assessing the effects of anti-inflammatory treatments. There is no single test that can be used to quantify airway inflammation, and a range of different specimens and markers of airway inflammation should be considered[64,65]. The 'exhaled breath profile' of several markers reflecting airway inflammation and oxidative stress is a promising approach for monitoring and management of patients with COPD[65]. Exhaled NO has been studied in greatest detail. In normal cigarette smokers and most patients with COPD, exhaled NO levels are lower than normal[66], whereas, in asthma, levels are high in patients not treated with inhaled corticosteroids. An elevated level of NO in patients with COPD therefore indicates coexistent asthma and predicts a response to corticosteroid therapy[67]. Exhaled interleukin-6 (IL-6) and leukotriene B$_4$ (LTB$_4$) have been found in the exhaled breath condensate of cigarette smokers, and increased LTB$_4$ and 8-isoprostane, a marker of oxidative stress, were measured in the exhaled breath of patients with exacerbations of COPD[68,69].

Sputum examination

Routine culture of sputum is not necessary and sputum analysis for presence of airway inflammation is not made routinely in clinical practice.

In stable bronchitis, sputum is mucoid, and microscopic examination reveals a predominance of macrophages or neutrophils, with few bacteria. During an exacerbation, the sputum becomes grossly purulent, primarily due to an influx of neutrophils, but may also have some pathogens (Gram-positive diplococci or fine Gram-negative pleomorphic rods).

The pathogens most often cultured from the sputum are *Streptococcus pneumoniae*, *Haemophilus influenzae*, *Moraxella catarrhalis*.

The analysis of induced sputum is increasingly performed as a means of assessing airway inflammation, but this is not a routine measurement for patients with COPD[70–72]. Sputum induction by the inhalation of nebulized hypertonic saline has been demonstrated to be a relatively safe and effective method of enabling sputum expectoration[73,74]. Sputum processing generally consists of selecting the solid mucinous portion of sputum, which is liquefied by reduction with dithiothreitol (DTT), and using the cellular portion to produce cytospins for light microscopy, while employing the supernatant for analysis of soluble proteins and mediators. In response to the expanding volume of sputum research, the European Respiratory Society has compiled a report on standardization of sputum induction and processing methodology[75].

Bronchoalveolar lavage and biopsy

Studies with bronchoalveolar lavage and mucosal bronchial biopsy are important mechanistic studies for the evaluation of anti-inflammatory therapies for asthma and COPD[76]. A European Respiratory Society Task Force has issued guidelines for measurements of acellular components and standardization of bronchoalveolar lavage[77], while the reproducibility of endobronchial biopsy has been established[78]. Fluticasone has been shown to lack effects on neutrophils and CD8+ T cells in biopsies from patients with COPD, but to have subtle effects on mast cells[79].

Imaging

Chest X-ray

COPD is a functional diagnosis so that chest radiographs can only suggest this diagnosis (Figure 3.22 and 3.23). The chest radiograph is essential, both for its value in excluding other pulmonary disorders that may produce the same respiratory symptoms and for showing overdistention of the lungs or the specific findings of emphysema. In mild COPD, the plain chest X-ray is usually normal.

Chronic bronchitis is not diagnosed by chest X-ray, but there are radiographic signs which can suggest the diagnosis: bronchial wall thickening, prominent lung markings, and tubular shadows or

Figure 3.22   Chest X-rays in COPD

Chest X-ray is rarely itself diagnostic for COPD – but is valuable in excluding alternative diagnoses and for detecting complications (infection, pneumothorax, malignancy, heart failure, pulmonary embolism)

Mild COPD
Chest X-ray is usually normal

Chronic bronchitis
- 'Dirty lung'
- Increased lung markings
- Bronchial wall thickening

Emphysema
- Hyperinflation ───────────────→
- Oligemia
- Loss of fine vasculature markings, especially at the periphery of the lung where there is rapid tapering of vascular markings
- Bulla: areas of translucency surrounded by thin wall

Hyperinflation
- Large volume hyperlucent lungs – darker
- Low, flat diaphragm on lateral film/PA
- Thin heart shadow
- Enlarged retrosternal air space on the lateral view

Pulmonary hypertension and *cor pulmonale*
- Hilar vasculature becomes prominent
- Descending branch of right pulmonary artery > 20 mm
- Cardiomegaly – reflecting right ventricular hypertrophy

'tramlines' amidst a 'dirty lung'. Hyperinflation leads to large-volume lungs, a low and flat diaphragm, a thin heart shadow, and an enlarged retrosternal air space.

Emphysema, when mild, may not be detectable on chest X-ray, although the triad of overinflation, oligemia and bullae comprises the lung arterial deficiency pattern, most often associated with emphysema. Increased lung markings may resemble the 'dirty lung' appearance seen in chronic bronchitis. Overinflation is best seen by flattening of the diaphragms with a concavity of the superior surface of the diaphragm, and can also be seen by an increase in the width of the retrosternal air space, but this is less sensitive. When emphysema is prominent, there is loss of fine vascular markings, especially at the periphery of the lung, and bullae (areas of translucency surrounded by a thin wall) may appear.

Cor pulmonale causes increasing width of the cardiac shadow in serial chest radiographs, especially if accompanied by encroachment of the cardiac shadow on the retrosternal space. Useful screens for pulmonary hypertension[13] are the width of the descending branch of the right pulmonary artery of > 20 mm, and the hilar cardiothoracic ratio. When

cor pulmonale occurs, the hilar vasculature may become prominent, and the heart may enlarge, especially in the anteroposterior direction.

With *infections*, there may be localized infiltrates in the lungs; these should disappear with antibiotic treatment. Some features on the chest X-ray are *not* consistent with a diagnosis of uncomplicated COPD and should raise the possibility of an alternative diagnosis: a persistent localized infiltrate or persistent atelectasis, hilar node enlargement, parenchymal nodules or masses, pleural disease, and interstitial infiltrates.

Computerized tomography

High-resolution computerized tomography (CT) is defined as thin-section CT (1–2 mm collimation scans) (Figure 3.24), while spiral (helical) CT provides continuous scanning when the patient is moved through the CT gantry. High-resolution CT is useful in studies on patients with COPD to assess the extent of airway, interstitial and vascular disease[80], as well as detecting bronchiectasis[81] and early cancerous lesions. High-resolution CT is sufficiently sensitive to monitor longitudinal changes in

Figure 3.23   Chest X-rays in COPD

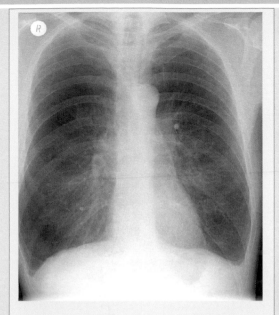

Findings typical of advanced emphysema
Large-volume lungs with thin heart shadow and flattened hemidiaphragms bilaterally. Note the increased transradiancy in the upper lobes with attenuated vascular markings.

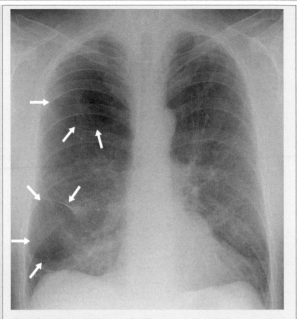

Emphysema with two bullae
The upper bulla is seen as a transradiant avascular area in the right upper lobe with the wall visualized as a thin curvilinear inferior border (arrows). A further bulla is seen within the right lower lobe.

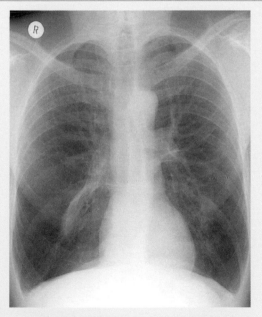

α_1- antitrypsin deficiency and panacinar emphysema
Chest X-ray shows large volume lungs with low flat diaphragms. Both lower zones are hypertransradiant and the vessels within these zones are reduced in size. Distribution of these changes is typical of panacinar emphysema.

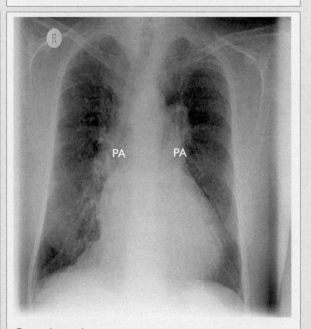

Cor pulmonale
Chronic airflow obstruction with bilateral enlarged pulmonary arteries (PA) in keeping with pulmonary hypertension. Cardiomegaly is present with the transverse cardiac dimension > 50% of the transverse lung dimension.

Photographs by courtesy of Dr Zelena Aziz and Professor David M. Hansell, Royal Brompton Hospital, London, UK.

Figure 3.24   Computerized tomography (CT) imaging

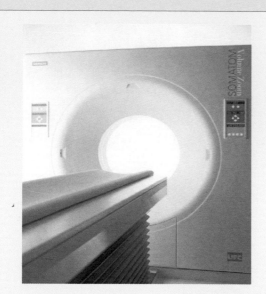
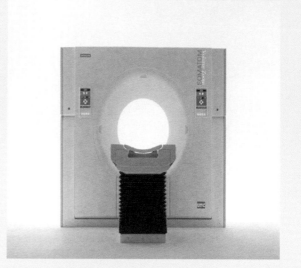

Siemens Somatom Volume Zoom CT Scanner

Pictures by courtesy of Siemens, Erlangen, Germany

X-ray generator

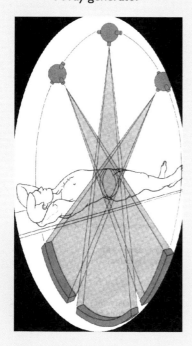

Data acquisition

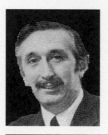

Godfrey
Hounsfield

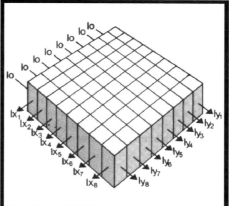

CT measures the attenuation of X-rays in:

Hounsfield Units (HU)
- Water = 0 HU
- Air = -1000 HU
- Bone = +1000 HU

Voxel dimension = length x width x thickness

Figure 3.25   High-resolution computerized tomography appearances in COPD

CT feature	Pathophysiology
Bronchial wall thickening	**Chronic bronchitis**
Ground-glass attenuation with nodular component	**Respiratory bronchiolitis with interstitial lung disease** **Inflammation** in and around bronchioles with accumulation of macrophages in alveoli
Reticular pattern	**Interstitial fibrosis**
Mosaic attenuation pattern of lung parenchyma at end expiration	**Obstruction** of bronchioles causing regional underventilation with reduced perfusion
Multiple small round areas of low attenuation, with decreased Hounsfield units (HU), in the secondary pulmonary lobule Several mm (< 1 cm) in diameter, surrounded by normal lung parenchyma Upper lobe predominance	**Centrilobular emphysema** Generally caused by cigarette smoking
Peripheral variant of centrilobular emphysema Areas of low attenuation in the subpleural regions of the lung and adjacent to interlobular septa and pulmonary vessels	**Paraseptal emphysema** Prone to lead to bulla and pneumothorax
Uniform destruction of the secondary pulmonary lobule gives homogeneous 'black lung' Paucity of vascular markings Diffuse distribution in lower lobes	**Panacinar (panlobular) emphysema** May be asscociated with α_1-antitrypsin deficiency
Thin-walled, focal areas of avascularity Bulla are > 1 cm in diameter Bulla tend to involve upper lobes	**Bulla**
Vascular pruning, enlarged pulmonary artery Mosaic attenuation	**Pulmonary hypertension**

Table developed in consultation with Professor David M. Hansell, Royal Brompton Hospital, London.

the extent of emphysema[82–84], and it has been shown that annual changes in lung density and percentage of low attenuation area are detectable with inspiratory high-resolution CT[85]. Inflammatory infiltration of the lung parenchyma is associated with ground-glass attenuation; bronchiolitis can be visualized as parenchymal micronodules. Bronchial wall thickening may occur, and emphysema is visible as areas of decreased attenuation[86–90] (Figures 3.25 and 3.26).

In a recent major publication, progression from ground-glass attenuation with parenchymal micronodules (respiratory bronchiolitis with interstitial

Figure 3.26   High-resolution computerized tomography in COPD

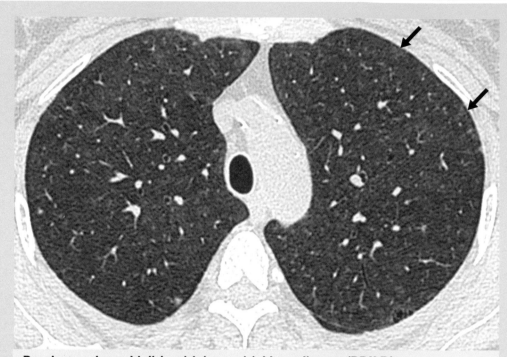

Respiratory bronchiolitis with interstitial lung disease (RBILD)
Ill-defined white nodules are arrowed, representing accumulation of macrophages in the interstitium and respiratory bronchiolitis.

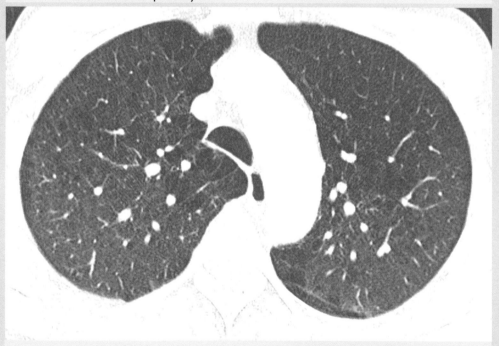

Centrilobular emphysema
'Moth-eaten' appearance of lung with multiple patchy black areas (lower attenuation corresponding to lung destruction and centrilobular emphysema).

Photographs by courtesy of Dr Graham Robinson and Professor David M. Hansell, Royal Brompton Hospital, London. (*Continued*)

Figure 3.26 *(Continued)* **High-resolution computerized tomography in COPD**

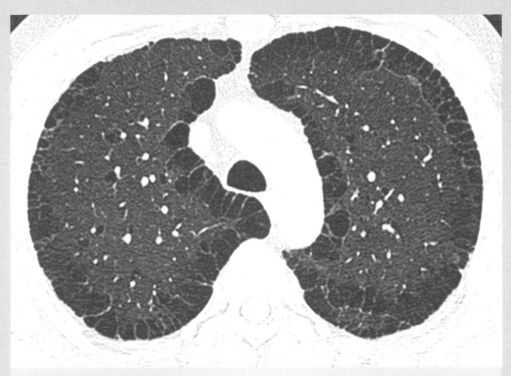

Paraseptal emphysema
Multiple sub-pleural air spaces with hairline-thin walls.

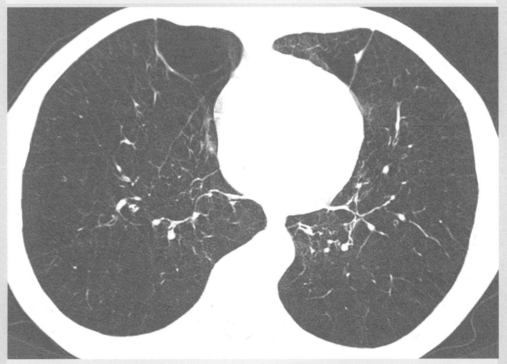

Panacinar emphysema
Large areas of ill-defined low attenuation due to panacinar parenchyma destruction.

lung disease) to emphysema has been demonstrated in a group of 111 smokers who were studied over a mean period of 5 years[87,91]. Smoking causes a variety of high-resolution CT changes within the small airways and interstitium in COPD[92,93].

It appears that subtle changes in progression of lung disease related to α_1-AT deficiency may be more readily detected with CT imaging than with pulmonary function testing[94–96]. Following α_1-AT augmentation therapy, annual CT has proved useful in disease assessment[97,98]. Nevertheless, there are considerable challenges in the standardization of CT and in the development of methodology for image processing and analysis.

Computerized tomography can resolve the pulmonary parenchyma much better than a standard roentgenogram[86]. High-resolution CT uses between 1.0 mm and 2.0 mm collimation rather than the standard 10 mm collimation used in conventional CT. CT may be used to quantitate the amount of air trapping by comparing images during inspiration and full expiration[99]. The diagnosis of emphysema on the basis of pathologic changes is frequently best made on CT scans of the chest, but a CT scan should be performed if there is any suspicion of malignancy or if surgical treatment is planned.

A CT scan of the thorax is useful for demonstrating emphysema, where typical appearances are:

- Areas of low attenuation and bullae
- Attenuation and pruning of the vascular tree
- Abnormal vascular configurations

A CT scan of the lungs may be indicated as the disease progresses:

- Most patients with COPD are heavy smokers and a small carcinoma may be difficult to diagnose on a plain chest radiograph. It may be impossible to distinguish between a simple infectious exacerbation of COPD and the appearance of malignancy on a plain radiograph.

- Complications of COPD such as pulmonary thromboembolism and pulmonary artery thrombosis can be detected by a CT with contrast injection – especially using spiral CT.

- CT scans can distinguish centrilobular (centriacinar) from panacinar emphysema – but this may not be useful in management for the moment.

- Bronchiectasis can be diagnosed on CT scans and this may be a feature in patients with severe disease.

- CT scans are essential in the selection of patients for lung volume reduction surgery in order to see the distribution of emphysema.

Electrocardiography

COPD influences the electrical events of the heart:

- Lung hyperinflation has an insulating effect and diminishes the transmission of electrical potentials to the ECG leads

- The heart descends to a lower position within the thorax

- COPD may result in right ventricular hypertrophy (QRS right-axis deviation) and dilation, as well as right atrial enlargement (P wave right-axis deviation)

P waves:

- P pulmonale constitutes tall, peaked P waves (in standard leads II, III and AVF) in association with P wave right-axis deviation.

QRS complex:

- QRS right-axis deviation is commonly directed to +90° in uncomplicated COPD.

- QRS right-axis deviation increases from +90° towards +180° with the development of pulmonary hypertension.

- Right bundle branch block may be complete or incomplete and may occur transiently with increased oxygen desaturation.

Increasing severity of COPD:

- Progressive QRS right-axis deviation
- Progressive P wave right-axis deviation

Features of *cor pulmonale*:

- R or R' greater than or equal to the S wave in V_1

- R wave less than the amplitude of the S wave in V_6

- QRS right-axis deviation greater than +180° without right bundle branch block.

An ECG is also useful for detecting coexistent ischemic heart disease.

Echocardiography and esophageal cardiography

- Two-dimensional echocardiography, and pulsed Doppler techniques with echocardiography to estimate mean pulmonary arterial pressure are other methods to assess pulmonary hypertension and right ventricular function[100–102]. Left ventricular size and performance are generally normal in patients with COPD in the absence of other associated cardiac abnormalities.

- Esophageal cardiography appears to be more sensitive and correctly diagnosed *cor pulmonale* in 24 of 25 COPD patients in one study[101], but is impractical for routine use.

- Patients with *cor pulmonale* may have the following echocardiographic features:

  - Right ventricular size increased, with an inlet diameter of > 4 cm

  - Moderate-to-severe tricuspid regurgitation, with right ventricular (RV)–right atrial (RA) pressure drop of > 35 mmHg

  - Delayed onset of right ventricular filling of > 80 ms from end ejection.

Miscellaneous

Exercise testing

Some patients with mild COPD may have little or no disturbance of blood gases at rest and hypoxia only appears on exercise. In others with more marked disease, the decision as to whether to recommend supplemental oxygen should be made with the help of an objective evaluation of the degree of effort limitation. There are several exercise protocols, such as the progressive ergometer stress test, the 6-min walk test[104], and the incremental shuttle walking test, involving walking around two markers 10 meters apart[105,106]. These may be useful to monitor progress, and are generally part of pulmonary rehabilitation programs. Oxygenation should be checked by pulse oximetry or arterial blood gases during exercise.

Six-min walk test In this test, the patient is encouraged to walk as far as possible at his or her own pace for 6 min and the total distance measured is noted[104]. In a more advanced version of this test, the patient is fitted with a pulse oximeter and oxygen saturation is measured throughout the test. The distance covered correlates well with lung function and diffusing capacity but not with oxygen saturation during the walk. In a typical COPD patient with an FEV_1 of about 1 l or 40% predicted, the 6-min walk distance would be about 400 meters. There is considerable inter-subject variability, which depends on emotional state, expectations and motivation. It is a valuable and simple index for following progression of the disease in the individual patient. The American Thoracic Society has published recent guidelines for the 6-min walk test, since this is an important component in the functional assessment of patients with COPD[104,105]. The 6-min walk test is performed indoors on a long flat straight corridor of at least 30 meters in length, and the use of a treadmill is not recommended. In a recent review, it was found that the 6-min walk test is easy to administer and more reflective of activities of daily living than other walk tests[106].

Incremental shuttle walk test This is similar to the 6-min walk test but involves walking round two markers set 10 meters apart and is easier to conduct in a hospital setting[107,108] (Figure 3.27). The 12-level incremental shuttle-walking test provokes a symptom-limited maximal performance exercise but it uses an audio signal from a tape cassette to guide the speed of walking of the patient back and forth between two traffic cones on a 10-meter course[109,110]. The shuttle-walking test has an incremental and progressive structure to assess functional capacity, and maximum heart rates are significantly higher than for the 6-min walk test. The endurance shuttle walk test also uses a 10-meter course, but has an externally controlled constant walking speed[108].

Health status: health-related quality of life

COPD may have a major impact on the patient's quality of life. Validated questionnaires, such as the St. George's Respiratory Disease Questionnaire specifically designed for patients with COPD, quantify symptoms and the impact of the disease on daily living[111,112]. Quality-of-life questionnaires assess the overall impact of COPD on daily living and may be more sensitive than physiological measurements in assessing the severity of disease and its response to treatment, but they are time-consuming to perform. They are very useful in clinical trials of COPD therapies, however.

Health status has become a major evaluation for patients with COPD[113]. The St. George's

Figure 3.27   The incremental shuttle walk test

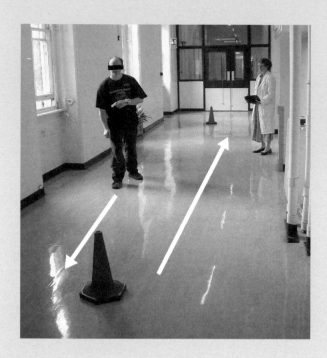

The incremental shuttle walk test involves the patient moving between two traffic cones placed 9 meters apart, each being inset 0.5 m to give a 10-m course. The patient moves in time with prerecorded bleeps generated by a microcomputer on a tape cassette or CD-ROM (available from Dr M.D.L. Morgan at Glenfield Hospital, Leicester, UK). The speed gradually increases from slow walking to jogging. The subject should continue until unable to maintain the required speed without becoming unduly breathless. The patient is monitored by pulse oximetry. For details, see Singh SJ, Morgan MDL, *et al. Thorax* 1992;47:1019–24

Respiratory Questionnaire is a standardized self-completed questionnaire for measuring health-related quality of life in airways disease[114,115]. The St. George's Respiratory Questionnaire and the Chronic Respiratory Disease Questionnaire are validated questionnaires for patients with COPD[111]. The final version has 76 items divided into three sections: 'symptoms', 'activity' and 'impacts', and provides a total score. Scores range from 0 (perfect health) to 100 (worst possible state), with a four-point change in score considered a worthwhile treatment effect. The St. George's Respiratory Questionnaire and the Chronic Respiratory Disease Questionnaire have been found equivalent in a comparative study[116]. Generic questionnaires have a place in COPD studies, but are relatively insensitive, and include the Sickness Impact Profile and SF-36[117].

Sleep studies: pulse oximetry and polysomnography

Many patients with COPD underventilate during sleep, causing ventilation/perfusion imbalance or respiratory failure[118]. Sleep studies should be performed if hypoxemia or right heart failure develops in the presence of relatively mild airflow limita-

tion, and if sleep apnea is present on history (see Chapter 7). Screening by overnight monitoring of oxygenation on pulse oximetry can be performed[119].

- Monitoring for nocturnal desaturation is only necessary in COPD patients who do not meet the criteria for long-term oxygen therapy, but whose clinical assessment suggests the effects of intermittent hypoxemia, such as pulmonary hypertension, erythrocytosis or mental status changes.

- This approach is valid since nocturnal hypoxemia alone does not impair survival in COPD patients[120] and administering supplemental nocturnal oxygen for sleep desaturation in patients with a daytime arterial P_{O_2} above 60 mmHg does not reduce mortality[121].

Body mass index and fat-free mass

Assessment of nutritional status in patients with more severe COPD is increasingly performed (Figure 3.28), since systemic disease and weight loss are important factors in the prognosis of COPD[122–125]. Body weight and height are used to calculate the body mass index (BMI). Fat-free mass

Figure 3.28 Assessment of body composition

Components

body cell mass		
lipid		
extracellular water		
	intracellular water	
	protein	
minerals		

fat-free mass

fat	lipid
	water
	protein
	minerals

Parameters

- Weight
- Height
- Body mass index (BMI) $= \dfrac{\text{Weight}}{(\text{height})^2}$

- Fat-free mass (FFM)
- Fat-free mass index $= \dfrac{\text{FFM}}{(\text{height})^2}$

Skin-fold anthropometry

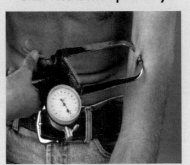

Dual-energy X-ray absorptiometry (DEXA) scan

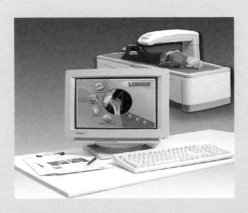

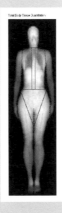

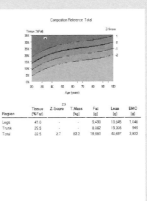

Photograph of DPX-L bone densitometer by permission of Lunar Radiation Corporation (Madison, WI). The scanner performs multiple transverse scans from head to toes with 1-cm intervals. The radiation dose is < 0.1 mSV and the scanning lasts approximately 15 min. Bone mineral content (BMC), fat mass (FM) and lean mass are derived according to computer algorithms provided by the manufacturer. Fat-free mass (FFM) is the sum of BMC and lean mass.

Bioimpedance analysis (BIA)

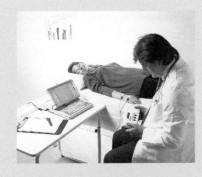

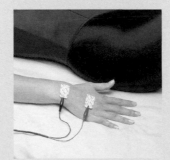

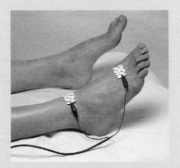

Photograph of Bodystat 1500 bioimpedance analyzer by permission of Bodystat LD (Xitron, San Diego, CA). Electrodes are attached to the right wrist/hand and right ankle/foot, with the patient supine. The principle of BIA is that conductivity is higher in FFM, since this contains body fluids and electrolytes.

Figure 3.29   Tests of muscle strength

Hand grip dynamometer

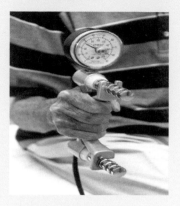

Hanten WP. *J Hand Ther* 1999;
12:193–200

Nasal sniff test

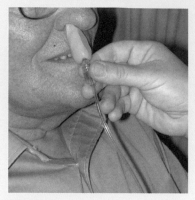

Methodology for the assessment
of sniff pressure is reviewed in
Am J Respir Crit Med 2002;
166:533–4

Quadriceps twitch test following external stimulation

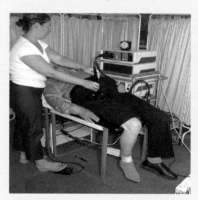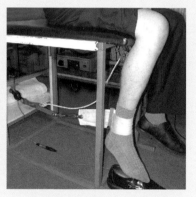

For details, see Polkey MI. *Muscle and Nerve* 1996;19:549–55

(FFM) corresponds to those body compartments containing water, protein and minerals. FFM can readily be measured by the techniques of dual-energy X-ray absorptiometry (DEXA) scanning or bioelectrical impedance analysis (BIA)[126,127]. The treatment of nutritional depletion is covered in Chapter 7.

Muscle testing

An American Thoracic Society/European Respiratory Society statement has recently been made on respiratory muscle testing[47]. Figure 3.29 illustrates tests of handgrip strength and quadriceps strength, as well as the nasal sniff test. Cellular adaptations in the diaphragm have been reported in COPD[128,129], and skeletal muscle apoptosis can occur in conjunction with cachexia in COPD[9,130], with weakness and dysfunction of voluntary skeletal muscle[8,131,132]. Mid-thigh muscle cross-sectional area is found to be a predictor of mortality to assess muscle wasting in COPD[133]. Muscle fibers have been classified on the basis of staining for myofibrillar ATPase as well as

Figure 3.30   Classification of muscle fiber type   107

Classification scheme	Motor unit type			
	Slow-twitch fatigue-resistant (S)	Fast-twitch fatigue-resistant (FFR)	Fast-twitch fatigue-intermediate (FFInt)	Fast-twitch fatiguable (FF)
Metabolic enzyme staining	slow-twitch oxidative (SO)	fast-twitch oxidative, glycolytic (FOG)	?	fast-twitch glycolytic (FG)
pH lability of myofibrillar ATPase staining	I	IIa	IIx	IIb
Myosin heavy chain (MHC) immunoreactivity	MHC_{slow}	MHC_{2A}	MHC_{2X}	MHC_{2B}

Adapted from *Am J Respir Crit Care Med* 1999;159:S1–40

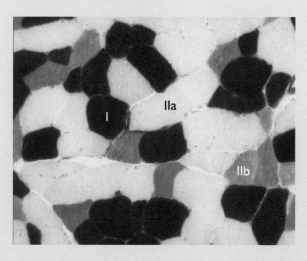

Quadriceps biopsy with myofibrillar ATPase stain to demonstrate representative muscle fiber types

glycolytic and oxidative enzymes (Figure 3.30), while immunoreactivity for myosin heavy chain (MHC) isoforms can be performed.

Patients with advanced COPD have been reported to have a significantly reduced proportion of type I fibers in the vastus laterallis, with an increased proportion of type IIb fibers[134].

NATURAL HISTORY, STAGES OF SEVERITY, MONITORING, PROGNOSIS AND DEATH

Natural history

So far, no intervention except for smoking cessation has been shown to reduce the rate of loss of lung function in COPD[135]. Studies on the natural history of COPD involve monitoring post-bronchodilator FEV_1 in considerable numbers of patients over a number of years. Four major studies have recently been performed on effects of inhaled corticosteroids on the longitudinal decline in post-bronchodilator FEV_1 over 3 years in patients with mild[136,137] or moderate-to-severe COPD[138,139] (*see* Figure 5.52). Effects on FEV_1 were modest and only present in the first few months, and inhaled corticosteroids failed to affect the rate of loss of lung function over 3 years. However, in moderate-to-severe COPD, inhaled corticosteroids are effective in preventing exacerbations, and cause some improvement in health status.

The clinical course of COPD is characterized by presentation with a productive cough, initially more prominent in the morning. There is insidious onset of breathlessness, initially on exercise but later at rest. These symptoms become progressive (increasing over time) and persistent (present every day), and worse during respiratory infections. Acute exacerbations of COPD occur with increasing frequency, especially in winter. The onset of chronic respiratory failure is heralded by hypoxia on exercise, which later occurs during sleep, and eventually is present at rest by day. Chronic respiratory failure is associated with pulmonary hypertension and *cor pulmonale*, manifested as right-sided heart failure. Patients with chronic respiratory failure are vulnerable to exacerbations of COPD and terminal acute respiratory failure.

Stages of COPD severity

COPD is arbitrarily classified into levels of severity, and the levels of post-bronchodilator FEV_1 employed to stage COPD patients in the GOLD guidelines are shown in Figure 3.14. Since COPD typically results from cigarette smoke causing irreversible damage to the alveoli and smaller airways, there is at present no chance of completely curing the disease. COPD usually follows a slow but progressive downhill course over many years.

Decline in lung function

Patients with COPD usually show an accelerated annual decline in forced expiratory volume in 1 second (FEV_1), often greater than 50 ml/year, compared to the normal decline of approximately 20 ml/year), although this is variable between patients. The classic studies of Fletcher and Peto[140]

established that only 10–20% of cigarette smokers are susceptible to long-term exposure to cigarette smoke (Figure 3.14). The decline in function occurs along a slowly accelerating curvilinear path. In most persons, the loss is assumed to occur uniformly, although there are generally insufficient data to be certain of this. Mortality is related to the number of cigarettes smoked[141]. Quitting smoking results in a return to the normal rate of decline in lung function and is the only treatment that has so far been able to reduce the rate of decline in patients with COPD. These results have been confirmed in the more recent Lung Health Study in the USA[135,142]. Some patients with COPD have a low baseline COPD and may have a normal rate of decline in lung function, but eventually reach a point where they become symptomatic. Rising airway bacteria load as well as changes in bacteria species are associated with airway inflammation and accelerated decline in FEV_1[143].

Horse-race effect

A direct relationship between initial FEV_1 level and the slope of FEV_1 decline is known as the 'horse-race effect'; this term describes the observation that the horse leading in the middle of the race is most likely to win the race[144]. An individual with low initial lung function is more likely to proceed to lower lung function over time.

Smoking cessation

After the cessation of smoking, there is a minor improvement in lung function in the first year, but lung function lost as a result of smoking is not regained[135,142]. However, the rate of decline of lung function with increasing age in former smokers slows to that seen in non-smokers of the same age[145,146]. To date, only smoking cessation has altered the natural history of lung function loss in COPD[135,142]. If the patient stops smoking, the rate of decline of lung function is substantially slowed, but the natural history with continued smoking is of inevitable loss of lung function.

Prognosis

The prognosis of patients with COPD who have mild airflow limitation is favorable if they can give up smoking; survival in a group with initial post-bronchodilator FEV_1 of ≥ 50% of predicted was only slightly worse than in a group of smokers without airflow obstruction[147]. The prognosis is generally poor in patients with severe COPD, especially if it is accompanied by hypoxia and hypercapnia, although domiciliary long-term oxygen therapy and non-invasive ventilation are beneficial[148–150]. Advanced age, $FEV_1 < 50\%$ predicted, and comorbidities such as chronic renal failure and *cor pulmonale* are associated with poor prognosis[151,152]. However, follow-up studies have shown that some patients with severe COPD may survive for periods of as long as 15 years[147,153–155].

Death

Death generally occurs as a result of some medical complication of COPD, such as an overwhelming pneumonia, retained secretions with atelectasis and pneumonia, pneumothorax, cardiac arrhythmia, or pulmonary embolism. Assiduous and thoughtful management and facilitation of patient entry into the medical care system when they are acutely ill are all important in giving individuals with COPD the maximum possible length and quality of life. This is especially relevant for patients with end-stage COPD who have significantly impaired quality of life and emotional well-being, which is relatively poorly treated[156,157]. Recommendations for end-of-life care on the intensive care unit are available from an ethics viewpoint[158] as well as clinical management[159].

REFERENCES

1. O'Donnell DE, Revill SM, Webb KA. Dynamic hyperinflation and exercise intolerance in chronic obstructive pulmonary disease. *Am J Respir Crit Care Med* 2001;164:770–7

2. O'Donnell DE, Webb KA. Exertional breathlessness in patients with chronic airflow limitation. The role of lung hyperinflation. *Am Rev Respir Dis* 1993;148:1351–7

3. Bestall JC, Paul EA, Garrod R, Garnham R, Jones PW, Wedzicha JA. Usefulness of the Medical Research Council (MRC) dyspnoea scale as a measure of disability in patients with chronic obstructive pulmonary disease. *Thorax* 1999;54:581–6

4. American Thoracic Society. Standards for the diagnosis and care of patients with chronic obstructive pulmonary disease. *Am J Respir Crit Care Med* 1995;152:S77–120

5. Rennard SI, Daughton DM. Cigarette smoking and disease. In Elias JA, Fishman JA, Grippi MA, Kaiser L, Senior RM, eds. *Pulmonary Diseases and Disorders*. New York: McGraw Hill, 1997:697–708

6. British Thoracic Society. BTS guidelines for the management of chronic obstructive pulmonary disease. *Thorax* 1997;52 (Suppl 5)

7. National Institutes of Health (NIH), National Heart Lung and Blood Institute (NHLBI), World Health Organisation (WHO). Global Initiative for Chronic Obstructive Lung Disease (GOLD): Global Strategy for the Diagnosis, Management, and Prevention of Chronic Obstructive Pulmonary Disease. NHLBI/WHO Workshop Report. www.goldcopd.com/workshop/index.html. 2001

8. Engelen MP, Schols AM, Does JD, Wouters EF. Skeletal muscle weakness is associated with wasting of extremity fat-free mass but not with airflow obstruction in patients with chronic obstructive pulmonary disease. *Am J Clin Nutr* 2000;71:733–8

9. Agusti AG, Sauleda J, Miralles C, Gomez C, Togores B, Sala E, et al. Skeletal muscle apoptosis and weight loss in chronic obstructive pulmonary disease. *Am J Respir Crit Care Med* 2002;166:485–9

10. Schols AM, Slangen J, Volovics L, Wouters EF. Weight loss is a reversible factor in the prognosis of chronic obstructive pulmonary disease. *Am J Respir Crit Care Med* 1998;157:1791–7

11. van Ede L, Yzermans CJ, Brouwer HJ. Prevalence of depression in patients with chronic obstructive pulmonary disease: a systemic review. *Thorax* 1999;54:688–92

12. Anonymous. Blue bloater: pink puffer. *Br Med J* 1968;2:677

13. Matthay RA, Niederman MS, Wiedemann HP. Cardiovascular–pulmonary interaction in chronic obstructive pulmonary disease with special reference to the pathogenesis and management of *cor pulmonale*. *Med Clin North Am* 1990;74:571–618

14. Klinger JR, Hill NS. Right ventricular dysfunction in chronic obstructive pulmonary disease. Evaluation and management. *Chest* 1991;99:715–23

15. Farber MO, Roberts LR, Weinberger MH, Robertson GL, Fineberg NS, Manfredi F. Abnormalities of sodium and water handling in chronic obstructive lung disease. *Arch Intern Med* 1982;142:1326–30

16. Wedzicha JA, Seemungal TA, MacCallum PK, et al. Acute exacerbations of chronic obstructive pulmonary disease are accompanied by elevations of plasma fibrinogen and serum IL-6 levels. *Thromb Haemost* 2000;84:210–15

17. Prescott E, Almdal T, Mikkelsen KL, Tofteng CL, Vestbo J, Lange P. Prognostic value of weight change in chronic obstructive pulmonary disease: results from the Copenhagen City Heart Study. *Eur Respir J* 2002;20:539–44

18. Schols AM, Soeters PB, Mostert R, Pluymers RJ, Wouters EF. Physiologic effects of nutritional support and anabolic steroids in patients with chronic obstructive pulmonary disease. A placebo-controlled randomized trial. *Am J Respir Crit Care Med* 1995;152:1268–74

19. Schols AM, Soeters PB, Dingemans AM, Mostert R, Frantzen PJ, Wouters EF. Prevalence and characteristics of nutritional depletion in patients with stable COPD eligible for pulmonary rehabilitation. *Am Rev Respir Dis* 1993;147:1151–6

20. Wouters EF. Nutrition and metabolism in COPD. *Chest* 2000;117(5 Suppl 1):274–80S

21. Schols AM, Mostert R, Soeters PB, Wouters EF. Body composition and exercise performance in patients with chronic obstructive pulmonary disease. *Thorax* 1991;46:695–9

22. Catterall JR, Calverley PM, MacNee W, *et al.* Mechanism of transient nocturnal hypoxemia in hypoxic chronic bronchitis and emphysema. *J Appl Physiol* 1985;59:1698–703

23. Douglas NJ, Flenley DC. Breathing during sleep in patients with obstructive lung disease. *Am Rev Respir Dis* 1990;141:1055–70

24. Fletcher EC, Miller J, Divine GW, Fletcher JG, Miller T. Nocturnal oxyhemoglobin desaturation in COPD patients with arterial oxygen tensions above 60 mmHg. *Chest* 1987;92:604–8

25. Catterall JR, Douglas NJ, Calverley PM, *et al.* Transient hypoxia during sleep in chronic obstructive pulmonary disease is not a sleep apnea syndrome. *Am Rev Respir Dis* 1983;128:24–9

26. Crystal RG, Brantly ML, Hubbard RC, Curiel DT, States DJ, Holmes MD. The alpha 1-antitrypsin gene and its mutations. Clinical consequences and strategies for therapy. *Chest* 1989;95:196–208

27. Mahadeva R, Lomas DA. Genetics and respiratory disease. 2. Alpha 1-antitrypsin deficiency, cirrhosis and emphysema. *Thorax* 1998;53:501–5

28. Bush A, Cole P, Hariri M, *et al.* Primary ciliary dyskinesia: diagnosis and standards of care. *Eur Respir J* 1998;12:982–8

29. Sugiyama Y. Diffuse panbronchiolitis. *Clin Chest Med* 1993;14:765–72

30. Fletcher C, Peto R, Tinker CM, Speizer FE. *The Natural History of Chronic Bronchitis and Emphysema.* New York: Oxford University Press, 1976

31. Peto R, Speizer FE, Cochrane AL, *et al.* The relevance in adults of air-flow obstruction, but not of mucus hypersecretion, to mortality from chronic lung disease. Results from 20 years of prospective observation. *Am Rev Respir Dis* 1983;128:491–500

32. Anthonisen NR, Wright EC, Hodgkin JE. Prognosis in chronic obstructive pulmonary disease. *Am Rev Respir Dis* 1986;133:14–20

33. Burrows B, Earle RH. Course and prognosis of chronic obstructive lung disease. A prospective study of 200 patients. *N Engl J Med* 1969;280:397–404

34. Hansen EF, Phanareth K, Laursen LC, Kok-Jensen A, Dirksen A. Reversible and irreversible airflow obstruction as predictor of overall mortality in asthma and chronic obstructive pulmonary disease. *Am J Respir Crit Care Med* 1999;159:1267–71

35. Niewoehner DE, Kleinerman J, Rice DB. Pathologic changes in the peripheral airways of young cigarette smokers. *N Engl J Med* 1974;291:755–8

36. Emerman CL, Cydulka RK. Use of peak expiratory flow rate in emergency department evaluation of acute exacerbation of chronic obstructive pulmonary disease. *Ann Emerg Med* 1996;27:159–63

37. Rebuck DA, Hanania NA, D'Urzo AD, Chapman KR. The accuracy of a handheld portable spirometer. *Chest* 1996;109:152–7

38. Hoppin FG. Pulmonary function tests for diagnosis and evaluation of COPD. In Cherniack NS, ed. *Chronic Obstructive Pulmonary Disease.* Philadelphia: WB Saunders, 1991:363–72

39. O'Donnell DE. Assessment of bronchodilator efficacy in symptomatic COPD: is spirometry useful? *Chest* 2000;117(Suppl 2):42–7S

40. Newton MF, O'Donnell DE, Forkert L. Response of lung volumes to inhaled salbutamol in a large population of patients with severe hyperinflation. *Chest* 2002;121:1042–50

41. O'Donnell DE, Lam M, Webb KA. Spirometric correlates of improvement in exercise performance after anticholinergic therapy in chronic obstructive pulmonary disease. *Am J Respir Crit Care Med* 1999;160:542–9

42. Belman MJ, Botnick WC, Shin JW. Inhaled bronchodilators reduce dynamic hyperinflation during exercise in patients with chronic obstructive pulmonary disease. *Am J Respir Crit Care Med* 1996;153:967–75

43. Bates DV. *Respiratory Function in Disease.* Philadelphia: WB Saunders, 1989:172–87

44. Symonds G, Renzetti AD Jr, Mitchell MM. The diffusing capacity in pulmonary emphysema. *Am Rev Respir Dis* 1974;109:391–4

45. Hughes JMB. Diffusing capacity (transfer factor) for carbon monoxide. In Hughes JMB, Pride NB, eds. *Lung Function Tests. Physiology, Principles and Clinical Applications*. London: WB Saunders, 1999:93–106

46. Miller A, Thornton JC, Warshaw R, Anderson H, Teirstein AS, Selikoff IJ. Single breath diffusing capacity in a representative sample of the population of Michigan, a large industrial state. Predicted values, lower limits of normal, and frequencies of abnormality by smoking history. *Am Rev Respir Dis* 1983;127:270–7

47. American Thoracic Society. ATS/ERS Statement on respiratory muscle testing. *Am J Respir Crit Care Med* 2002;166:518–624

48. Clark CJ, Cochrane LM, Mackay E, Paton B. Skeletal muscle strength and endurance in patients with mild COPD and the effects of weight training. *Eur Respir J* 2000;15:92–7

49. Bernard S, LeBlanc P, Whittom F, *et al*. Peripheral muscle weakness in patients with chronic obstructive pulmonary disease. *Am J Respir Crit Care Med* 1998;158:629–34

50. Gea JG, Pasto M, Carmona MA, Orozco-Levi M, Palomeque J, Broquetas J. Metabolic characteristics of the deltoid muscle in patients with chronic obstructive pulmonary disease. *Eur Respir J* 2001;17:939–45

51. Laurell CB, Eriksson S. The electrophoretic alpha 1-globulin pattern of serum in alpha 1-antitrypsin deficiency. *Scand J Clin Lab Invest* 1963;15:132–40

52. Hubbard RC, Crystal RG. Antiproteases. In Crystal RG, West JB, eds. *The Lung*. New York: Raven Press, 1991:1775–87

53. McElvaney NG, Crystal RG. Inherited susceptibility of the lung to proteolytic injury. In Crystal RG, West JB, Barnes PJ, Weibel ER, eds. *The Lung: Scientific Foundations*. Philadelphia: Lippincott-Raven, 1997:2537–53

54. Sandford AJ, Weir TD, Spinelli JJ, Pare PD. Z and S mutations of the alpha1-antitrypsin gene and the risk of chronic obstructive pulmonary disease. *Am J Respir Cell Mol Biol* 1999;20:287–91

55. Tarjan E, Magyar P, Vaczi Z, Lantos A, Vaszar L. Longitudinal lung function study in heterozygous PiMZ phenotype subjects. *Eur Respir J* 1994;7:2199–204

56. Poller W, Meisen C, Olek K. DNA polymorphisms of the alpha 1-antitrypsin gene region in patients with chronic obstructive pulmonary disease. *Eur J Clin Invest* 1990;20:1–7

57. Kalsheker NA, Watkins GL, Hill S, Morgan K, Stockley RA, Fick RB. Independent mutations in the flanking sequence of the alpha-1-antitrypsin gene are associated with chronic obstructive airways disease. *Dis Markers* 1990;8:151–7

58. Samilchuk E, D'Souza B, Voevodin A, Chuchalin A, al Awadi S. TaqI polymorphism in the 3' flanking region of the PI gene among Kuwaiti Arabs and Russians. *Dis Markers* 1997;13:87–92

59. Donahoe M, Rogers RM. Laboratory evaluation of the patient with chronic obstructive pulmonary disease. In Cherniack NS, ed. *Chronic Obstructive Pulmonary Disease*. Philadelphia: WB Saunders, 1991:373–86

60. Wedzicha JA, Cotes PM, Empey DW, *et al*. Serum immunoreactive erythropoietin in hypoxic lung disease with and without polycythemia. *Clin Sci* 1985;69:413–22

61. Smith JR, Landau SA. Smokers' polycythemia. *N Engl J Med* 1978;298:413–22

62. Belman MJ. Exercise in patients with chronic obstructive pulmonary disease. *Thorax* 1993;48:936–46

63. Mulloy E, McNicholas WT. Ventilation and gas exchange during sleep and exercise in severe COPD. *Chest* 1996;109:387–94

64. Kharitonov SA, Barnes PJ. Clinical aspects of exhaled nitric oxide. *Eur Respir J* 2000;16:781–92

65. Kharitonov SA, Barnes PJ. Exhaled markers of pulmonary disease. *Am J Respir Crit Care Med* 2001;163:1693–722

66. Maziak W, Loukides S, Culpitt S, Sullivan P, Kharitonov SA, Barnes PJ. Exhaled nitric oxide in chronic obstructive pulmonary disease. *Am J Respir Crit Care Med* 1998;157:998–1002

67. Papi A, Romagnoli M, Baraldo S, *et al*. Partial reversibility of airflow limitation and increased exhaled NO and sputum eosinophilia in chronic obstructive pulmonary disease. *Am J Respir Crit Care Med* 2000;162:1773–7

68. Carpagnano GE, Kharitonov SA, Foschino-Barbaro MP, Resta O, Gramiccioni E, Barnes PJ. Increased inflammatory markers in the exhaled breath condensate of cigarette smokers. *Eur Respir J* 2003;21:589–93

69. Biernacki WA, Kharitonov SA, Barnes PJ. Increased leukotriene B4 and 8-isoprostane in exhaled breath condensate of patients with exacerbations of COPD. *Thorax* 2003;58:294–8

70. Pin I, Gibson PG, Kolendowicz R, *et al*. Use of induced sputum cell counts to investigate airway inflammation in asthma. *Thorax* 1992;47:25–9

71. Gibson PG, Girgis-Gabardo A, Morris MM, Mattoli S, Kay JM, Dolovich J. Cellular characteristics of sputum from patients with asthma and chronic bronchitis. *Thorax* 1989;44:693–9

72. Keatings VM, Collins PD, Scott DM, Barnes PJ. Differences in interleukin-8 and tumor necrosis factor-alpha in induced sputum from patients with chronic obstructive pulmonary disease or asthma. *Am J Respir Crit Care Med* 1996;153:530–4

73. Vlachos-Mayer H, Leigh R, Sharon RF, Hussack P, Hargreave FE. Success and safety of sputum induction in the clinical setting. *Eur Respir J* 2000;16:997–1000

74. Fahy JV. A safe, simple, standardized method should be used for sputum induction for research purposes. *Clin Exp Allergy* 1998;28:1047–9

75. European Respiratory Society Task Force. Standardised methodology of sputum induction and processing. *Eur Respir J* 2002;20(Suppl 37):1–55s

76. Robinson D. Bronchoalveolar lavage as a tool for studying airway inflammation in asthma. *Eur Respir Rev* 1998;8:1072–4

77. Haslam PL, Baughman RP, eds. Report of European Respiratory Society (ERS) Task Force: Guidelines for measurement of acellular components and recommendations for standardization of bronchoalveolar lavage (BAL). *Eur Respir Rev* 1999;9:25–157

78. Faul JL, Demers EA, Burke CM, Poulter LW. The reproducibility of repeat measures of airway inflammation in stable atopic asthma. *Am J Respir Crit Care Med* 1999;160:1457–61

79. Hattotuwa KL, Gizycki MJ, Ansari TW, Jeffery PK, Barnes NC. The effects of inhaled fluticasone on airway inflammation in chronic obstructive pulmonary disease: a double-blind, placebo-controlled biopsy study. *Am J Respir Crit Care Med* 2002;165:1592–6

80. Muller NL, Coxson H. Chronic obstructive pulmonary disease. 4. Imaging the lungs in patients with chronic obstructive pulmonary disease. *Thorax* 2002;57:982–5

81. O'Brien C, Guest PJ, Hill SL, Stockley RA. Physiological and radiological characterisation of patients diagnosed with chronic obstructive pulmonary disease in primary care. *Thorax* 2000;55:635–42

82. Cosio MG, Snider GL. Chest computed tomography: is it ready for major studies of chronic obstructive pulmonary disease? *Eur Respir J* 2001;17:1062–4

83. Cleverley JR, Muller NL. Advances in radiologic assessment of chronic obstructive pulmonary disease. *Clin Chest Med* 2000;21:653–63

84. Ferretti GR, Bricault I, Coulomb M. Virtual tools for imaging of the thorax. *Eur Respir J* 2001;18:381–92

85. Soejima K, Yamaguchi K, Kohda E, *et al*. Longitudinal follow-up study of smoking-induced lung density changes by high-resolution computed tomography. *Am J Respir Crit Care Med* 2000;161:1264–73

86. Bergin C, Muller N, Nichols DM, *et al*. The diagnosis of emphysema. A computed tomographic-pathologic correlation. *Am Rev Respir Dis* 1986;133:541–6

87. Remy-Jardin M, Edme JL, Boulenguez C, Remy J, Mastora I, Sobaszek A. Longitudinal follow-up study of smoker's lung with thin-section CT in correlation with pulmonary function tests. *Radiology* 2002;222:261–70

88. Remy-Jardin M, Remy J, Gosselin B, Becette V, Edme JL. Lung parenchymal changes secondary to cigarette smoking: pathologic-CT correlations. *Radiology* 1993;186:643–51

89. Nakano Y, Muro S, Sakai H, *et al*. Computed tomographic measurements of airway dimensions and emphysema in smokers. Correlation with lung function. *Am J Respir Crit Care Med* 2000;162:1102–8

90. Coxson HO, Rogers RM, Whittall KP, *et al*. A quantification of the lung surface area in emphysema using computed tomography. *Am J Respir Crit Care Med* 1999;159:851–6

91. Remy-Jardin M, Remy J, Boulenguez C, Sobaszek A, Edme JL, Furon D. Morphologic effects of cigarette smoking on airways and pulmonary parenchyma in healthy adult volunteers: CT evaluation and correlation with pulmonary function tests. *Radiology* 1993;186:107–15

92. Hansell DM. Small airways diseases: detection and insights with computed tomography. *Eur Respir J* 2001;17:1294–313

93. King GG, Muller NL, Pare PD. Evaluation of airways in obstructive pulmonary disease using high-resolution computed tomography. *Am J Respir Crit Care Med* 1999;159:992–1004

94. Dowson LJ, Guest PJ, Stockley RA. Longitudinal changes in physiological, radiological, and health status measurements in alpha(1)-antitrypsin deficiency and factors associated with decline. *Am J Respir Crit Care Med* 2001;164:1805–9

95. Dowson LJ, Guest PJ, Hill SL, Holder RL, Stockley RA. High-resolution computed tomography scanning in alpha1-antitrypsin deficiency: relationship to lung function and health status. *Eur Respir J* 2001;17:1097–104

96. Desai SR, Ryan SM, Colby TV. Smoking-related interstitial lung diseases: histopathological and imaging perspectives. *Clin Radiol* 2003;58:259–68

97. Dirksen A, Friis M, Olesen KP, Skovgaard LT, Sorensen K. Progress of emphysema in severe alpha1-antitrypsin deficiency as assessed by annual CT. *Acta Radiol* 1997;38:826–32

98. Dirksen A, Dijkman JH, Madsen F, et al. A randomized clinical trial of alpha-1-antitrypsin augmentation therapy. *Am J Resp Crit Care Med* 1999;160:1468–72

99. Knudson RJ, Standen JR, Kaltenborn WT, et al. Expiratory computed tomography for assessment of suspected pulmonary emphysema. *Chest* 1991;99:1357–66

100. Dabestani A, Mahan G, Gardin JM, et al. Evaluation of pulmonary artery pressure and resistance by pulsed Doppler echocardiography. *Am J Cardiol* 1987;59:662–8

101. Tramarin R, Torbicki A, Marchandise B, Laaban JP, Morpurgo M. Doppler echocardiographic evaluation of pulmonary artery pressure in chronic obstructive pulmonary disease. A European multicentre study. Working Group on Noninvasive Evaluation of Pulmonary Artery Pressure. European Office of the World Health Organization, Copenhagen. *Eur Heart J* 1991;12:103–11

102. Sajkov D, Cowie RJ, Bradley JA, Mahar L, McEvoy RD. Validation of new pulsed Doppler echocardiographic techniques for assessment of pulmonary hemodynamics. *Chest* 1993;103:1348–53

103. Mittal SR, Jain SC, Sharma SK. The role of electrocardiographic criteria for the diagnosis of right ventricular hypotherapy in chronic obstructive pulmonary disease. *Int J Cardiol* 1986;11:165–73

104. Enright PL, Sherrill DL. Reference equations for the six-minute walk in healthy adults. *Am J Respir Crit Care Med* 1998;158:1384–7

105. American Thoracic Society. ATS statement: Guidelines for the six-minute walk test. *Am J Respir Crit Care Med* 2002;166:111–17

106. Solway S, Brooks D, Lacasse Y, Thomas S. A qualitative systematic overview of the measurement properties of functional walk tests used in the cardiorespiratory domain. *Chest* 2001;119:256–70

107. Singer SJ, Morgan MD, Hardman AE. Comparison of oxygen uptake during a conventional treadmill test and the shuttle walking test in chronic airflow limitation. *Eur Respir J* 1994;7:2016–20

108. Revill SM, Morgan MD, Singh SJ, Williams J, Hardman AE. The endurance shuttle walk: a new field test for the assessment of endurance capacity in chronic obstructive pulmonary disease. *Thorax* 1999;54:213–22

109. Singh SJ, Morgan MD, Scott S, Walters D, Hardman AE. Development of a shuttle walking test of disability in patients with chronic airways obstruction. *Thorax* 1992;47:1019–24

110. Dyer CA, Singh SJ, Stockley RA, Sinclair AJ, Hill SL. The incremental shuttle walking test in elderly people with chronic airflow limitation. *Thorax* 2002;57:34–8

111. Jones PW. Quality of life, symptoms and pulmonary function in asthma: long-term treatment with nedocromil sodium examined in a controlled multicentre trial. *Eur Resp J* 1994;7:55–62

112. Spencer S, Calverley PM, Sherwood BP, Jones PW. Health status deterioration in patients with chronic obstructive pulmonary disease. *Am J Respir Crit Care Med* 2001;163:122–8

113. Jones PW, Mahler DA. Key outcomes in COPD: health-related quality of life. Proceedings of an expert round table held July 20–22, 2001, Boston, Massachusetts, USA. *Eur Respir Rev* 2002;12

114. Jones PW, Quirk FH, Baveystock CM. The St George's Respiratory Questionnaire. *Respir Med* 1991;85(Suppl B):25–31

115. Jones PW. Health status measurement in chronic obstructive pulmonary disease. *Thorax* 2001;56:880–7

116. Rutten-van Molken MP, Roos B, van Noord JA. An empirical comparison of the St George's respiratory questionnaire (SGRQ) and the chronic respiratory disease questionnaire (CRQ) in a clinical trial setting. *Thorax* 1999;54:995–1003

117. Engstrom CP, Persson LO, Larsson S, Sullivan M. Health-related quality of life in COPD: why both disease-specific and generic measures should be used. *Eur Respir J* 2001;18:69–76

118. Brown LK. Sleep-related disorders and chronic obsructive pulmonary disease. *Respir Care Clin N Am* 1998;4:493–512

119. Weitzenblum E, Chaout A, Charpentier C, et al. Sleep-related hypoxaemia in chronic obstructive pulmonary disease: causes, consequences and treatment. *Respiration* 1997;64:187–93

120. Connaughton JJ, Catterall JR, Elton RA, Stradling JR, Douglas NJ. Do sleep studies contribute to the management of patients with severe chronic obstructive pulmonary disease? *Am Rev Respir Dis* 1988;138:341–4

121. Fletcher EC, Luckett RA, Goodnight-White S, Miller CC, Qian W, Costarangos-Galarza C. A double-blind trial of nocturnal supplemental oxygen for sleep desaturation in patients with chronic obstructive pulmonary disease and a daytime PaO2 above 60 mmHg. *Am Rev Respir Dis* 1992;145:1070–6

122. Wouters EF. Chronic obstructive pulmonary disease: systemic effects of COPD. Thorax 2002;57:1067–70

123. Agusti AGN, Noguera A, Sauleda J, Sala E, Pons J, Busquets X. Systemic effects of chronic obstructive pulmonary disease. *Eur Respir J* 2003;21:347–60

124. Schols AM. Pulmonary cachexia. *Int J Cardiol* 2002;85:101–10

125. Schols AM, slangen J, Volovics L, Wouters EF. Weight loss is a reversible factor in the prognosis of chronic obstructive pulmonary disease. *Am J Respir Crit Care Med* 1998;157:1791–7

126. Engelen MP, Schols AM, Heidendal GA, Wouters EF. Dual-energy X-ray absorptiometry in the clinical evaluation of body composition and bone mineral density in patients with chronic obstructive pulmonary disease. *Am J Clin Nutr* 1998;68:1298–303

127. Schols AM, Wouters EF, Soeters PB, Westerterp KR. Body composition by bioelectrical-impedance analysis compared with deuterium dilution and skinfold anthropometry in patients with chronic obstructive pulmonary disease. *Am J Clin Nutr* 1991;53:421–4

128. Levine S, Kaiser L, Leferovich J, Tikunov B. Cellular adaptations in the diaphragm in chronic obstructive pulmonary disease. *N Engl J Med* 1997;337:1799–806

129. Polkey MI, Kyroussis D, Hamnegard CH, Mills GH, Green M, Moxham J. Diaphragm strength in chronic obstructive pulmonary disease. *Am J Respir Crit Care Med* 1996;154:1310–17

130. Reid MB. COPD as a muscle disease. *Am J Respir Crit Care Med* 2001;164:1101–2

131. Gosselink R, Troosters T, Decramer M. Peripheral muscle weakness contributes to exercise limitation in COPD. *Am J Respir Crit Care Med* 1996;153:976–80

132. American Thoracic Society/European Respiratory Society. Skeletal muscle dysfunction in chronic obstructive pulmonary disease. *Am J Respir Crit Care Med* 1999;159 (part 2):S1–40

133. Marquis K, Debigare R, Lacasse Y, *et al.* Midthigh muscle cross-sectional area is a better predictor of mortality than body mass index in patients with chronic obstructive pulmonary disease. *Am J Respir Crit Care Med* 2002;166:809–13

134. Whittom F, Jobin J, Simard P-M, *et al.* Histochemical and morphological characteristics of the vastus laterallis muscle in COPD patients. *Med Sci Sports Exerc* 1998;30:1467–74

135. Scanlon PD, Connett JE, Waller LA, *et al.* Smoking cessation and lung function in mild-to-moderate chronic obstructive pulmonary disease. The Lung Health study. *Am J Respir Crit Care Med* 2000;161:381–90

136. Pauwels RA, Lofdahl CG, Laitinen LA, *et al.* Long-term treatment with inhaled budesonide in persons with mild chronic obstructive pulmonary disease who continue smoking. European Respiratory Society Study on Chronic Obstructive Pulmonary Disease. *N Engl J Med* 1999;340:1948–53

137. Vestbo J, Sorensen T, Lange P, Brix A, Torre P, Viskum K. Long-term effect of inhaled budesonide in mild and moderate chronic obstructive pulmonary disease: a randomised controlled trial. *Lancet* 1999;353:1819–23

138. Burge PS, Calverley PM, Jones PW, Spencer S, Anderson JA, Maslen TK. Randomised, double blind, placebo controlled study of fluticasone propionate in patients with moderate to severe chronic obstructive pulmonary disease: the ISOLDE trial. *Br Med J* 2000;320:1297–303

139. Lung Health Study Research Group. Effect of inhaled triamcinolone on the decline in pulmonary function in chronic obstructive pulmonary disease. *N Engl J Med* 2000;343:1902–9

140. Fletcher C, Peto R. The natural history of chronic airflow obstruction. *Br Med J* 1977;1:1645–8

141. Doll R, Peto R, Wheatley K, Gray R, Sutherland I. Mortality in relation to smoking: 40 years' observations on male British doctors. *Br Med J* 1994;309:901–11

142. Anthonisen NR, Connett JE, Kiley JP, *et al.* Effects of smoking intervention and the use of an inhaled anticholinergic bronchodilator on the rate of decline of FEV1. The Lung Health Study. *J Am Med Assoc* 1994;272:1497–505

143. Wilkinson TM, Patel IS, Wilks M, Donaldson GC, Wedzicha JA. Airway bacterial load and FEV1 decline in patients with chronic obstructive pulmonary disease. *Am J Respir Crit Care Med* 2003;167:1090–5

144. Burrows B, Knudson RJ, Camilli AE, Lyle SK, Lebowitz MD. The 'horse-racing effect' and predicting decline in forced expiratory volume in one second from screening spirometry. *Am Rev Respir Dis* 1987;135:788–93

145. US Department of Health and Human Services. The health consequences of smoking. Chronic obstructive lung disease. *Report of the Surgeon General* 1984;1–541

146. Camilli AE, Burrows B, Knudson RJ, Lyle SK, Lebowitz MD. Longitudinal changes in forced expiratory volume in one second in adults. Effects of smoking and smoking cessation. *Am Rev Respir Dis* 1987;135:794–9

147. Anthonisen NR. Prognosis in chronic obstructive pulmonary disease: results from multicenter clinical trials. *Am Rev Respir Dis* 1989;140:S95–9

148. Medical Research Council Working Party. Long term domiciliary oxygen therapy in chronic bronchitis and emphysema. Report of the Medical Research Council Working Party. *Lancet* 1981;1:681–6

149. Nocturna Oxygen Therapy Trial Group. Continuous or nocturnal oxygen therapy in hypoxemic chronic obstructive lung disease: a clinical trial. *Ann Intern Med* 1980;93:391–8

150. Cooper CB, Waterhouse J, Howard P. Twelve year clinical study of patients with hypoxic cor pulmonale given long term domiciliary oxygen therapy. *Thorax* 1987;42:105–10

151. Antonelli Inc, Fuso L, De Rosa M, *et al*. Co-morbidity contributes to predict mortality of patients with chronic obstructive pulmonary disease. *Eur Respir J* 1997;10:2794–800

152. Incalzi RA, Fuso L, De Rosa M, *et al*. Electrocardiographic signs of chronic cor pulmonale: a negative prognostic finding in chronic obstructive pulmonary disease. *Circulation* 1999;99:1600–5

153. Traver GA, Cline MG, Burrows B. Predictors of mortality in chronic obstructive pulmonary disease. A 15-year follow-up study. *Am Rev Respir Dis* 1979;119:895–902

154. Kanner RE, Renzetti AD, Stanish WM. Predictions of survival in subjects with chronic airflow limitation. *Am J Med* 1983;174:249–55

155. Kanner R, Renzetti AD. Predictions of spirometic changes and mortality in the obstructive airways disorders. *Chest* 1984;85:15–17s

156. Gore JM, Brophy CJ, Greenstone MA. How well do we care for patients with end stage chronic obstructive pulmonary disease (COPD)? A comparison of palliative care and quality of life in COPD and lung cancer. *Thorax* 2000;55:1000–6

157. Claessens MT, Lynn J, Zhong Z, *et al*. Dying with lung cancer or chronic obstructive pulmonary disease: insights from SUPPORT. Study to Understand Prognoses and Preferences for Outcomes and Risks of Treatments. *J Am Geriatr Soc* 2000;48(Suppl 5):S146–53

158. Truog RD, Cist AF, Brackett SE, *et al*. Recommendations for end-of-life care in the intensive care unit: The Ethics Committee of the Society of Critical Care Medicine. *Crit Care Med* 2001;29:2332–48

159. Curtis JR, Rubenfeld GD, eds. *Managing Death in the Intensive Care Unit*. Oxford: Oxford University Press, 2001

4

Smoking cessation

CONTENTS

SUMMARY

Smoking cessation is the single most beneficial management step for patients with COPD, and the only intervention that reduces the accelerated decline in lung function. It is necessary to reduce personal exposure to cigarette smoke, occupational dusts and chemicals, and indoor and outdoor air pollutants.

Tobacco control policies are required at international, national and local levels to reduce smoking in public forums, to reduce cigarette advertising, and to give strong non-smoking messages. The WHO recognizes the importance of preventing smoking as well as smoking cessation within the Tobacco Free Initiative (TFI) in the recently released *Draft Framework Convention on Tobacco Control* (FCTC) (3rd March, 2003).

Even brief counselling has some effect in enabling smoking cessation. All health-care professionals should *ask* their patients about cigarette smoking at every opportunity, and *advise* all smokers to quit, then *assess* their willingness to quit, *assist* them to give up, and *arrange* follow-up contact.

Nicotine addiction is the major problem, and treatment should be directed at dealing with this addictive state. Nicotine replacement may be given as gum, sublingual tablet or lozenge, by nasal spray, by transdermal patch and by inhalation. Caution must be taken in patients with cardiovascular disease.

Bupropion slow-release facilitates smoking cessation when given with counselling and nicotine replacement, as has been shown to be effective in smokers with COPD. Care must be taken since bupropion has a propensity to cause seizures.

The majority of patients have several attempts at giving up, so smoking cessation may need to be repeatedly attempted. Abrupt quitting is more successful than gradual reduction, but, even after an intensive smoking cessation program, the majority of patients are still smoking 1 year later.

PUBLIC HEALTH MEASURES

The WHO Draft Framework Convention on Tobacco Control (FCTC) is a new legal instrument to address issues such as tobacco advertising and promotion, agricultural diversification, smuggling, taxes and subsidies[1].

Comprehensive tobacco control policies and programs with clear, consistent and repeated non-smoking messages should be delivered through every feasible channel. This should involve health-care providers, national and international health organizations, schools, radio, TV, internet and print media.

Legislation and agreement are required to restrict tobacco advertising via TV, cinema, print, and sporting events. Warnings on cigarette packs should be larger and include photographs of smoking-related pathology.

National and local campaigns should be undertaken to reduce exposure to tobacco smoke in public forums. Legislation to establish smoke-free hospitals, schools, universities, restaurants, transport, public facilities and work environments should be encouraged by government officials and public health workers. Smoke-free homes should be encouraged.

Smoking prevention and cessation programs should target all ages, including young children, females and males, adolescents, young adults, and pregnant women. The US Public Health Service clinical practice guideline *Treating Tobacco Use and Dependence* gives important recommendations for the organization and implementation of smoking cessation measures (Figure 4.1). Furthermore, the guideline recommends a five-step program to help health professionals enable their patients to stop

---

Figure 4.1   US Public Health Service Guideline on Treating Tobacco Use and Dependence

Major findings and recommendations

1. Tobacco dependence is a chronic condition that warrants repeated treatment until long-term or permanent abstinence is achieved.

2. Effective treatments for tobacco dependence exist and all tobacco users should be offered these treatments.

3. Clinicians and health-care delivery systems must institutionalize the consistent identification, documentation and treatment of every tobacco user at every visit.

4. Brief tobacco dependence treatment is effective and every tobacco user should be offered at least brief treatment.

5. There is a strong dose–response relationship between the intensity of tobacco dependence counselling and its effectiveness.

6. Three types of counselling were found to be especially effective: practical counselling, social support as part of treatment, and social support arranged outside of treatment.

7. Five first-line pharmacotherapies for tobacco dependence – bupropion slow-release (SR), nicotine gum, nicotine inhaler, nicotine nasal spray and nicotine patch – are effective and at least one of these medications should be prescribed in the absence of contraindications.

8. Tobacco dependence treatments are cost-effective relative to other medical and disease prevention interventions.

US Public Health Service Report.
Treating Tobacco Use and Dependence: A Clinical Practice Guideline.
J Am Med Assoc 2000;283:3244–54

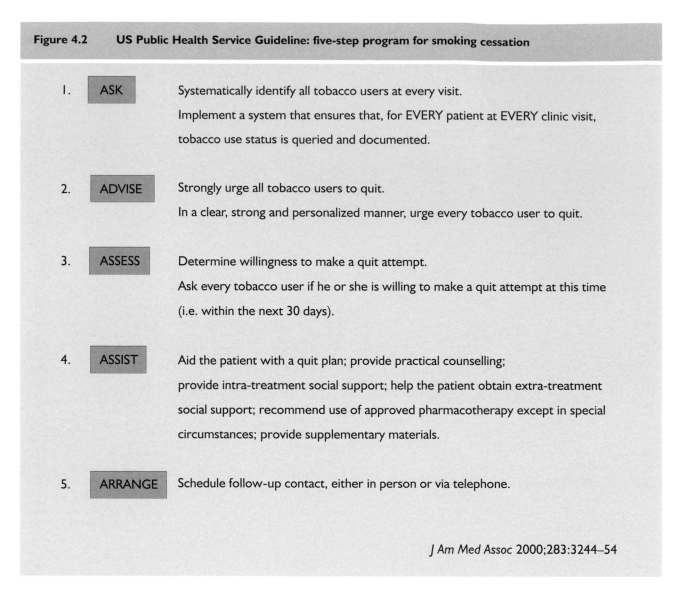

Figure 4.2   US Public Health Service Guideline: five-step program for smoking cessation

1. **ASK**   Systematically identify all tobacco users at every visit.

    Implement a system that ensures that, for EVERY patient at EVERY clinic visit,

    tobacco use status is queried and documented.

2. **ADVISE**   Strongly urge all tobacco users to quit.

    In a clear, strong and personalized manner, urge every tobacco user to quit.

3. **ASSESS**   Determine willingness to make a quit attempt.

    Ask every tobacco user if he or she is willing to make a quit attempt at this time

    (i.e. within the next 30 days).

4. **ASSIST**   Aid the patient with a quit plan; provide practical counselling;

    provide intra-treatment social support; help the patient obtain extra-treatment

    social support; recommend use of approved pharmacotherapy except in special

    circumstances; provide supplementary materials.

5. **ARRANGE**   Schedule follow-up contact, either in person or via telephone.

J Am Med Assoc 2000;283:3244–54

smoking[2]. This involves the steps Ask, Advise, Assess, Assist and Arrange (Figure 4. 2).

Important documents on smoking cessation in the UK have been the Health Education Authority (HEA) Smoking Cessation Guidelines[3–5] and the government Tobacco White Paper[6]. There are a number of helpful meta-analyses and reviews on pharmacotherapy, mainly nicotine replacement and bupropion slow-release to assist in smoking cessation[7–15].

COUNSELLING

Counselling delivered by physicians and other health professionals significantly increases rates of quitting over self-initiated strategies[16–18]. Even a brief (3-minute) period of counselling to urge a smoker to

quit results in smoking cessation rates of 5–10%[19]. At the very least, this should be carried out for every smoker at every visit to a health professional[4].

However, there is a strong dose–response relationship between counselling intensity and cessation success[20,21]. Ways to make the treatment more intense include increasing the length of the treatment session, the number of treatment sessions, and the number of weeks over which the treatment is delivered. With more complex interventions (for example, controlled clinical trials that include skills training, problem solving, and psychosocial support), quit rates can reach 20–30%[20]. In one multicenter, controlled clinical trial, a combination of physician advice, group support, skills training, and nicotine replacement therapy achieved a quit rate of 35% at 1 year and 22% at 5 years[22]. Both individual and

Figure 4.3   Advice to patients on how to stop smoking

1. DATE:
   Set a realistic quit date and time and stick to it

2. THERAPY:
   Understand the potential benefits of
   • Smoking cessation classes and counselling
   • Bupropion
   • Nicotine replacement therapy

3. SUPPORT:
   • Obtain the help of local professionals
   • Assess the books, internet sites, videos, and educational materials available
   • Assess natural remedies, acupuncture, hypnosis and other methods available

4. USEFUL ACTIONS:
   Dispose of all unused cigarettes, ashtrays, matches and lighters from home, work, coats and bags
   Wash and dry clean your clothes to get rid of the smell of smoke
   Tell your friends, family and work colleagues that you are stopping smoking
   Ask people not to smoke around you
   Visit the dentist for teeth cleaning and oral hygiene
   Know the health hazards of smoking
   Change your lifestyle and routine: new activities, hobbies and sports
   Eat healthily and exercise
   Understand the costs of smoking
   Plan a series of rewards with the money you save
   Avoid difficult situations such as after alcohol
   When you want a cigarette, don't have 'just one' cigarette
   Have a strategy worked out for when you are tempted

group counselling are effective formats for smoking cessation. However, in patients hospitalized with COPD, a randomized trial found active intense counselling of little benefit[23]. Self-care methods are not as effective as formal intervention methods[24]. Nursing interventions with advice and counselling have been shown in a meta-analysis to be effective[18].

Education is important since it provides basic information about the addictive nature of smoking and the risks of continuing. Describe the benefits and methods of quitting, and the techniques that optimize success. Outline the nature, time course and symptoms of withdrawal, and techniques for dealing with withdrawal. Explain that any return to smoking, including even a single puff, increases the likelihood of a relapse. For the individual patient who faces the often daunting task of giving up smoking, recommendations on advice are given in Figure 4.3, with useful information available on the internet given in Figure 4.4.

Support and encourage the patient in the quit attempt. Indicate that effective cessation treatments are now available and, in fact, half of all people who smoked have now quit. Communicate your confidence in the patient's ability to quit. Communicate care and concern. Ask how the patient feels about smoking and whether they want to quit, expressing concern along with the ability and willingness to help. Be open to the patient's fears of quitting. Encourage the patient to talk about the quitting process. Talk to the patient about the reasons why they want to quit, the difficulty encountered while quitting, the success the patient has achieved, and their concerns and worries about quitting. In the

Figure 4.4   Selected internet information on smoking cessation

Tobacco websites

World Health Organization (WHO) Tobacco Free Initiative (TFI)   http://www5.who.int/tobacco

American Lung Association (ALA)   http://www.lungusa.org/tobacco

Journal of American Medical Association (JAMA)
    Publishes useful patient pages on smoking cessation   http://www.ama-assn.org/public/
    journals/patient/index.htm

Smoking cessation websites

USA

Action on Smoking and Health (ASH) USA   http://www.ash.org/

The Arizona Smokers' Helpline   http://www.ashline.org/

The QuitNet   http://www.quitnet.com/
    The original quit smoking site from Boston University

Europe and UK

Stop-tabac.ch Smoking Cessation Program   http://www.stop-tabac.ch/
    University of Geneva multi-lingual website

NHS Smoking Helpline   http://www.givingupsmoking.co.uk
    UK Department of Health's website

Action on Smoking and Health (ASH) UK   http://www.ash.org.uk/
    Useful factsheets for smoking cessation

quitsmokinguk.com   http://www.quitsmoking.com
    Online community for quitting smokers

context of a smoking cessation clinic, social support interventions may be of benefit[25].

Psychology stages for patients going through the process of smoking cessation are given in Figure 4.5. Most individuals go through several psychology stages before they commit to and carry out smoking cessation. It is helpful for the health professional to assess a patient's readiness to quit in order to decide appropriate action. If the patient is not ready to quit, the health professional should provide brief intervention to promote motivation to quit. Alternatively, if the patient is ready to quit, then smoking cessation support should be arranged.

Behavior therapy involves recognition of danger signals likely to be associated with the risk of relapse[26]; these include being around other smokers, being under time pressure, getting into an argument, drinking alcohol, and negative moods. In addition, therapy can be given to enhance the skills needed to handle these situations, such as learning to anticipate and avoid a particular stress. Aversive therapy using such techniques as rapid smoking have not been demonstrated to be effective[27]. However, group therapy is clearly more effective than no or minimal intervention or self-help[28].

Telephone counselling appears to be effective when used alone or when augmenting smoking

Figure 4.5   Smoking cessation: psychology stages

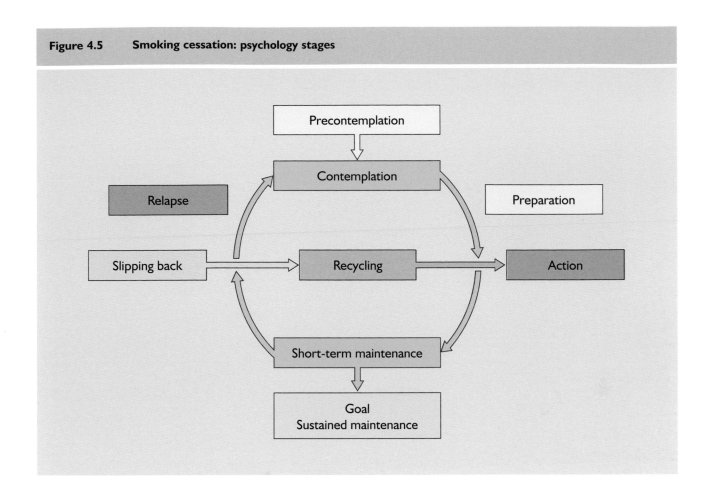

cessation programs[29,30]. Self-administered methods of smoking cessation have the potential to reach a large population of cigarette smokers, through use of manuals that encourage self-administered behavioral treatments and self-administered nicotine therapy[24,31].

Hypnosis and acupuncture may be helpful in some patients, but a meta-analysis of controlled trials did not find hypnotherapy to be effective[8,32], and there has been failure to convincingly demonstrate the efficacy of acupuncture[33,34]. A review of randomized controlled trials on the effects of exercise on smoking cessation found a positive effect in only one of eight studies, and recommends further trials with larger sample sizes[35,36].

NICOTINE REPLACEMENT PRODUCTS

Nicotine addiction

Nicotine is the chief naturally occurring plant alkaloid found in tobacco leaves (see structure in Figure 4.6). Nicotine has stimulatory activity at the autonomic ganglia of the parasympathetic and sympathetic systems, on nicotinic cholinergic receptors at the neuromuscular junctions with skeletal muscle, and on central nervous system (CNS) receptors. It is believed that binding to CNS nicotine receptors causes release of dopamine, endorphins and catecholamines, which give the sensation of well-being and decrease anxiety. The majority of cigarette smokers develop a degree of nicotine addiction.

Forms of nicotine replacement

Every effort should be made to tailor the choice of nicotine replacement therapy to the individual's culture and lifestyle in order to improve adherence[37–39]. In particular, the level of nicotine dependence can be assessed in the patient using the Fagerström Tolerance Questionnaire[40]. Treatment with nicotine replacement is generally employed for between 6 and 12 weeks (3 months), with a gradual withdrawal during this period. If abstinence has not been achieved within 12 weeks, then treatment should be reviewed. Nicotine is readily absorbed through skin and mucous membranes, and Figure 4.6 demonstrates a range of nicotine replacement products. Nicotine products are generally available over the counter (OTC)[7].

Nicotine skin (transdermal) patches

These comprise a highly effective nicotine product[41–47]. The patch is generally favored over the gum because it requires less training for effective use,

---

Figure 4.6   Nicotine replacement products

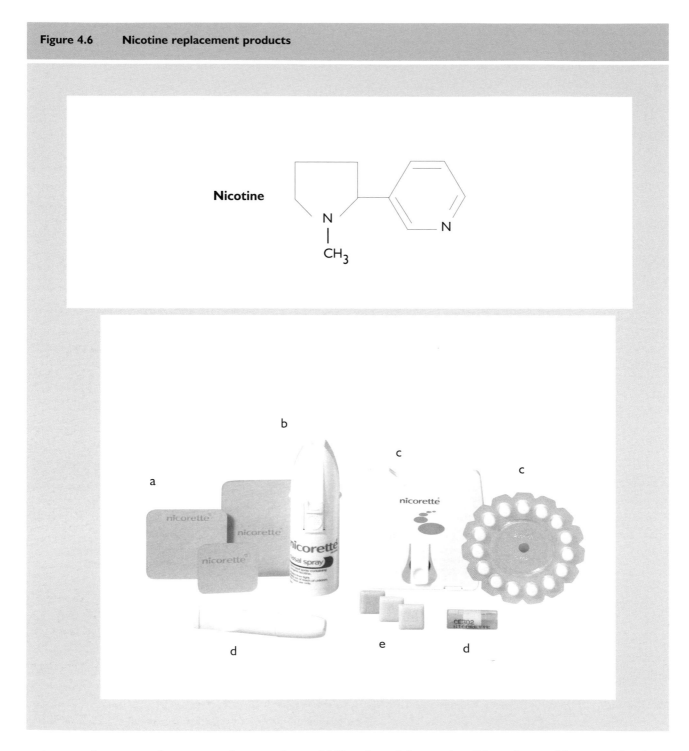

A range of nicotine replacement products are shown. (a) Transdermal skin patches; (b) nasal spray; (c) microtablets for sublingual use; (d) inhalator with a cartridge containing nicotine; (e) chewing gum. Photographs by courtesy of Pharmacia.

ensures up to 16 hours of nicotine replacement after a single application, and is associated with fewer compliance problems. However, skin patches cannot give nicotine rapidly in order to meet a strong craving.

Patches are self-adhesive and flesh-colored and should be applied on waking to dry, non-hairy skin on the hip, upper arm or trunk. Removal is performed within 16 hours, generally before going to bed, since night-time nicotine may cause sleep disturbance[9]. Nicotine skin patches can cause skin irritation and need to be rotated to different locations. They should not be placed on broken or diseased skin. Each day, patches should be placed on a different skin area, avoiding using the same area for 7 days, in order to minimize skin irritation.

Patches are available ranging in content from 5, 10 to 15 mg or, alternatively, 7, 14 to 21 mg of nicotine. The 21-mg patch is reckoned to give as much nicotine as ten cigarettes a day. Clinicians should attempt to tailor nicotine patch dosage regimens to the intensity of cigarette smoking and degree of nicotine dependence. Patients should use the highest-dose skin patch for the first 4 weeks, and drop to progressively lower doses over an 8-week period. Where only two doses are available, the higher dose should be used for the first 4 weeks and the lower dose for the second 4 weeks.

Nicotine inhalators

The inhalators simulate the intake of nicotine from a cigarette[48–50]. Cartridges impregnated in nicotine are available that contain 10 mg nicotine and deliver 4 mg per use. They are placed in the plastic inhaler (inhalator) which resembles a cigarette holder. The patient draws on the inhalator and nicotine passes into the mouth and oropharynx. Shallow puffing or deep inhalations are equally effective. Initially, six to 12 cartridges should be employed daily for up to 8 weeks, with a gradual reduction over the next 4 weeks. The use of an inhalator provides oral and visual gratification, but less nicotine than from other systems, so they may be more useful in the smoker with low-level nicotine dependence.

Nasal nicotine spray

The spray gives a more rapid rise in plasma nicotine concentrations than with the gum or patch[51–57]. The nasal spray may be very effective in former heavy smokers when a patient has sudden cravings to smoke, although local irritation can be a problem for some patients. The patient should expect local irritant effects during the first few days, but these should pass. Nasal sprays can be used at up to two sprays per nostril per hour. Nicotine nasal spray can cause sneezing and watering eyes and so should not be used when driving or operating machinery.

Nicotine chewing gum

Gum is the most widely used nicotine product, and is especially useful for control of cravings. Side-effects have been reported in over 3000 users[58,59]. Nicotine gum users tend to return to the nicotine levels they were at before stopping smoking[60]. Sugar-free original, mint and fruit flavors are available at 2 mg and 4 mg, and contain a resin complex of nicotine polacrilex in a gum base. Individuals smoking more than 20 cigarettes a day may require the 4 mg gum, especially if they are highly nicotine-dependent smokers. Gum should be withdrawn gradually within 3 months. Eight to 12 pieces of gum many be used a day.

Each piece of gum should be chewed slowly in spells over about 30 minutes when the urge to smoke occurs. The patient needs to be advised that absorption occurs through the oral mucosa. For this reason, the patient should chew the gum slowly until it is malleable and the taste becomes strong. The gum should then be 'parked' against the inside of the cheek. When the taste fades, the patient should chew the gum again, and repeat this cycle over 20–30 minutes. This allows prolonged absorption of about half of the nicotine from the gum, and in a faster manner than from skin patches.

Continuous chewing produces secretions that are swallowed, but there is little nicotine absorption from the stomach, and nausea with gastric irritation may result. Acidic beverages, particularly coffee, juices and soft drinks, interfere with the absorption of nicotine. Thus the patient needs to avoid eating or drinking anything except water for 15 minutes before and during chewing.

The taste of nicotine gum can be unpleasant at first, although for most patients this only lasts a few days. For some elderly patients, compliance with gum may be poor due to social inacceptability. Finally, the gum can be tough to chew and cause jaw ache due to temporomandibular joint problems. It is possible that weight gain from smoking cessation can be decreased by use of nicotine gum[61].

Nicotine microtablets

Microtablets (as a cyclodextrin complex) should be placed under the tongue (sublingual), but not chewed or swallowed[62–65]. The tablets should be allowed to dissolve under the tongue, and not swallowed, sucked or chewed. Two mg are taken every hour in subjects who smoke 20 cigarettes or less daily, while individuals who smoke over 40 cigarettes a day can take 4 mg hourly, to a maximum of 80 mg daily.

Figure 4.7   Nicotine replacement products: cautions, contraindications and side-effects

Cautions and contraindications

- Severe cardiovascular disease: cardiac arrhythmias
  immediately post-myocardial infarction (MI)
  recent cerebrovascular accident (CVA)
  recent transient ischemic attack (TIA)
  peripheral vascular disease
- Hyperthyroidism and diabetes mellitus
- Untreated gastritis and peptic ulcer
- Pregnancy and breast feeding
- Renal and hepatic impairment
- Pheochromocytoma

Systemic side-effects

- Nausea and vomiting, dyspepsia, hiccups, gastrointestinal disturbances
- Dizziness and headache, insomnia, vivid dreams, anxiety, irritability, somnolence
- Influenza-like symptoms
- Palpitations, chest pain, blood pressure changes

Local side-effects

- Tablets and chewing gums: unpleasant taste, swollen tongue, throat irritation, aphthous ulceration

- Skin patches: local skin reactions, vasculitis
  Patches should not be placed on broken or damaged skin

- Inhalers: dry mouth, stomatitis, throat irritation, sinusitis, cough

- Nasal sprays: sneezing, nasal irritation, nose bleeds, watering eyes, ear sensations
  Avoid administering nasal sprays when driving or operating machinery

Nicotine lozenges

The lozenges are available in a mint flavor at 1 mg, and may be taken every 1–2 hours, with a maximum of 25 lozenges daily.

Efficacy

Nicotine replacement therapy is more effective when combined with counselling and behavior therapy, although nicotine patch or gum consistently increases smoking cessation rates, regardless of the level of additional behavioral or psychosocial interventions[2,7–9]. Numerous studies indicate that nicotine replacement therapy in any form reliably increases long-term smoking abstinence rates, when compared with placebo. Nicotine replacement therapy doubles long-term (6–12 month) abstinence rates[5]. Subjects taking nicotine replacement products should have stopped smoking.

Cautions

It is important to carefully assess the cautions and contraindications, as well as systemic and local side-effects of nicotine replacement therapy (Figure 4.7).

BUPROPION

Bupropion slow-release (SR) (amfebutamone) should be used as an adjunct to counselling and nicotine replacement therapy (Figures 4.8 and 4.9). Bupropion is an atypical antidepressant that helps smoking cessation[66–68]. Its mechanism of action may involve inhibition of dopamine reuptake on the mesolimbic dopaminergic system rather than its antidepressant effect.

There are three published pivotal trials:

- Bupropion SR was given at 100 mg, 150 mg or 300 mg per day for 7 weeks of treatment. At 1 year, rates of smoking cessation on bupropion were 19.6%, 22.9% and 23.1%, respectively, while the placebo treatment caused cessation in 12.4%[69].

- Bupropion SR given as a course, building up to 150 mg twice daily for 9 weeks with nicotine patches, caused smoking cessation rates at 12 months of 35.5%, compared with placebo at 15.6%[70].

Figure 4.8   Bupropion: indication, chemistry and dosage regimen

Indication

Adjunct to smoking cessation in combination with nicotine products and motivational support

Chemistry

Bupropion hydrochloride slow-release (SR) tablets, 150 mg

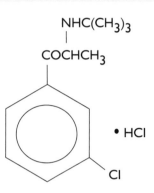

Dose

- Initiate treatment while patient is still smoking, initially 150 mg daily (1 tablet) for 6 days

- Increase to 150 mg twice daily on the 7th day, doses at least 8 h apart

  steady-state levels of bupropion achieved by second week

  ideally set target date to stop smoking in second week

- Discontinue if abstinence not achieved by 7 weeks

  maximum period of treatment 7–12 weeks

Figure 4.9   **Bupropion: contraindications, cautions and side-effects**

Contraindications

- Current seizure disorder or any history of seizure
- Hypersensitivity to bupropion
- Current treatment with Wellbutrin SR for depression – contains bupropion
- Bulimia/anorexia nervosa – high incidence of seizures
- Severe hepatic cirrhosis
- Bipolar disorder
- Concomitant administration of monoamine oxidase inhibitors (MAOIs)
- Known central nervous system tumor
- Abrupt withdrawal from alcohol or benzodiazepines

Seizures

Bupropion is associated with a dose-related risk of seizures;
these occur in approximately 1 in 1000 patients.

In patients at increased risk of seizures, bupropion should only be used after carefully assessing the potential risk–benefit, and a maximum dose of 150 mg daily should be used.

Patients at increased risk of seizures

- Concomitant medications known to lower seizure threshold
  antipsychotics, antidepressants, theophylline, systemic steroids, antimalarials, tramadol, quinolones, sedating antihistamines
- Alcohol abuse
- History of head trauma
- Diabetes treated with hypoglycemics or insulin
- Addiction to opiates, cocaine or stimulants
- Use of stimulants or anorectic products

Side-effects

- Dry mouth, nausea and vomiting, constipation
- Insomnia, dizziness, tremor, concentration disturbances
- Rash, urticaria, pruritus, sweating, flushing
- Taste disorder, tinnitus
- Tachycardia, hypertension, postural hypotension
- Seizures

Figure 4.10   The Lung Health Study (LHS)

1. Smoking cessation reduces rate of decline of FEV_1

    Anthonisen NR, *et al. J Am Med Assoc* 1994;272:1497–501

2. Multiple attempts to quit smoking, with relapses intervening, cause a lower rate of decline of FEV_1 than continuous smoking

    Murray RP, *et al. J Clin Epidemiol* 1998;51:317–26

3. Smoking cessation causes fewer respiratory symptoms

    Kanner RE, *et al. Am J Med* 1999;106:410–16

4. Continuous smokers with early COPD have a rate of decline in FEV_1 of about 60 ml/year.

    Smoking cessation causes half the rate of decline in FEV_1, to about 30 ml/year.

    This is a comparable rate of decline of FEV_1 to that in never-smokers

    Scanlon PD, *et al. Am J Respir Crit Care Med* 2000;161:381–90

5. Characteristics of subjects who quit smoking: no longer using nicotine gum at 1 year, few previous quit attempts, older subjects

    Murray RP, *et al. Preventive Med* 2000;30:392–400

6. Regular inhaled corticosteroid (triamcinolone 600 mg twice daily) for a mean of 40 months does not alter the rate of decline in FEV_1

    The Lung Health Study Research Group. *N Engl J Med* 2000;343:1902–9

7. Long-term follow-up after 11 years: 38% of continuing smokers had an FEV_1 of < 60%, compared with 10% of sustained quitters

    Anthonisen NR, *et al. Am J Respir Crit Care Med* 2002;166:675–9

8. Smoking cessation causes reduced cardiovascular and coronary artery disease

    Anthonisen NR, *et al. Am J Respir Crit Care Med* 2002;166:333–9

9. IL-13 and IL-4R polymorphisms are not associated with the rate of decline of FEV_1

    He JQ, *et al. Am J Respir Cell Mol Biol* 2003;28:379–85

10. Weight gain is a consequence of smoking cessation, and can be reduced with nicotine gum

    Nides M, *et al. Health Psychol* 1994;13:354–61
    O'Hara P, *et al. Am J Epidemiol* 1998;148:831–2

- Bupropion SR caused smoking abstinence rates of 16% compared with placebo rates of 9% at 26 weeks in 404 patients with mild to moderate COPD[71].

Bupropion is generally well tolerated apart from dry mouth and sleeplessness, but epileptic fits occur in approximately one in 1000 patients, predominantly those with previous epilepsy[13,72]. Patients at increased risk of seizures should only be treated with bupropion after carefully assessing the potential risk–benefit, and giving a maximum daily dose of 150 mg (Figure 4.10). For this reason, current recommendations are to initiate treatment with 150 mg of daily bupropion for 6 days, before increasing to 150 mg twice daily on the 7th day (Figure 4.8). Special consideration should be given when considering pharmacotherapy for people with medical contraindications, light smokers (fewer than ten cigarettes a day), and pregnant and adolescent smokers.

MISCELLANEOUS PHARMACOTHERAPY

- Clonidine is an α_2-adrenergic agonist with some efficacy, but side-effects (especially sedation) are common, so it is not recommended[8,73].

- The antidepressant, nortriptyline, has been shown to be beneficial in smoking cessation[68].

- Opioid antagonists such as naloxone and naltrexone have been studied as adjuncts for smoking cessation, but limited data from two trials with naltrexone are equivocal[74].

- There is no clear evidence that anxiolytics aid smoking cessation[75].

THE LUNG HEALTH STUDY

The Lung Health Study was a randomized, multicenter trial carried out from October 1986 to April 1994 to test the effectiveness of smoking cessation in early COPD. A total of 5887 patients with early COPD (FEV$_1$ of 55–90% predicted) were recruited from 14 centers in the USA and Canada. Figure 4.10 summarizes some of the key published findings[61,76–88]. A critical observation is that smoking cessation slows the rate of decline of FEV$_1$ in COPD (Figure 4.11)[76,79,89].

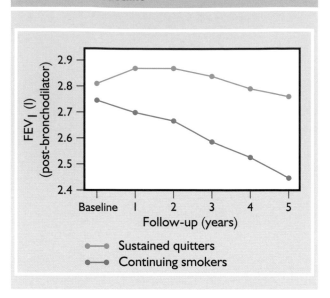

Figure 4.11   Smoking cessation effect on FEV$_1$ decline

Mean post-bronchodilator forced expiratory volume in 1 second (FEV$_1$) for participants in the smoking intervention and placebo group who were sustained quitters and continuous smokers. The two curves diverge sharply after baseline. Anthonisen NR, *et al. J Am Med Assoc* 1994;272:1497–505.

EFFECTS OF SMOKING CESSATION ON THE RESPIRATORY SYSTEM

The Lung Health Study documents that smoking cessation has beneficial effects on lung function over an 11-year period[76,77,79,82] and this is associated with decreased respiratory symptoms[78] and significant reductions in fatal and non-fatal cardiovascular and coronary artery disease[83]. A Finnish study has also documented beneficial effects of stopping smoking on lung function and mortality[90]. Smoking cessation reduces bronchoalveolar lavage total cell numbers within 1 month, while transient increases in albumin and hyaluronan occur[91], but alveolar macrophage fluorescence remains high up to 15 months after cessation[92]. Within 2 months of smoking cessation, there are decreased numbers of neutrophils and alveolar macrophages on bronchoscopy and bronchoalveolar lavage[93]. However, a more recent study has demonstrated ongoing inflammation in bronchoalveolar lavage and sputum in COPD patients who do not smoke, with increased mucosal eosinophils and sputum neutrophils[94].

OTHER RISK FACTORS FOR COPD

Occupational exposures

The emphasis should be on primary prevention, although secondary prevention through surveillance and early case detection is also important. Most occupationally induced respiratory disorders can be reduced through strategies aimed at reducing the burden of inhaled particles and gases:

- Strict control of airborne exposure in the workplace.

- Education of exposed workers, industrial managers, health-care professional and legislatures.

- Education on how cigarette smoking aggravates occupational lung disorders.

Indoor and outdoor air pollution

The concept of total personal exposure to contaminants may be more important than looking at separate components.

- Legislation on air quality is important at a national level.

- Patients at high risk should avoid vigorous exercise and going outside when air pollution is high.

- Adequate ventilation is required if solid fuels are used for cooking and heating.

- Respiratory protective equipment may be important in the workplace.

REFERENCES

1. Draft WHO framework convention on tobacco control. World Health Organisation, March 3, 2003. http://www5.who.int/tobacco.index.cfm

2. Tobacco Use and Dependence Clinical Practice Guideline Panel. A clinical practice guideline for treating tobacco use and dependence. *J Am Med Assoc* 2000;283:3244–54

3. Raw M, McNeill A, West R. Smoking cessation guidelines and their cost effectiveness. *Thorax* 1998;53(Suppl 5):S1–38

4. Britton J, Knox A. Helping people to stop smoking: the new smoking cessation guidelines [editorial]. *Thorax* 1999;54:1–2

5. West R, McNeill A, Raw M. Smoking cessation guidelines for health professionals: an update. Health Education Authority. *Thorax* 2000;55:987–99

6. *Smoking Kills – A White Paper*. London: The Stationery Office, 1998

7. Hughes JR, Goldstein MG, Hurt RD, Shiffman S. Recent advances in the pharmacotherapy of smoking. *J Am Med Assoc* 1999;281:72–6

8. Lancaster T, Stead L, Silagy C, Sowden A. Effectiveness of interventions to help people stop smoking: findings from the Cochrane Library. *Br Med J* 2000;321:355–8

9. Silagy C, Lancaster T, Stead L, Mant D, Fowler G. Nicotine replacement therapy for smoking cessation. *Cochrane Database Syst Rev* 2002:CD000146

10. Fagerstrom K. What is new with tobacco dependence? *Respiration* 2002;69:5–6

11. Silagy C, Mant D, Fowler G, Lodge M. Meta-analysis on efficacy of nicotine replacement therapies in smoking cessation. *Lancet* 1994;343:139–42

12. Henningfield JE. Nicotine medications for smoking cessation. *N Engl J Med* 1995;333:1196–203

13. Hays JT, Ebbert JO. Bupropion for the treatment of tobacco dependence: guidelines for balancing risks and benefits. *CNS Drugs* 2003;17:71–83

14. DeGraff AC Jr. Pharmacologic therapy for nicotine addiction. *Chest* 2002;122:392–4

15. Hilton A. Stopping smoking: the importance of nicotine addiction. *Thorax* 2000;55:256–7

16. Baillie AJ, Mattick RP, Hall W, Webster P. Meta-analytic review of the efficacy of smoking cessation interventions. *Drug Alcohol Rev* 1994;13:157–70

17. Silagy C, Stead LF. Physician advice for smoking cessation. *Cochrane Database Syst Rev* 2001: CD000165

18. Rice VH, Stead LF. Nursing interventions for smoking cessation. *Cochrane Database Syst Rev* 2000:CD001188

19. Wilson DH, Wakefield MA, Steven ID, Rohrsheim RA, Esterman AJ, Graham NM. 'Sick of Smoking': evaluation of a targeted minimal smoking cessation intervention in general practice. *Med J Aust* 1990;152:518–21

20. Kottke TE, Battista RN, DeFriese GH, Brekke ML. Attributes of successful smoking cessation interventions in medical practice. A meta-analysis of 39 controlled trials. *J Am Med Assoc* 1988;259:2883–9

21. Ockene JK, Kristeller J, Goldberg R, Amick TL, Pekow PS, Hosmer D, et al. Increasing the efficacy of physician-delivered smoking interventions: a randomized clinical trial. J Gen Intern Med 1991;6:1–8

22. Shimizu T. The future potential of eicosanoids and their inhibitors in paediatric practice. Drugs 1998;56:169–76

23. Pederson LL, Wanklin JM, Lefcoe NM. The effects of counseling on smoking cessation among patients hospitalized with chronic obstructive pulmonary disease: a randomized clinical trial. Int J Addict 1991;26:107–19

24. Viswesvaran C, Schmidt FL. A meta-analytic comparison of the effectiveness of smoking cessation methods. J Appl Psychol 1992;77:554–61

25. May S, West R. Do social support interventions ('buddy systems') aid smoking cessation? A review. Tob Control 2000;9:415–22

26. Irvin JE, Bowers CA, Dunn ME, Wang MC. Efficacy of relapse prevention: a meta-analytic review. J Consult Clin Psychol 1999;67:563–70

27. Hajek P, Stead LF. Aversive smoking for smoking cessation. Cochrane Database Syst Rev 2000: CD000546

28. Stead LF, Lancaster T. Group behaviour therapy programmes for smoking cessation. Cochrane Database Syst Rev 2000:CD001007

29. Lichtenstein E, Glasgow RE, Lando HA, Ossip-Klein DJ, Boles SM. Telephone counseling for smoking cessation: rationales and meta-analytic review of evidence. Health Educ Res 1996;11:243–57

30. Stead LF, Lancaster T, Perera R. Telephone counselling for smoking cessation (Cochrane Review). Cochrane Database Syst Rev 2003:CD002850

31. Curry SJ, Ludman EJ, McClure J. Self-administered treatment for smoking cessation. J Clin Psychol 2003;59:305–19

32. Abbot NC, Stead LF, White AR, Barnes J, Ernst E. Hypnotherapy for smoking cessation. Cochrane Database Syst Rev 2000:CD001008

33. White AR, Resch KL, Ernst E. A meta-analysis of acupuncture techniques for smoking cessation. Tob Control 1999;8:393–7

34. White AR, Rampes H, Ernst E. Acupuncture for smoking cessation. Cochrane Database Syst Rev 2002:CD000009

35. Ussher MH, Taylor AH, West R, McEwen A. Does exercise aid smoking cessation? A systematic review. Addiction 2000;95:199–208

36. Ussher MH, West R, Taylor AH, McEwen A. Exercise interventions for smoking cessation. Cochrane Database Syst Rev 2000:CD002295

37. Balfour D, Benowitz N, Fagerstrom K, Kunze M, Keil U. Diagnosis and treatment of nicotine dependence with emphasis on nicotine replacement therapy. A status report. Eur Heart J 2000;21:438–45

38. Jimenez-Ruiz C, Kunze M, Fagerstrom KO. Nicotine replacement: a new approach to reducing tobacco-related harm. Eur Respir J 1998;11:473–9

39. Tonnesen P, Mikkelsen KL. Smoking cessation with four nicotine replacement regimes in a lung clinic. Eur Respir J 2000;16:717–22

40. Heatherton TF, Kozlowski LT, Frecker RC, Fagerstrom KO. The Fagerstrom Test for Nicotine Dependence: a revision of the Fagerstrom Tolerance Questionnaire. Br J Addict 1991;86:1119–27

41. Tonnesen P, Norregaard J, Simonsen K, Sawe U. A double-blind trial of a 16-hour transdermal nicotine patch in smoking cessation. N Engl J Med 1991;325:311–15

42. Stapleton JA. Dose effects and predictors of outcome in a randomised trial of nicotine patches in general practice. Addiction 1995;106:421–7

43. Fagerstrom KO, Sachs DP. Medical management of tobacco dependence: a crtical review of nicotine skin patches. Current Pulmonol 1995;16:223–38

44. Sachs DP, Sawe U, Leischow SJ. Effectiveness of a 16-hour transdermal nicotine patch in a medical practice setting, without intensive group counseling. Arch Intern Med 1993;153:1881–90

45. Tonnesen P, Paoletti P, Gustavsson G, Russell MA, Saracci R, Gulsvik A, et al. Higher dosage nicotine patches increase one-year smoking cessation rates: results from the European CEASE trial. Eur Respir J 1999;13:238–46

46. Fiore MC, Smith SS, Jorenby DE, Baker TB. The effectiveness of the nicotine patch for smoking cessation. A meta-analysis. J Am Med Assoc 1994;271:1940–7

47. Fiscella K, Franks P. Cost-effectiveness of the transdermal nicotine patch as an adjunct to physicians' smoking cessation counseling. J Am Med Assoc 1996;275:1247–51

48. Tonnesen P, Norregaard J, Mikkelsen K, Jorgensen S, Nilsson F. A double-blind trial of a nicotine inhaler

for smoking cessation. *J Am Med Assoc* 1993;269:1268–71

49. Schneider NG, Olmstead R, Nilsson F, Mody FV, Franzon M, Doan K. Efficacy of a nicotine inhaler in smoking cessation: a double-blind, placebo-controlled trial. *Addiction* 1996;91:1293–306

50. Bolliger CT, Zellweger JP, Danielsson T, van B, X, Robidou A, Westin A, et al. Smoking reduction with oral nicotine inhalers: double blind, randomised clinical trial of efficacy and safety. *Br Med J* 2000;321:329–33

51. Russell MA. Nasal nicotine solution: a potential aid to giving up smoking? *Br Med J* 1983;286:683–4

52. Schneider NG, Lunell E, Olmstead RE, Fagerstrom KO. Clinical pharmacokinetics of nasal nicotine delivery. A review and comparison to other nicotine systems. *Clin Pharmacokinet* 1996;31:65–80

53. Johansson CJ, Olsson P, Bende M, Carlsson T, Gunnarsson PO. Absolute bioavailability of nicotine applied to different nasal regions. *Eur J Clin Pharmacol* 1991;41:585–8

54. Sutherland G, Stapleton JA, Russell MA, Jarvis MJ, Hajek P, Belcher M, et al. Randomised controlled trial of nasal nicotine spray in smoking cessation. *Lancet* 1992;340:324–9

55. Hjalmarson A, Franzon M, Westin A, Wiklund O. Effect of nicotine nasal spray on smoking cessation. A randomized, placebo-controlled, double-blind study. *Arch Intern Med* 1994;154:2567–72

56. Schneider NG, Olmstead R, Mody FV, Doan K, Franzon M, Jarvik ME, et al. Efficacy of a nicotine nasal spray in smoking cessation: a placebo-controlled, double-blind trial. *Addiction* 1995;90:1671–82

57. Blondal T, Gudmundsson LJ, Olafsdottir I, Gustavsson G, Westin A. Nicotine nasal spray with nicotine patch for smoking cessation: randomised trial with six year follow up. *Br Med J* 1999;318:285–8

58. Murray RP, Bailey WC, Daniels K, Bjornson WM, Kurnow K, Connett JE, et al. Safety of nicotine polacrilex gum used by 3,094 participants in the Lung Health Study. Lung Health Study Research Group. *Chest* 1996;109:438–45

59. Herrera N, Franco R, Herrera L, Partidas A, Rolando R, Fagerstrom KO. Nicotine gum, 2 and 4 mg, for nicotine dependence. A double-blind placebo-controlled trial within a behavior modification support program. *Chest* 1995;108:447–51

60. Murray RP, Nides MA, Istvan JA, Daniels K. Levels of cotinine associated with long-term ad-libitum nicotine polacrilex use in a clinical trial. *Addict Behav* 1998;23:529–35

61. Nides M, Rand C, Dolce J, Murray R, O'Hara P, Voelker H, et al. Weight gain as a function of smoking cessation and 2-mg nicotine gum use among middle-aged smokers with mild lung impairment in the first 2 years of the Lung Health Study. *Health Psychol* 1994;13:354–61

62. Molander L, Lunell E, Fagerstrom KO. Reduction of tobacco withdrawal symptoms with a sublingual nicotine tablet: a placebo controlled study. *Nicotine Tob Res* 2000;2:187–91

63. Molander L, Lunell E, Fagerstrom KO. Reduction of tobacco withdrawal symptoms with a sublingual nicotine tablet: a placebo-controlled study. *Nicotine Tob Res* 2000;2:187–91

64. Wallstrom M, Nilsson F, Hirsch JM. A randomized, double-blind, placebo-controlled clinical evaluation of a nicotine sublingual tablet in smoking cessation. *Addiction* 2000;95:1161–71

65. Fagerstrom KO, Tejding R, Westin A, Lunell E. Aiding reduction of smoking with nicotine replacement medications: hope for the recalcitrant smoker? *Tob Control* 1997;6:311–16

66. Haustein KO. Bupropion: pharmacological and clinical profile in smoking cessation. *Int J Clin Pharmacol Ther* 2003;41:56–66

67. Huibers MJ, Chavannes NH, Wagena EJ, van Schayck CP. Antidepressants for smoking cessation: a promising new approach? *Eur Respir J* 2000;16:379–80

68. Hughes JR, Stead LF, Lancaster T. Antidepressants for smoking cessation. *Cochrane Database Syst Rev* 2002:CD000031

69. Hurt RD, Sachs DP, Glover ED, Offord KP, Johnston JA, Dale LC, et al. A comparison of sustained-release bupropion and placebo for smoking cessation. *N Engl J Med* 1997;337:1195–202

70. Jorenby DE, Leischow SJ, Nides MA, Rennard SI, Johnston JA, Hughes AR, et al. A controlled trial of sustained-release bupropion, a nicotine patch, or both for smoking cessation. *N Engl J Med* 1999;340:685–91

71. Tashkin D, Kanner R, Bailey W, Buist S, Anderson P, Nides M, et al. Smoking cessation in patients with chronic obstructive pulmonary disease: a double-blind, placebo-controlled, randomised trial. *Lancet* 2001;357:1571–5

72. Holm KJ, Spencer CM. Bupropion: a review of its use in the management of smoking cessation. *Drugs* 2000;59:1007–24

73. Gourlay SG, Stead LF, Benowitz NL. Clonidine for smoking cessation. *Cochrane Database Syst Rev* 2000:CD000058

74. David S, Lancaster T, Stead LF. Opioid antagonists for smoking cessation. *Cochrane Database Syst Rev* 2001:CD003086

75. Hughes JR, Stead LF, Lancaster T. Anxiolytics for smoking cessation. *Cochrane Database Syst Rev* 2000:CD002849

76. Anthonisen NR, Connett JE, Kiley JP, Altose MD, Bailey WC, Buist AS, et al. Effects of smoking intervention and the use of an inhaled anticholinergic bronchodilator on the rate of decline of FEV_1. The Lung Health Study. *J Am Med Assoc* 1994;272:1497–505

77. Murray RP, Anthonisen NR, Connett JE, Wise RA, Lindgren PG, Greene PG, et al. Effects of multiple attempts to quit smoking and relapses to smoking on pulmonary function. Lung Health Study Research Group. *J Clin Epidemiol* 1998;51:1317–26

78. Kanner RE, Connett JE, Williams DE, Buist AS. Effects of randomized assignment to a smoking cessation intervention and changes in smoking habits on respiratory symptoms in smokers with early chronic obstructive pulmonary disease: the Lung Health Study. *Am J Med* 1999;106:410–6

79. Scanlon PD, Connett JE, Waller LA, Altose MD, Bailey WC, Sonia BA, et al. Smoking cessation and lung function in mild-to-moderate chronic obstructive pulmonary disease. The Lung Health Study. *Am J Respir Crit Care Med* 2000;161:381–90

80. Lung Health Study Research Group. Effect of inhaled triamcinolone on the decline in pulmonary function in chronic obstructive pulmonary disease. *N Engl J Med* 2000;343:1902–9

81. Ferguson AC, Whitelaw M, Brown H. Correlation of bronchial eosinophil and mast cell activation with bronchial hyperresponsiveness in children with asthma. *J Allergy Clin Immunol* 1992;90:609–13

82. Anthonisen NR, Connett JE, Murray RP. Smoking and lung function of Lung Health Study participants after 11 years. *Am J Respir Crit Care Med* 2002;166:675–9

83. Anthonisen NR, Connett JE, Enright PL, Manfreda J. Hospitalizations and mortality in the Lung Health Study. *Am J Respir Crit Care Med* 2002;166:333–9

84. He JQ, Connett JE, Anthonisen NR, Sandford AJ. Polymorphisms in the IL13, IL13RA1, and IL4RA genes and rate of decline in lung function in smokers. *Am J Respir Cell Mol Biol* 2003;28:379–85

85. O'Hara P, Connett JE, Lee WW, Nides M, Murray R, Wise R. Early and late weight gain following smoking cessation in the Lung Health Study. *Am J Epidemiol* 1998;148:821–30

86. Murray RP, Connett JE, Rand CS, Pan W, Anthonisen NR. Persistence of the effect of the Lung Health Study (LHS) smoking intervention over eleven years. *Prev Med* 2002;35:314–19

87. Murray RP, Istvan JA, Daniels K, Beaudoin CM. Alcohol and morbidity in the Lung Health Study. *J Stud Alcohol* 1998;59:250–7

88. Murray RP, Istvan JA, Voelker HT. Does cessation of smoking cause a change in alcohol consumption? Evidence from the Lung Health Study. *Subst Use Misuse* 1996;31:141–56

89. Pride NB. Smoking cessation: effects on symptoms, spirometry and future trends in COPD. *Thorax* 2001;56(Suppl 2):7–10

90. Pelkonen M, Notkola IL, Tukiainen H, Tervahauta M, Tuomilehto J, Nissinen A. Smoking cessation, decline in pulmonary function and total mortality: a 30 year follow up study among the Finnish cohorts of the Seven Countries Study. *Thorax* 2001;56:703–7

91. Skold CM, Blaschke E, Eklund A. Transient increases in albumin and hyaluronan in bronchoalveolar lavage fluid after quitting smoking: possible signs of reparative mechanisms. *Respir Med* 1996;90:523–9

92. Skold CM, Hed J, Eklund A. Smoking cessation rapidly reduces cell recovery in bronchoalveolar lavage fluid, while alveolar macrophage fluorescence remains high. *Chest* 1992;101:989–95

93. Rennard SI, Daughton D, Fujita J, Oehlerking MB, Dobson JR, Stahl MG, et al. Short-term smoking reduction is associated with reduction in measures of lower respiratory tract inflammation in heavy smokers. *Eur Respir J* 1990;3:752–9

94. Rutgers SR, Postma DS, ten Hacken NH, Kauffman HF, Der Mark TW, Ter GH, et al. Ongoing airway inflammation in patients with COPD who do not currently smoke. *Thorax* 2000;55:12–18

5

Drug therapy for stable COPD

CONTENTS

SUMMARY: GOLD PROPOSALS (2003) FOR COPD DRUG THERAPY (Figure 5.1)

- The Global Initiative for Chronic Obstructive Lung Disease (GOLD) strategy proposes a stepwise approach to pharmacological management of chronic COPD[1,2]; the incremental steps in treatment correspond to stages of increasing severity of COPD, as defined by symptoms and signs together with spirometry evaluation. Since COPD is usually progressive, the 'step-down' approach used in treatment of asthma is not usually applicable in COPD. The responses to treatment of individual patients are variable, and all patients with COPD should be monitored regularly with time.

- For COPD patients at GOLD Stages I–IV, it is appropriate to give inhaled short-acting anticholinergics (ipratropium bromide and oxitropium bromide) and/or short-acting β_2-agonists (salbutamol (Europe)/albuterol (US) and terbutaline) on an 'as required' basis for the relief of symptoms.

- At GOLD Stages II–IV, regular therapy with long-acting bronchodilators should be given, rather than with short-acting β_2-agonists. The once-daily anticholinergic, tiotropium bromide, or the long-acting β_2-agonists (LABAs) are modern convenient choices for regular therapy. Tiotropium bromide is inhaled once daily, while the LABAs salmeterol and formoterol are inhaled twice daily. Combining bronchodilators may improve efficacy for some patients, and this may cause less risk of side-effects than by increasing the dose of a single bronchodilator. Bronchodilators may have relatively small effects on FEV_1 compared to benefit in terms of symptoms and health-related quality of life.

- Theophylline slow-release (SR) may be used in refractory cases as both a bronchodilator and an anti-inflammatory. Theophylline is a reserve therapy because it has a narrow therapeutic ratio, and monitoring of serum theophylline levels is generally required.

- GOLD (2003) recommends regular treatment with inhaled corticosteroids for symptomatic patients with a postbronchodilator $FEV_1 < 50\%$ predicted and repeated exacerbations (e.g. three exacerbations in the past 3 years). Patients with a postbronchodilator FEV_1 of $< 50\%$ predicted have severe (stage III) or very severe (stage IV) COPD. However, regular treatment with inhaled corticosteroids does not modify the long-term decline of FEV_1 (natural history) of patients with COPD. An increased incidence of skin bruising and decreased bone density have been reported with higher doses of inhaled corticosteroids in COPD.

- Systemic steroids and antibiotics are only indicated as short courses to treat certain types of more severe exacerbations.

- Combined inhaled corticosteroids and LABAs within a single inhaler (Seretide®: salmeterol with fluticasone propionate; Symbicort®: formoterol with budesonide) have been shown to be more effective than the individual components, in terms of improved lung function and decreased exacerbations.

Figure 5.1   GOLD recommendations on therapy for patients with COPD of varying stages of severity

Stage (2003 update)	0 At risk	I Mild	II Moderate	III Severe	IV Very severe
Pre-bronchodilator FEV$_1$ (% predicted)	Normal	>80%	50–80%	30–50%	<30%

- Avoidance of risk factors **SMOKING CESSATION**
- Influenza vaccination

Short-acting bronchodilator if needed

- Add regular treatment with one or more long-acting bronchodilators, including tiotropium
- Pulmonary rehabilitation

Add regular treatment with inhaled corticosteroids if repeated exacerbations

- Long-term oxygen therapy (LTOT) if respiratory failure
- Consider surgical options

Based on GOLD global strategy (2003)
For clinical definitions of stages, refer to Figures 1.3 and 3.15

Figure 5.2 **Overview of COPD management**

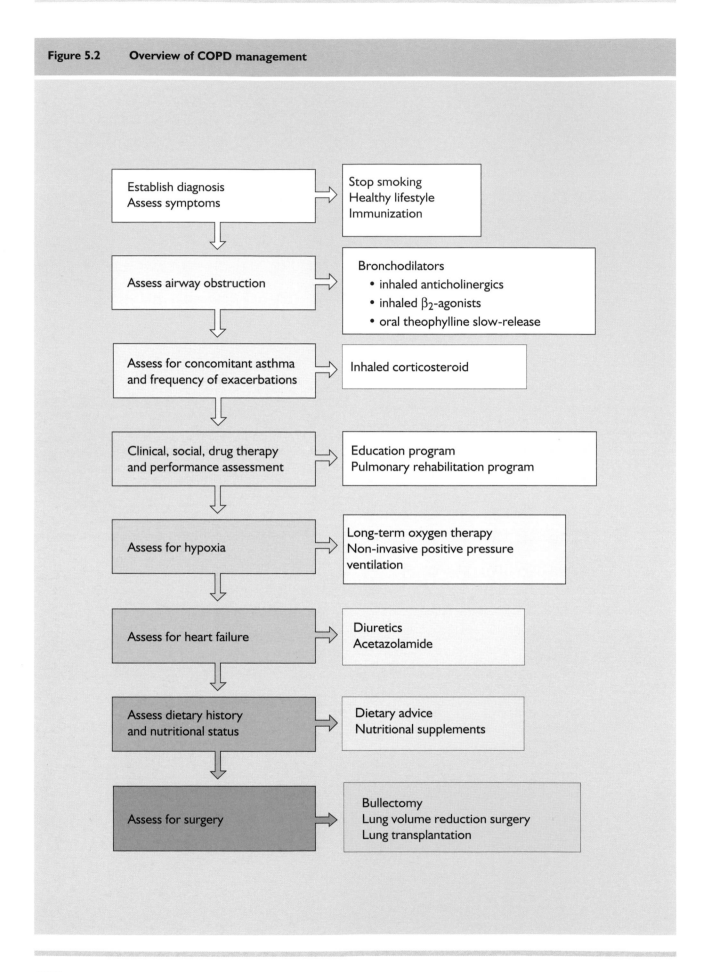

OVERVIEW OF COPD MANAGEMENT
(Figure 5.2)

Smoking cessation (Chapter 4), the adoption of a healthy lifestyle (limiting inhaled risk factors, adequate diet, regular exercise, and limited alcohol consumption), and annual vaccination against influenza are mandatory for all patients with COPD.

Pharmacotherapy is one element of care within a program that frequently involves a multi-disciplinary team of health-care professionals on a long-term basis. Bronchodilators are the mainstay of drug therapy for chronic COPD, and the most common agents used are inhaled anticholinergics and/or β2-agonists. Inhaled corticosteroids may be prescribed in severe COPD for patients with frequent exacerbations.

Health education, dietary advice and exercise training programs benefit patients with COPD, and are best used as components within a comprehensive pulmonary rehabilitation program (Chapter 6).

It is important to treat common complications of COPD such as respiratory failure, *cor pulmonale*, muscle wasting and cachexia. Oxygen therapy increases survival in patients with severe COPD and respiratory failure (Chapter 7), while diuretics may be needed to treat *cor pulmonale*. There are specific indications for surgical interventions such as bullectomy, lung volume reduction surgery, and lung transplantation (Chapter 7).

The COPD escalator

Instead of presenting the GOLD guidelines as steps, the principal therapeutic actions can be considered as an escalator, as proposed originally in the British Thoracic Society guidelines (Figure 5.3)[3]. Worsening

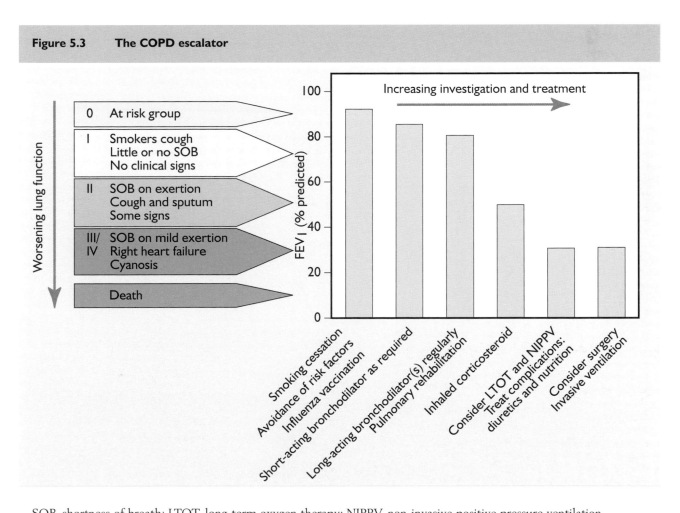

Figure 5.3   The COPD escalator

SOB, shortness of breath; LTOT, long-term oxygen therapy; NIPPV, non-invasive positive pressure ventilation
Adapted from the British Thoracic Society (BTS) Guidelines for the management of COPD (1997) in the light of the Global Initiative for Chronic Obstructive Lung Disease, GOLD (2001 and 2003 update).

lung function and increased levels of symptoms require progressive escalation of more investigation and treatment. If the patient with established COPD continues smoking, then the prognosis is generally poor, and COPD is a common cause of mortality (Chapters 1 and 7).

Principles of bronchodilator therapy

Spirometry

Appropriate therapy for a COPD patient depends upon diagnosis and assessment of the severity of disease in the individual patient. Stage II COPD patients have a post-bronchodilator FEV_1 of 50–80% predicted, confirming that airflow limitation is not fully reversible. COPD patients generally have fixed non-reversible airways obstruction. Bronchodilator reversibility is present if the FEV_1 improves by > 200 ml and > 12% from the pre-bronchodilator value.

The mainstay of COPD therapy

It is a paradox that COPD is defined primarily by the presence of fixed irreversible airways obstruction – yet bronchodilators are the mainstay of therapy. Although bronchodilators may only cause a modest improvement in FEV_1, they may cause considerable improvement in symptoms, in exercise response and health-related quality of life.

Close monitoring

The clinical severity and response to treatment of an individual patient change and therapy should be monitored closely. Each treatment regimen needs to be patient-specific and take account of the frequency and severity of exacerbations as well as the presence of complications of COPD. The choice between short-acting and long-acting β_2-agonists, anticholinergic, theophylline or combination therapy depends on individual responses, ability to use inhalers and side-effects.

Stage I COPD

The GOLD strategy states that short-acting β_2-agonists and short-acting anticholinergics taken by inhalation are generally equipotent, but some studies suggest that anticholinergics are more likely to be effective in a given clinical setting[4,5].

Stages II–IV COPD

In long-term studies in chronic COPD, regular long-acting β_2-agonists have been shown to be more convenient and effective than short-acting bronchodilators. The updated GOLD guidelines of 2003 recommend tiotropium bromide alongside long-acting β_2-agonists as first-line maintenance therapy for COPD patients at stages II–IV.

Types of bronchodilators (Figure 5.4)

- *The short-acting β_2-agonists*, salbutamol and terbutaline, are generally used as additional treatments when required for symptom control.

- *The short-acting anticholinergics*, ipratropium bromide and oxitropium bromide, need to be inhaled up to 4 times per day.

- *The long-acting anticholinergic*, tiotropium bromide, is a once-daily inhaled agent that has unique kinetic selectivity for M_1 and M_3 muscarinic receptors[6,7].

- *The combined bronchodilator*, Combivent®, contains a short-acting β_2-agonist (salbutamol) with a short-acting anticholinergic (ipratropium bromide) in a single inhaler.

- *The long-acting inhaled β_2-agonists*, salmeterol and formoterol, are long-acting inhaled bronchodilators and are useful bronchodilators for regular treatment. They may be combined with a corticosteroid (salmeterol/fluticasone and formoterol/budesonide).

- *The combination of long-acting β_2-agonists with tiotropium bromide* is potentially useful, as demonstrated in recent clinical trials[8,9].

- *Oral β_2-agonists and theophylline* are occasionally useful as reserve therapies. Monitoring of serum therapeutic levels is mandatory for methylxanthines due to their variable metabolism and tendency for adverse events (low toxic therapeutic dose ratio). The long-acting oral β_2-agonist bambuterol may also be useful in some patients.

Figure 5.4   Commonly used bronchodilator drugs

Drug	Inhaler (μg)	Nebulizer (mg)	Oral (mg)	Duration of action (hours)
Anticholinergics				
Ipratropium bromide	20, 40 (MDI)	0.25, 0.5	–	6–8
Oxitropium bromide	100 (MDI)	–	–	7–9
Tiotropium bromide	18 (DPI)	–	–	24+
β$_2$-agonists				
Salbutamol (albuterol)	100, 200 (MDI/DPI)	2.5, 5.0	4	4–6
Terbutaline	250, 500 (DPI)	5, 10	5	4–6
Formoterol	12, 24 (MDI/DPI)	–	–	12+
Salmeterol	50, 100 (MDI/DPI)	–	–	12+
Methylxanthines*				
Aminophylline slow-release (SR)	–	–	200, 600	variable, up to 24
Theophylline (SR)	–	–	100, 600	variable, up to 24

MDI, metered dose inhaler, DPI, dry power inhaler.
*Methylxanthines require careful dose titration with monitoring of plasma levels and side-effects.

Types of inhalers

Inhaled therapy for patients with COPD is generally preferred, although attention to effective drug delivery and training in inhaler technique is essential.

The major type of inhaler used in COPD for many years has been the pressurized metered dose inhaler (Figure 5.5). These generally contain a drug substance in the presence of a propellant within an aluminum canister, which is released as an aerosol via a valve stem through an atomizing nozzle, with flash evaporation of rapidly moving propellant droplets. Under the terms of the Montreal Protocol on Substances that Deplete the Ozone Layer, chlorofluorocarbon (CFC) propellants have been replaced largely by the non-CFC propellant hydrofluoroalkane-134A (HFA). Whereas drugs were generally in suspension in CFC propellants, drugs may be in solution in HFA formulations[10]. With smaller particle size, more of the drug is delivered to the central and peripheral airways, as opposed to the oropharynx. Pressurized metered dose inhalers have the major drawback of needing coordinated actuation with inspiration (hand–breath coordination), and this may be difficult for frail and elderly patients with COPD. All patients should be carefully

| Figure 5.5 | Pressurized metered dose inhaler (pMDI) (top), with spacer (bottom) |

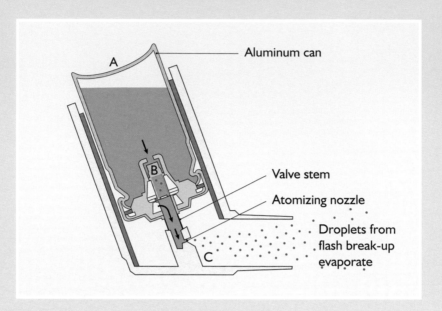

The pMDI consists or a canister reservoir (A), which contains the medication mixed under pressure with a propellant.

Hydrofluoroalkanes (HFAs) have now replaced chlorofluorocarbons (CFCs).

The mixture is released into a metering chamber (B) and expelled through a valve and then via a mouthpiece (C) as a fine spray.

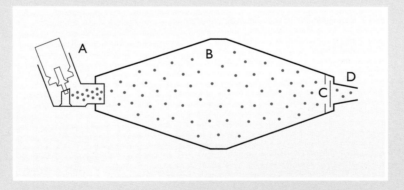

The drug is discharged from the pMDI (A) into the large-volume plastic spacer (B), and inhaled by the patient through a one-way inspiratory valve (C) via a mouthpiece (D).

educated and checked in inhaler technique supplied by the manufacturer; there is commonly the need to shake the inhaler before use and to hold breath for up to 10 seconds after inhaling to total lung capacity. Some patients may actuate the pressurized metered dose inhalers in the mouth while breathing in through the nose. There can be airway reactions to the propellants used.

To improve the effectiveness of pressurized metered dose inhalers in patients with poor inhalation technique, it is recommended that they are actuated into large-volume plastic spacer or reservoir devices. Spacers provide a space between the inhaler and mouth, reducing the velocity of the aerosol and subsequent impaction on the oropharynx and allowing more time for evaporation of the propellant.

Breath-activated multi-dose dry-powder inhalers (Figure 5.6) have been developed. Turbohaler® (AstraZeneca) is one of the first of these devices and has been employed with budesonide, formoterol, and the combination of these drugs. The Turbohaler® has a dosing wheel that scrapes off the required dose from a reservoir of dry powder. Dry-powder inhalers have the major advantage of being breath-actuated, thus not requiring hand–breath coordination. However, most dry-powder inhalers are flow rate-dependent, so that optimal performance may require the patient to use maximal inspiratory effort. The GlaxoSmithKline Accuhaler® or Diskus® has multiple unit doses prepackaged in foil blisters. Tiotropium bromide is administered by placing capsules of dry powder into the Handihaler®.

Figure 5.6   Dry powder inhalers: (a) Turbo(u)haler®; (b) Accuhaler® or Diskus®

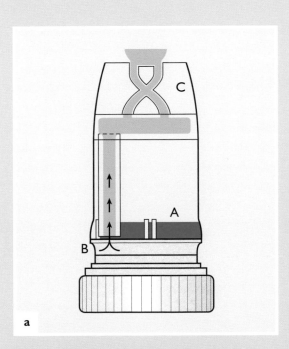

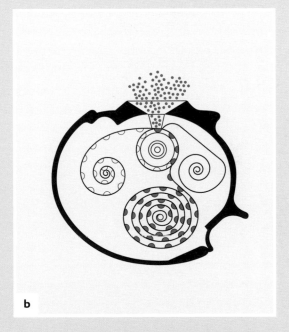

Drug is stored in a reservoir (A) and a metered dose is scraped out by rotating the base.

Inspired air (B) carries the powder to the mouthpiece (C) where it is further broken up.

Cog-wheel dose indicator with last 20 doses marked in red.

Manufactured by Astra Zeneca.

The powder is contained in small blisters attached to a strip; the backing is then peeled off, so that the drug is dispersed through the mouthpiece by the inspired air.

Manufactured by GlaxoSmithKline.

ANTICHOLINERGICS

Summary

- **GOLD:** The Global Initiative for Chronic Obstructive Lung Disease (GOLD, 2003 udpate) strategy emphasizes the role of bronchodilators in symptomatic management of stages I–IV COPD.

- **Anticholinergic drugs:** Ipratropium bromide and oxitropium bromide are short-acting inhaled anticholinergic drugs. Tiotropium bromide is a novel long-acting anticholinergic that is inhaled once daily and is recommended for regular use in COPD of stages II–IV (postbronchodilator FEV_1 of < 80%).

- **Pharmacology:** The anticholinergic drugs are quaternary ammonium derivatives that bind to muscarinic receptors of M_1, M_2 and M_3 subtypes. Tiotropium bromide has kinetic selectivity for M_1 and M_3 receptors.

- **Adverse events:** Dry mouth is commonly reported, and these drugs should be used with caution in patients with glaucoma, prostatism and those vulnerable to potential systemic anticholinergic side-effects.

- **Overall conclusion:** For regular use in patients with COPD, tiotropium bromide is more effective and convenient than ipratropium or oxitropium bromide.

Figure 5.7   Botanical origins of anticholinergic therapy

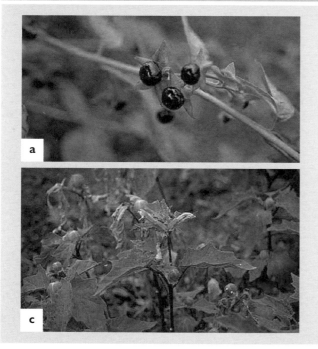
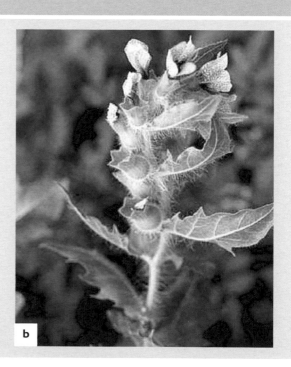

(a) The black berries of *Atropa belladonna* (deadly nightshade) contain the deadly plant alkaloid, atropine. Atropine is a competitive antagonist to acetylcholine at muscarinic receptor sites, M_1, M_2 and M_3. Atropine, when taken orally, causes blocked vagal innervation of the heart (tachycardia), decreased mucus secretion and bronchial smooth muscle relaxation in the respiratory system, mydriasis (pupillary dilation), decreased salivation with dry mouth, decreased gut mobility and acid secretion, bladder wall relaxation, and decreased sweating. (b) *Hyoscyamus niger* is the plant source of scopolamine (hyoscine) that was employed by the notorious Dr Crippen to murder his wife in London in 1910. (c) *Datura stramonium* (thorn-apple or jimsonweed) is the source of stramonium which was inhaled to alleviate respiratory disorders. Reproduced by permission of Henriette Kress (www.iblio.org/herbmed).

History (Figure 5.7)

Herbal remedies have been used since ancient times to treat human disease, and some of these plant extracts contain anticholinergic agents[11–16]. Ayurvedic medicine sources from India at around AD450 describe the use of thorn-apple extracts for their bronchial relaxant effects.

Atropine and scopolamine represent parent anticholinergic agents, and are alkaloids found in *Datura* species (thorn-apple) as well as *Atropa belladonna* (deadly nightshade). In the nineteenth century, army medical officers serving in India introduced the smoking of *Datura* to Britain, and recommended use of *Datura* for patients with bronchial complaints.

Since the late 1970s, inhaled ipratropium bromide (4 times a day) and oxitropium bromide (3 times a day) have been introduced. Combivent® is a useful combination of salbutamol and ipratropium bromide in a single inhaler (Figure 5.8). Tiotropium bromide (Spiriva® administered from the Handihaler®) is marketed by Boehringer-Ingelheim and Pfizer.

Molecular structures (Figure 5.9)

The parent compounds for anticholinergic therapy are the plant alkaloids atropine and scopolamine. Atropine methylnitrate, ipratropium bromide, oxitropium bromide and tiotropium bromide share a quaternary ammonium structure[6,17,18]. Quaternary ammonium compounds are poorly absorbed from respiratory or pharyngeal mucosal surfaces, and they have minimal oral bioavailability, ensuring that systemic anticholinergic effects are kept to a minimum.

Figure 5.8   Inhaled anticholinergic therapy

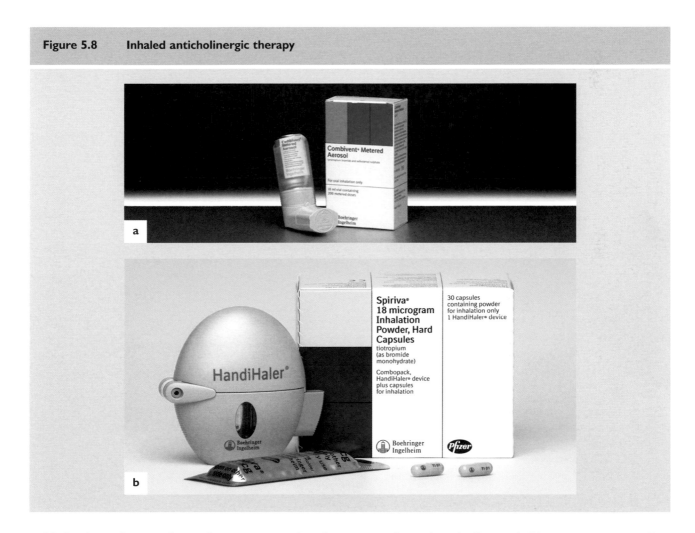

(a) Combivent® metered aerosol, containing combined ipratropium bromide and salbutamol; (b) tiotropium (Spiriva®) capsules containing dry powder are administered via the HandiHaler®. Photographs reproduced by permission of Boehringer-Ingelheim.

145

Figure 5.9   Structure of anticholinergics

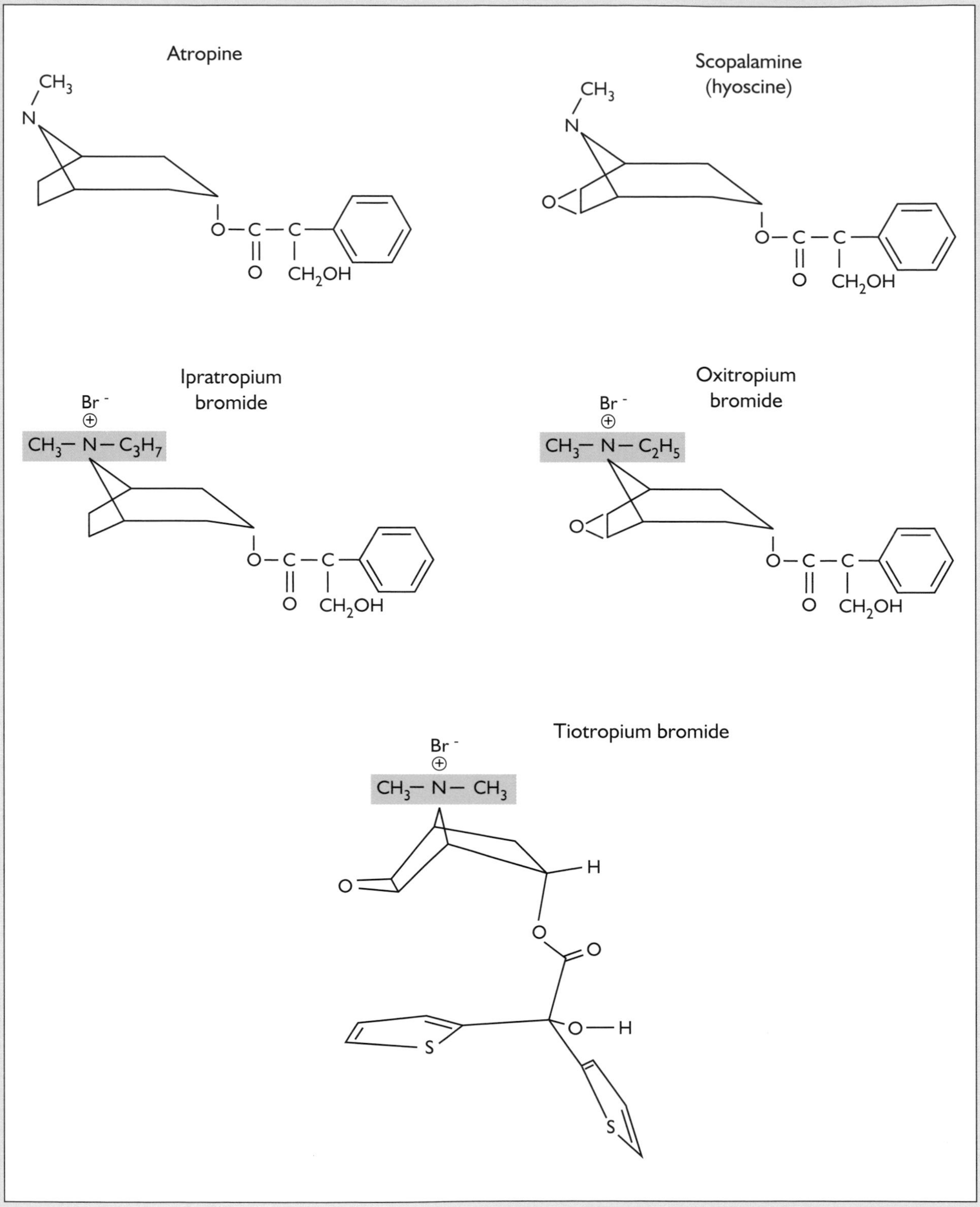

Unlike the plant alkaloids, atropine and scopolamine, modern synthetic anticholinergic drugs contain a positively charged quaternary nitrogen moiety, which ensures that the molecule has local action without systemic absorption. The quaternary nitrogen moiety is highlighted in green.

Parasympathetic nervous system

The autonomic nervous system is the involuntary unconscious control mechanism of the body that regulates visceral functions (Figure 5.10). The parasympathetic system is finely regulated and controls day-to-day respiratory, cardiac, gastrointestinal and bladder function; some of these activities have been termed the SLUD syndrome of salivation, lacrimation, urination and defecation. In contrast, the sympathetic system is a 'flight or fright' alarm system that prepares the body for maximal acute bodily function, and affects bronchial smooth muscle as well as blood flow.

The anatomies of the parasympathetic and sympathetic nervous systems are very different (Figures 5.11 and 5.12). Parasympathetic nerve fibers arise craniosacrally, with the vagus nerve arising from the brain stem as the tenth cranial nerve, and a smaller parasympathetic innervation leaving the sacral portion of the spinal cord. The vagus (wanderer) innervates most of the organs of the thorax and abdomen, and is involved in the parasympathetic innervation of the airways. Preganglionic fibers leave the brain stem in the vagus nerve; there is a local synapse in the pulmonary autonomic plexus around the airway wall, and a short postganglionic fiber leads to airways smooth muscle and mucus glands. Cholinergic control of the airways involves innervation of bronchial smooth muscle, causing vagal tone, as well as innervation of submucosal glands to cause mucus secretion and discharge (Figure 5.13). Cholinergic pathways may be activated by inflammatory mediators and inhaled irritants such as cigarette smoke. The nerve impulses then pass via Aδ- and C-fibers to parasympathetic ganglia.

Normal airways have a small degree of vagal cholinergic tone, but, because the airways are patent, this has no perceptible effect and may reduce airflow minimally (Figure 5.14). When the airways are irreversibly narrowed in COPD, vagal cholinergic tone has a much greater effect on airway resistance for geometric reasons; when this increased constriction is relieved by an anticholinergic drug, there is a perceptible improvement in airflow.

Muscarinic receptors (M_1–M_3)

Muscarinic receptors have been divided into five subtypes based on drug selectivity, but now confirmed by molecular cloning. There are muscarinic receptors of types M_1, M_2 and M_3 in human airways[19,20] (Figure 5.15).

- M_1 receptors are localized within parasympathetic ganglia and their blockade results in reduced reflex bronchoconstriction. Ganglionic transmission is mediated by both nicotinic receptors (N) and M_1 receptors in a facilitatory role.

- M_2 receptors located at cholinergic nerve terminals inhibit the release of acetylcholine, thus acting as autoreceptors.

- M_3 receptors mediate the bronchoconstrictor and the action of mucus secretion of acetylcholine in human airways. The most important effects of anticholinergics appear to be mediated through blockage of M_3 receptors.

Ipratropium bromide and oxitropium bromide have activity against M_1, M_2 and M_3 receptors. Anticholinergics act as muscarinic receptor antagonists, inhibiting cholinergic reflex bronchoconstriction, reducing vagal cholinergic tone, and decreasing mucus secretion.

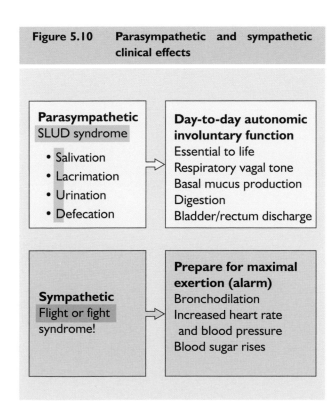

Figure 5.10   Parasympathetic and sympathetic clinical effects

Parasympathetic
SLUD syndrome
- Salivation
- Lacrimation
- Urination
- Defecation

Day-to-day autonomic involuntary function
Essential to life
Respiratory vagal tone
Basal mucus production
Digestion
Bladder/rectum discharge

Sympathetic
Flight or fight syndrome!

Prepare for maximal exertion (alarm)
Bronchodilation
Increased heart rate and blood pressure
Blood sugar rises

Anticholinergics oppose parasympathetic effects
β_2-adrenoreceptor agonists are sympathomimetics.

Figure 5.11   Schematic diagram of parasympathetic and sympathetic innervation of the lungs

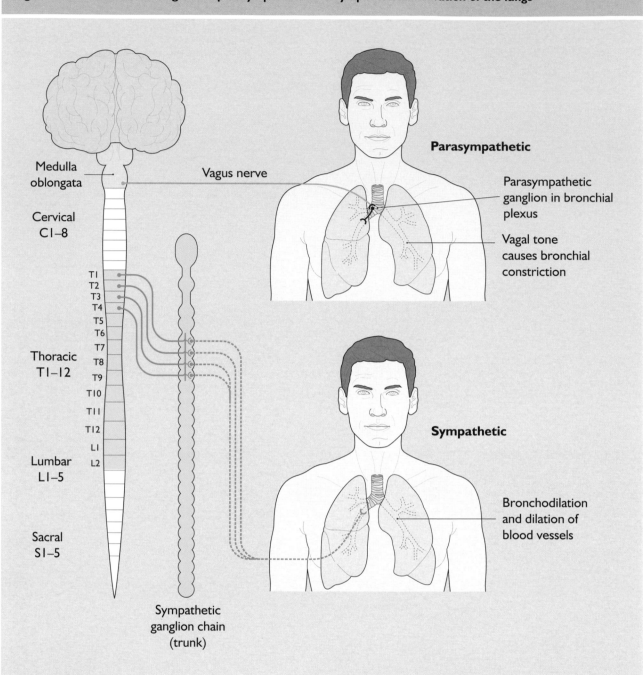

This schematic representation shows the brain, brain stem (containing the medulla oblongata) and spinal cord on the left-hand side of the figure.

Parasympathetic   Parasympathetic nerves are craniosacral in origin. The central brain stem nuclei of the vagus nerve (cranial nerve X) are located in the medulla oblongata, and the vagus passes down the neck to innervate major organs in the thorax and abdomen. The vagus nerve has synapses in the ganglia of the bronchial plexus, and a short postsynaptic neuron then maintains vagal tone (constriction) of airway smooth muscle.

Sympathetic   Sympathetic innervation has thoracolumbar origins from the spinal cord. The synapses of the sympathetic nerves which innervate the lungs are largely located in the two sympathetic ganglion chains (or trunks) that lie on either side of the spinal cord, resting on the posterior thoraco-abdominal wall. The relatively long postsynaptic sympathetic neuron passes to bronchial smooth muscle and innervates vascular smooth muscle. Activity of the sympathetic nervous system in 'fright, fight and flight' causes bronchodilation.

Figure 5.12   Anatomy of parasympathetic and sympathetic innervation of the bronchi

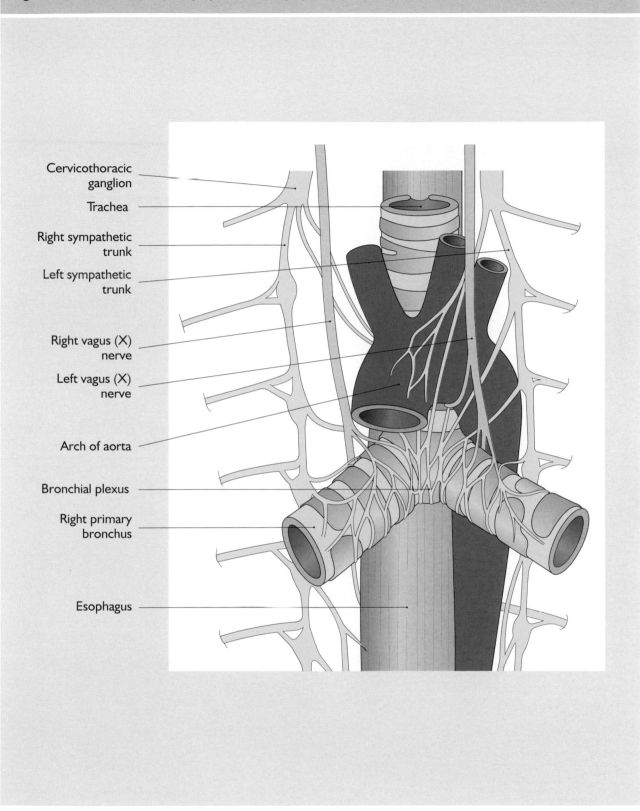

A detail is shown of the parasympathetic and sympathetic innervation of the main bronchi. The left vagus nerve differs from the right vagus nerve in having a recurrent laryngeal branch. Note that the vagus and sympathetic innervations merge with the bronchial plexus.

Figure 5.13   Cholinergic control of the airways

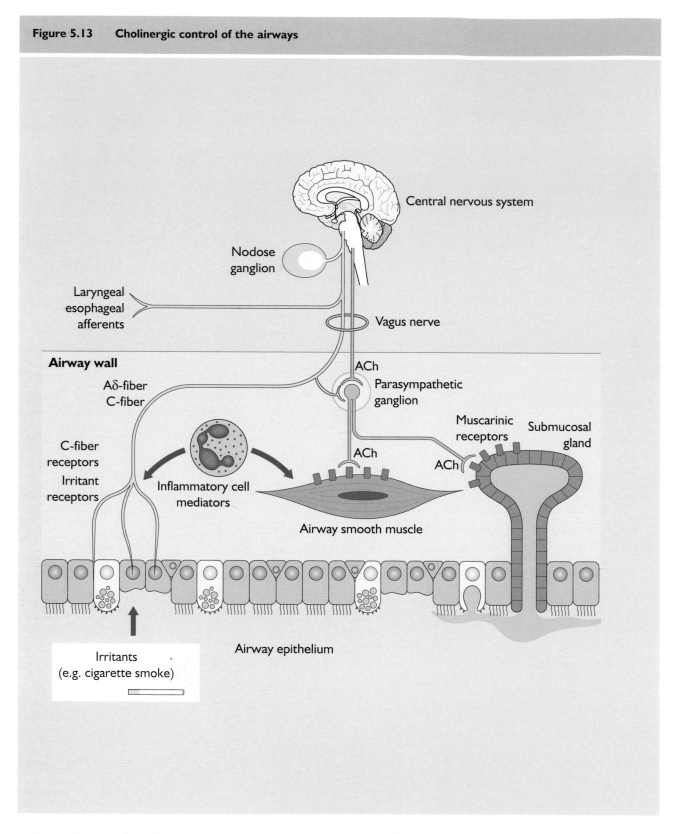

The mechanism of vagally mediated reflex bronchoconstriction is induced by irritants and non-specific stimuli acting on irritant receptors. Pre- and postganglionic parasympathetic nerves release acetylcholine (ACh). Preganglionic nerve fibers from the vagus nerve relay in parasympathetic ganglia in the airway wall, and short postganglionic pathways release ACh to cause bronchoconstriction and mucus secretion. Cholinergic afferent pathways may be activated by inflammatory mediators and cigarette smoke which act on C-fiber receptors.

Figure 5.14 Anticholinergics and vagal tone in COPD

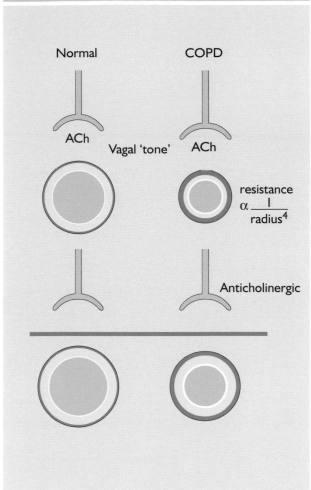

Figure 5.15 Muscarinic receptor subtypes

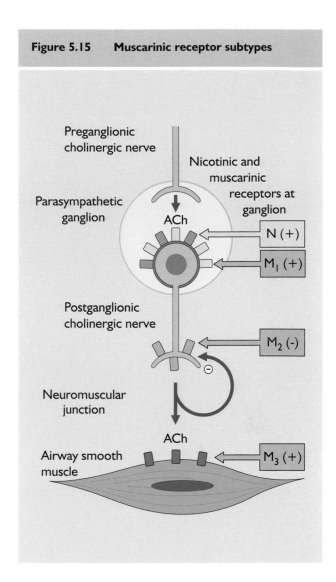

Normally, there is a certain amount of cholinergic vagal tone. This is exaggerated in COPD because of geometric factors related to the fixed narrowing of the airways, so that airway resistance improves to a greater extent than in normal airway with an anticholinergic drug. ACh, acetylcholine.

M_1 receptors are localized in parasympathetic ganglia and augment ganglionic transmission. M_2 receptors are at cholinergic nerve terminals and inhibit acetylcholine (ACh) release, whereas M_3 receptors are in muscle (and mucus glands) and mediate bronchoconstriction (and mucus secretion). Ganglionic transmission is mediated by both nicotinic receptors (N) and M_1 receptors in a facilitatory role.

Tiotropium bromide is a long-acting anticholinergic drug that has unique kinetic selectivity for M_1 and M_3 muscarinic receptors[6,7,17,18,21–24]. Tiotropium has similar affinity for the five types of muscarinic receptors, M_1–M_5. In the airways, tiotropium has a high affinity and dissociates very slowly from M_1 and M_3 receptors in human lung, but dissociates more rapidly from M_2 receptors; it produces long-term blockade of cholinergic neural bronchoconstriction in human airway smooth muscle[25–27].

M_3 action on airway smooth muscle

M_3 receptor (Figure 5.16)

Acetylcholine causes bronchoconstriction by stimulation of M_3 receptors on the surface membrane of airway smooth muscle cells[28,29]. The M_3 receptor is a serpentine receptor with seven transmembrane domains, a member of the seven-transmembrane family of receptors.

Figure 5.16   Human M$_3$ muscarinic receptor

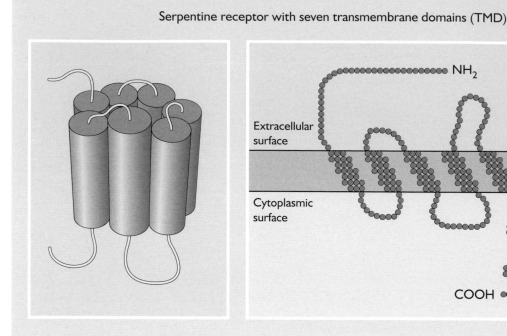

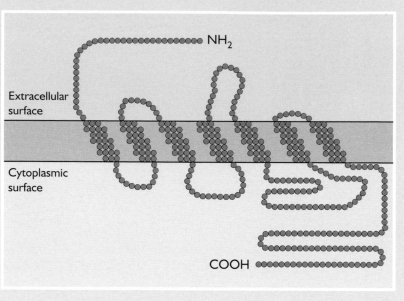

Serpentine receptor with seven transmembrane domains (TMD)

The human M$_3$ muscarinic receptor is a seven-transmembrane domain serpentine receptor with an external amino terminal and a cytoplasmic carboxyl terminal.

Signalling (Figure 5.17)

The M$_3$ receptor is a G protein-coupled receptor (GPCR), the G protein being a heterotrimer, consisting of αq, β and γ subunits[30]. On receptor activation, GTP binds to the Gαq subunit, that stimulates phospholipase Cβ (PLCβ). PLCβ cleaves phosphoinositol bisphosphate (PIP$_2$) into inositol triphosphate (IP$_3$) and diacyl glycerol (DAG). IP$_3$ interacts with receptors on the endoplasmic reticulum (ER) and causes calcium release into the cytoplasm. Liberated calcium binds calmodulin which activates myosin light chain kinase (MLCK).

Smooth muscle contraction (Figure 5.18)

Myosin is a hexamer consisting of two asymmetric heavy chains (200 and 240 kDa), with a pair of 17 kDa light chains and a pair of 20 kDa light chains[31]. The head has actin attachment sites and two domains of the calcium-stimulated magnesium-dependent ATPase. Contraction of airway smooth muscle requires an increase in cytosolic calcium, generally through an influx of calcium from ER

stores. Calcium in smooth muscle cells binds calmodulin and activates MLCK, which causes phosphorylation of myosin light chain 20 kDa and facilitates actin–myosin interaction, cross-bridge cycling and smooth muscle contraction.

Clinical physiology

(1) *Bronchodilation* Relaxation of airway smooth muscle tone causes an increase in FEV$_1$, but in COPD these changes are generally small (< 10%). Bronchodilator efficacy in COPD is generally assessed as the FEV$_1$ measured by spirometry. Tiotropium has been shown to consistently and significantly improve key lung function measures in long-term studies in patients with COPD[5,32–35].

(2) *Decreased hyperinflation* Reduced dynamic hyperinflation with a reduction in residual volume (RV) and functional residual capacity (FRC) may contribute to symptomatic benefits[36], since this makes breathing more comfortable and dyspnea is lessened[37]. There are

Figure 5.17   Cholinergic mechanism of smooth muscle contraction

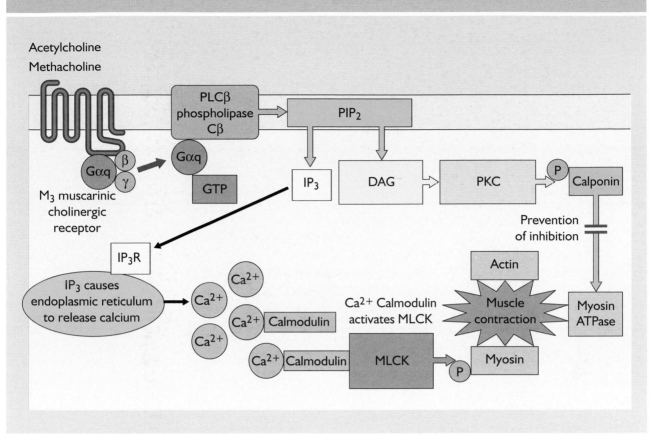

Acetylcholine binding to the M₃ muscarinic receptor results in guanosine triphosphate (GTP) binding to the Gαq subunit. GTP-bound Gαq stimulates phospholipase Cβ (PLCβ), which cleaves phosphoinositol bisphosphate (PIP₂) into inositol triphosphate (IP₃) and diacyl glycerol (DAG). IP₃ interacts with IP₃ receptors (IP₃R) on the endoplasmic reticulum (ER) and evokes Ca²⁺ release from the ER into the cytosol. Liberated Ca²⁺ binds calmodulin, forming a complex that activates myosin regulatory light chain kinase (MLCK). Phosphorylation (P) of myosin by MLCK facilitates interaction between actin and myosin and contraction. In addition, DAG activates protein kinase C (PKC), in an alternate mechanism of smooth muscle contraction. Adapted from Figure 4B of Johnson EN, Druey KM. *J Allergy Clin Immunol* 2002;109:592–602.

preliminary reports of promising effects of tiotropium on dynamic hyperinflation[38], and there is improvement in inspiratory capacity[39].

(3) *Symptoms* Symptomatic improvement may be greater than changes in FEV₁, especially in moderate to severe COPD[5,40], and tiotropium causes improvement in dyspnea[40].

(4) *Exercise tolerance* Improved exercise performance may be a conspicuous feature of bronchodilator usage in COPD[41], with tiotropium improving endurance and quality of life[42,43].

(5) *Mucociliary clearance* improvements occur. Anticholinergics have no detrimental effect on mucociliary clearance.

(6) *Respiratory muscle function* Improved muscle function is unlikely at the doses of anticholinergic therapy used clinically.

(7) *Natural history* There is no evidence that anticholinergic bronchodilators modify the rate of decline in lung function (FEV₁) in COPD[44].

Clinical indications

Occasional use of short-acting inhaled bronchodilators, on an 'as required' or 'on demand' basis are

Figure 5.18   Formation of actin–myosin cross-bridges

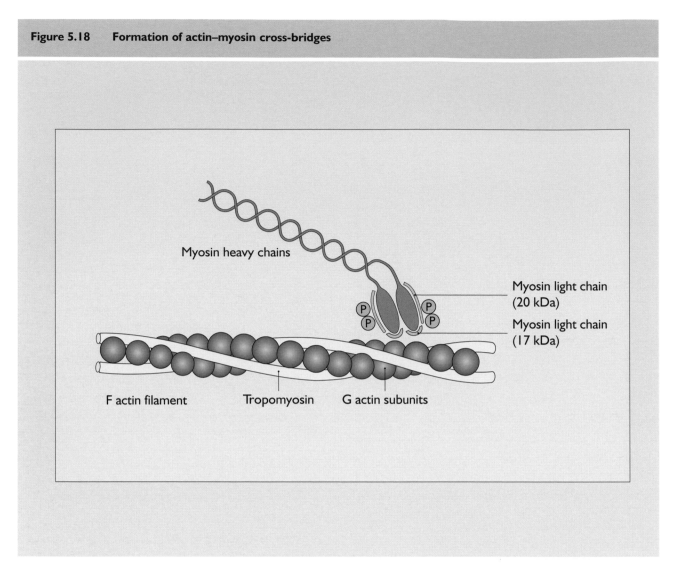

Adapted from Anderson GP, Rabe KF. In Hansel TT, Barnes PJ, eds. *New Drugs for Asthma, Allergy and COPD*. Basel: Karger, 2001.

recommended for Stage I (mild), Stage II (moderate), Stage III (severe) and Stage IV (very severe) COPD in the GOLD guidelines (2003 update). Regular treatment with long-acting inhaled bronchodilators is recommended for Stages II–IV COPD. Tiotropium bromide and/or long-acting β_2-agonists are generally more convenient and effective for regular maintenance treatment than ipratropium or oxitropium bromide.

Dosage and administration

Ipratropium bromide, oxitropium bromide and tiotropium bromide are inhaled, since they are topically active, and are absorbed very little from the gut.

Inhaler systems and dosage

- *Ipratropium bromide* is usually given by a metered dose inhaler or dry powder inhaler at 20 or 40 µg per actuation. A nebulizer formulation is also available. Ipratropium bromide is generally given at 40–80 µg three to four times daily.

- *Oxitropium bromide* is usually given by a metered dose inhaler or dry powder inhaler at 100 µg per actuation. A nebulizer formulation is also available. Oxitropium bromide is generally given at 200 µg two to three times daily.

- *Combivent®* is a combination bronchodilator inhaler containing an anticholinergic (ipratropium bromide, 20 μg) and short-acting β2-agonist (salbutamol, 100 μg)[45]. Combivent® is generally given as two inhalations four times a day.

- *Duovent® and Berodual®* are combination bronchodilators that contain an anticholinergic (ipratropium bromide) and short-acting β2-agonist (fenoterol). Duovent® is only available in a few countries. Berodual® is available more widely but is not marketed in North America or the UK.

- *Tiotropium bromide* (Spiriva®) is given in capsules, each capsule containing 22.5 μg tiotropium bromide monohydrate, equivalent to 18 μg tiotropium. Tiotropium is inhaled once a day from the HandiHaler®, a specialized dry powder inhalation system[46].

Pharmacokinetics

Ipratropium, oxitropium and tiotropium bromide are quaternary ammonium compounds which are poorly absorbed from the gastrointestinal tract. Following inhalation of ipratropium and oxitropium, uptake into the plasma is minimal, a peak blood concentration being obtained within 3 h after inhalation, with excretion via the kidneys.

Tiotropium bromide provides a bronchodilator effect exceeding 24 h with a plasma steady-state concentration of approximately 2 pg/ml, and a terminal half-life of 5–6 days that is independent of the dose[23]. It has been calculated that this concentration would occupy < 5% of systemic muscarinic receptors, perhaps accounting for the very low incidence of systemic side-effects. After chronic once-daily inhalation by COPD patients, pharmacokinetic steady state was reached after 2–3 weeks, with no accumulation thereafter. The pharmacokinetics and tissue distribution of tiotropium in the rat and dog have also been described[47].

Clinical studies

Ipratropium and oxitropium bromide

Ipratropium and oxitropium bromide have a slower onset of action than β2-agonists, with a peak effect being obtained between 30 and 90 min, and the bronchodilation being sustained for 6–8 h[48]. This limited duration of action may mean, however, that bronchodilation is not provided throughout the night. Ipratropium bromide has a duration of 6–8 h, while oxitropium is claimed to maintain bronchodilation for at least 8 h[48], although this could be due to the higher dose of oxitropium[17]. On the basis of the duration of action, ipratropium bromide is given four times daily, while oxitropium bromide is given three times daily. Oxitropium bromide is extensively used to treat COPD in Japan[49]. When using the FEV_1 as the outcome, the dose–response relationship of ipratropium bromide is relatively flat[50]. This is also true for the dose relationship with toxicity. There is a dose response for oxitropium bromide up to 400 μg[51,52], and effects last up to 8 h after inhalation.

A range of comparative clinical studies have been performed with ipratropium bromide:

(1) *Salbutamol* Ipratropium bromide causes greater and longer-term bronchodilation than salbutamol in severe COPD[53]. A number of studies have been performed with a combination of ipratropium bromide with salbutamol (Combivent®) in a single inhaler, compared with ipratropium and salbutamol given alone[45,54,55] (Figure 5.19). These studies have found ipratropium to be superior to salbutamol in terms of effects on FEV_1;

(2) *Salmeterol* Ipratropium causes similar maximal bronchodilation to salmeterol, but has a shorter duration of action[56,57]. Salmeterol and ipratropium have similar effects on arterial blood gases in stable COPD[58] and on exertional dyspnea[59];

(3) *Formoterol* Formoterol has been found to be more effective than ipratropium in terms of lung function[60];

(4) *Theophylline* Ipratropium bromide has greater acute bronchodilating effects than theophylline[61]. The combination of ipratropium bromide, salbutamol and theophylline is superior to these agents given alone[62].

Combivent® and Duovent®

There are large-scale clinical studies with the pressurized metered dose inhaler Combivent® that demonstrate the superiority of the combination (ipratropium bromide with salbutamol) over the individual elements (ipratropium bromide alone and salbutamol alone)[45,63,64] (Figure 5.19). The benefits

Figure 5.19   Ipratropium compared with salbutamol and Combivent® in patients with COPD

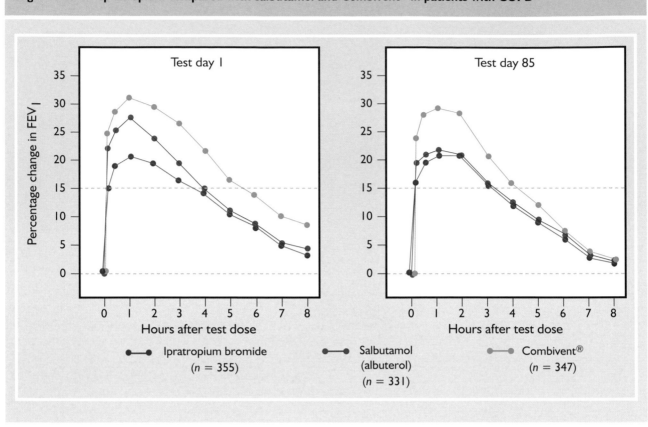

Adapted from Figure 1, Wilson *et al. Eur Respir Rev* 1996;6:286–9. Data are integrated from two pivotal clinical trials.

of nebulized combination ipratropium bromide and salbutamol have also been identified[54,55].

A series of clinical studies have been performed to characterize the role of Duovent® (ipratropium bromide plus fenoterol) in COPD[65–72], although Duovent® is available only in a limited number of countries.

Tiotropium bromide

The published clinical trial experiences with tiotropium are summarized in Figure 5.20.

Single-dose studies   Single-dose relationships of tiotropium bromide have been determined with nebulized doses of up to 160 μg in patients with COPD[73,74] (Figure 5.21) as well as doses of up to 80 μg from a dry powder inhaler in asthma[75].

One-week study   A 7-day study in patients with COPD demonstrated that approximately 70% of the bronchodilator effect of tiotropium is obtained after two doses, and that the FEV_1 steady state is reached within 48 h[76].

4-week study A 4-week study of tiotropium, at doses of up to 36 μg given daily at noon, found comparable responses at doses from 9 to 36 μg, representing a flat dose–response curve, with little dose dependency in terms of spirometric outcomes[77]. On this basis, a dose of 18 μg was selected for use in long-term studies, since the 36 μg dose increased the incidence of dry mouth without significantly increasing FEV_1.

13-week studies (interim reports from the 1-year studies) The Dutch Tiotropium Study Group has reported interim results at 13 weeks of a 1-year study with 288 patients with COPD, in which tiotropium at 18 μg from the Handihaler® administered once daily was significantly more effective than ipratropium administered four times daily[78]. The US Tiotropium Study Group reported 13-week interim results of a multicenter study, but compared tiotropium with placebo, and found significant improvements in lung function (FEV_1 and PEF), symptoms, as-needed albuterol/salbutamol usage and physician global assessment[79].

Figure 5.20	Clinical studies with tiotropium bromide in COPD			

Reference	Administration	Study	Treatment arms	Total number of subjects
Maesen et al. Eur Respir J 1993;6:1031–6	single-dose escalation	single-dose open escalation and bronchodilation (FEV$_1$ and sGAW) in COPD	tiotropium (nebulizer) 10, 20, 40, 80, 160 µg no placebo	6
Maesen et al. Eur Respir J 1995;8:1506–13	single-dose dose response COPD	randomized placebo-controlled cross-over design to study dose response of single doses on bronchodilation (FEV$_1$) in COPD	tiotropium (DPI) 10, 20, 40, 80 µg placebo	35
O'Connor et al. Am J Respir Crit Care Med 1996;154:876–80	single-dose dose response asthma	single-dose study on methacholine-induced bronchoconstriction in asthma	tiotropium (DPI) 10, 40, 80 µg placebo	12
van Noord et al. Eur Respir J 2002;19:639–44	1-week	pharmacodynamic steady state in COPD: FEV$_1$ steady state is reached within 48 h, with continued improvements beyond 1 week	tiotropium (Handihaler® DPI) 18 µg once daily vs. ipratropium 40 µg q.i.d.	31
Littner et al. Am J Respir Crit Care Med 2000;161:1136–42	4-week	29-day study of dose response in stable patients with COPD parallel group multicenter, placebo-controlled	tiotropium 0,4.5,9,18, 36 µg parallel group placebo	169
van Noord et al. Thorax 2000;55:289–94	*13-week	tiotropium inhaled at 18 µg once daily is more effective than ipratropium 40 µg q.i.d.	tiotropium 18 µg once daily vs. ipratropium 40 µg q.i.d.	288
Casaburi et al. Chest 2000;118:1294–302	*13-week	spirometric efficacy in a 13-week study in COPD	tiotropium 18 µg once daily vs. ipratropium 40 µg q.i.d.	279 + 191
Vincken et al. Eur Respir J 2002;19:209–16	1-year long-term efficacy	1-year comparative tiotropium vs. ipratropium study in COPD: lung function, dyspnea, health status, exacerbations, hospitalizations	tiotropium 18 µg once daily vs. ipratropium 40 µg q.i.d.	356 + 179
Casaburi et al. Eur Respir J 2002;19:217–24 Tashkin and Kesten. Chest 2003;123:1441–9	1-year long-term efficacy	placebo-controlled study in COPD: lung function, dyspnea, health status, exacerbations, hospitalizations	tiotropium 18 µg once daily vs. placebo	921
Donohue et al. Chest 2002;122:47–55 Donohue et al. Respir Med 2003;97:1014–20 Brusasco et al. Thorax 2003;58:399–404	two 6-month studies comparison of tiotropium with salmeterol	6-month placebo-controlled studies, double-blind, double-dummy parallel-group studies in COPD	tiotropium 18 µg once daily salmeterol 50 µg twice daily vs. placebo	1207

FEV$_1$, forced expiratory volume in 1 s; DPI, dry powder inhaler; *Interim reports from 1-year studies.

Figure 5.21   Single-dose study with tiotropium in COPD

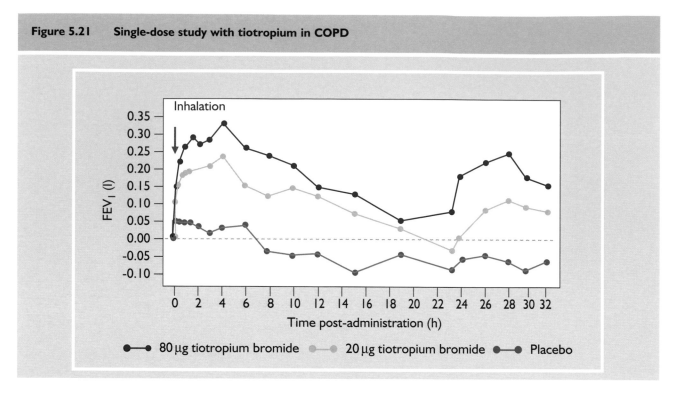

Increase in adjusted mean improvement in FEV$_1$ from test day baseline. Adapted from Figure 1, Maesen FPV *et al. Eur Respir J* 1995;8:1506–13.

Figure 5.22   One-year studies with tiotropium: effects on lung function

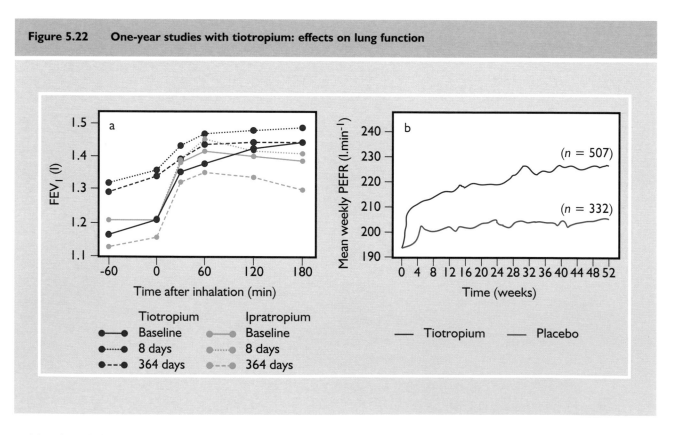

(a) Adapted from Vincken *et al. Eur Respir J* 2002;19:209–16.   (b) Adapted from Casaburi *et al. Eur Respir J* 2002;19:217–24.

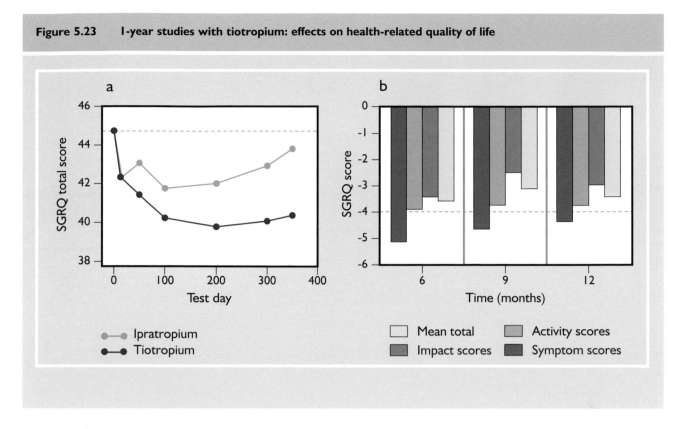

Figure 5.23   1-year studies with tiotropium: effects on health-related quality of life

Expressed as the St. George's Respiratory Questionnaire (SGRQ) score. A lower score indicates an improvement in health status, and a 4-point improvement is recognized as a clinically meaningful response. (a) Effects on mean SGRQ total score for tiotropium and ipratropium groups; (b) effects on SGRQ score measured at 6, 9 and 12 months for tiotropium (placebo not shown). (a) Adapted from Figure 4, Vincken *et al. Eur Respir J* 2002;19:209–16. (b) Adapted from Figure 4, Casaburi *et al. Eur Respir J* 2002;19:217–24.

1-year studies Two 1-year studies with tiotropium bromide in moderate-to-severe COPD have demonstrated significant improvement in lung function, and symptoms[5,40] (Figure 5.22). These studies confirm that the positive effects seen in 4- and 13-week studies are extended to 1 year, and suggest that tolerance does not occur in this period[80]. There were convincing effects on health-related quality of life, expressed as the St. George's Respiratory Questionnaire score (Figure 5.23). It is important to note that tiotropium was effective in long-term treatment of patients with COPD without regard to the magnitude of the short-term response at the start of treatment[32]. Hence, it is not possible to predict efficacy with tiotropium on the basis of a single administration. In the 1-year studies with tiotropium, less than half the patients had an exacerbation over the 1 year, with only about 10% of exacerbations requiring hospitalization[5,40]. Hence, tiotropium may decrease the incidence and severity of exacerbations of COPD.

Comparison with salmeterol In two 6-month randomized, double-blind, double-dummy, parallel-group studies, tiotropium 18 µg once daily was compared with salmeterol 50 µg twice daily[33–35]. Tiotropium was found to be superior to salmeterol in key lung function measures.

Side-effects (Figure 5.24)

Extensive experience has shown inhaled anticholinergics to be a remarkably safe class of drug. Inhaled delivery with virtually no systemic absorption means that systemic adverse effects are very uncommon. However, COPD patients are older and more likely to have co-morbidities than patients with asthma. Nevertheless, geriatric patients can use anticholinergics at the recommended dose.

• Dry mouth and cough are the most common adverse effects, seen in up to 15% of subjects receiving tiotropium. This incidence of dry mouth is higher than that seen with

Figure 5.24   Side-effects of anticholinergics

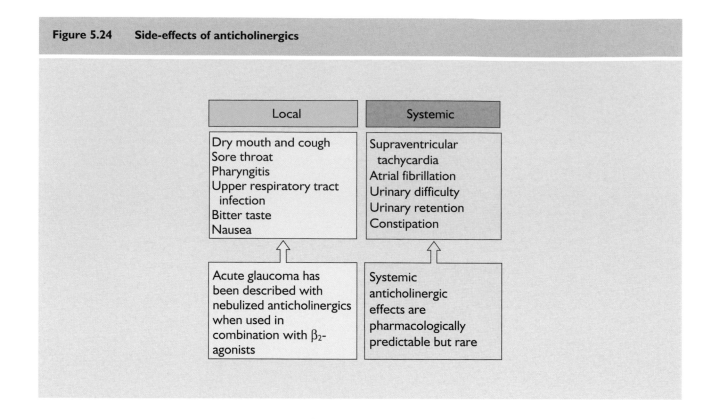

ipratropium bromide[78], but mostly mild. Dry mouth may theoretically be associated with dental caries.

- A bitter metallic taste has been reported by some patients.

- Paradoxical (inhalation) bronchoconstriction is usually due to additives in the nebulizer solution.

- Immediate hypersensitivity reactions may occur.

- Glaucoma may occur with nebulized drug when used without a mouthpiece in elderly patients, probably due to a direct effect on the eye. To avoid narrow-angle glaucoma, always avoid getting tiotropium in the eyes. Anticholinergics may cause eye pain, blurred vision, visual halos and conjunctival and corneal congestion (redness).

- Pharyngitis and increased upper respiratory infections may occur.

- Systemic effects are very rare, but theoretical possibilities are urinary retention, prostatic complications, constipation, tachycardia or palpitations.

- Headache, nervousness, irritation, dizziness may occur.

- Mucociliary clearance is unaffected by anticholinergics, although mucus secretion may be decreased.

- The incidence of respiratory infections is unaffected.

Future studies

It is likely that tiotropium, used alone or in combination with other bronchodilators, will emerge as an important maintenance treatment for patients with moderate (Stage II), severe (Stage III), and very severe (Stage IV) COPD. Although tiotropium bromide looks very promising as a regular bronchodilator therapy for COPD, additional studies as well as postmarketing experience will be of interest[81], including comparative studies with other bronchodilators, combination with other bronchodilators and corticosteroids, and long-term studies on decline in lung function (FEV_1). In addition, it is important to perform comparative studies on lung hyperinflation and exercise tolerance, effects on prevention and treatment of exacerbations, and potential efficacy in severe oral steroid-dependent asthma.

β₂-AGONISTS

Summary

GOLD Bronchodilators are the cornerstone of drug treatment of chronic stable COPD and comprise principally the inhaled anticholinergics and/or β₂-agonists[1].

Molecular mechanism The mode of action of β₂-agonists is well understood at the level of the molecular interactions with the β₂-adrenoceptor and the subsequent cell signalling events that mediate bronchodilation.

Short-acting The most frequently utilized short-acting β₂-agonists are salbutamol (albuterol) and terbutaline. Salbutamol and terbutaline have similar effects, causing rapid onset of bronchodilation for 4–6 h. Short-acting β₂-agonists may be used in mild COPD (GOLD Stage I) as well as moderate (GOLD Stage II), severe COPD (GOLD Stage III) and very severe (GOLD Stage IV). Short-acting β₂-agonists (salbutamol and terbutaline) should be used on an 'as-needed' basis to treat respiratory symptoms.

Long-acting The long-acting β₂-agonists salmeterol and formoterol are useful bronchodilators for maintenance use in Stages II–IV COPD, but differ in their pharmacology. Salmeterol has delayed onset as a bronchodilator compared to formoterol and is a partial rather than full agonist, while both agents cause bronchodilation for more than 12 h, enabling twice-daily dosing. There is increasing evidence that long-acting β₂-agonists are useful as regular bronchodilators in chronic COPD, since they improve lung function, symptoms, health-related quality of life and exercise performance. In addition, formoterol may also be effective on an as-needed basis. The efficacy of long-acting β₂-agonists has been demonstrated in numerous studies in COPD, both alone and in comparison with ipratropium bromide, oxitropium bromide, tiotropium bromide, and theophylline treatment[82–88].

Combinations Combined long-acting β₂-agonists and corticosteroids in single inhalers are effective for more severe patients with COPD that have frequent exacerbations.

Side-effects Side-effects are usually only a problem if excessive doses of β₂-agonists are used, although caution is required when employing β₂-agonists in patients with certain cardiac and thyroid disorders.

History (Figure 5.25)

The plant ma huang (*Ephedra sinica*) has been used in traditional Chinese medicine for the treatment of asthma for over 5000 years[11,89,90]. Ephedra is a shrub-like plant that grows in many desert regions, although *Ephedra sinica* is found especially in Northern China and Mongolia. The crude powdered stem of *Ephedra sinica* is rich in ephedrine, a plant-derived compound with similar properties to adrenaline, and can be taken as a tea.

It was not until 1900 that Solis-Cohen used 'adrenal substances' to treat asthma, with the successful use of adrenaline (epinephrine) for asthma attacks reported in 1903. Chemically synthesized β-selective isoprenaline was introduced in 1948, while the selective β₂-agonist salbutamol (albuterol) was introduced as a bronchodilator in

| Figure 5.25 | Botanical origin of β₂-agonists |

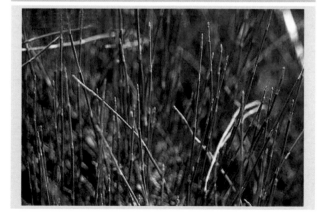

Ephedra sinica, Chinese desert herb.. Reproduced by permission of Henriette Kress (www.iblio.org/herbmed).

1969, with terbutaline following in 1974. The long-acting β_2-agonists salmeterol and formoterol became available as inhaled agents in clinical practice in the 1990s.

Molecular structures (Figure 5.26 and 5.27)

β_2-Agonists are sympathomimetic bronchodilators that are catecholamine derivatives. A catecholamine consists of a benzene ring, with hydroxyl groups at positions 3 and 4, and an amine side-chain attached at position 1. Salbutamol (albuterol) and terbutaline are very similar in structure. Formoterol and salmeterol each contain the saligenin head, which is similar to the catechol ring found within the endogenous

neurotransmitters, noradrenaline and adrenaline. However, formoterol and salmeterol differ in their molecular structure and properties, the major structural difference being that salmeterol contains a lipophilic 12-carbon side-chain.

Sympathetic nervous system (Figure 5.10)

The autonomic nervous system is the involuntary unconscious control mechanism of the body that regulates visceral functions. The sympathetic system is a 'flight or fight' alarm system that prepares for maximal acute bodily function. β_2-Agonists are sympathomimetic bronchodilators which are generally inhaled to localize activity to the airways. In

| Figure 5.26 | Molecular structures of natural catecholamines |

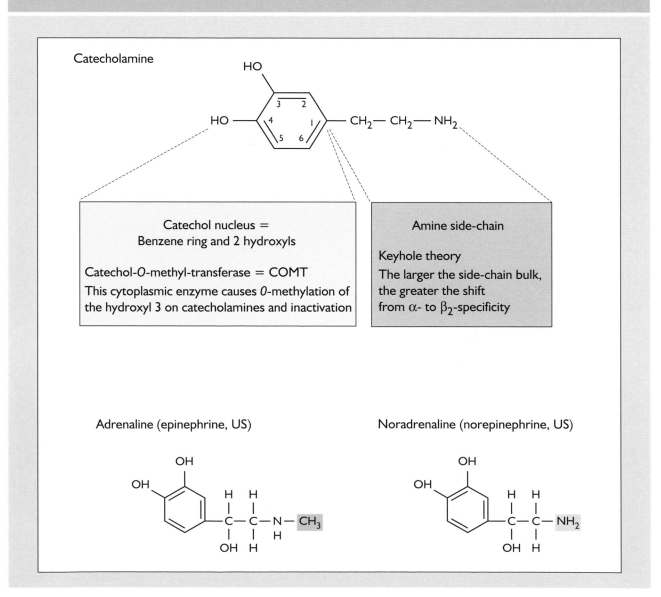

Figure 5.27   Molecular structures of β₂-agonists

Salbutamol = albuterol (US)

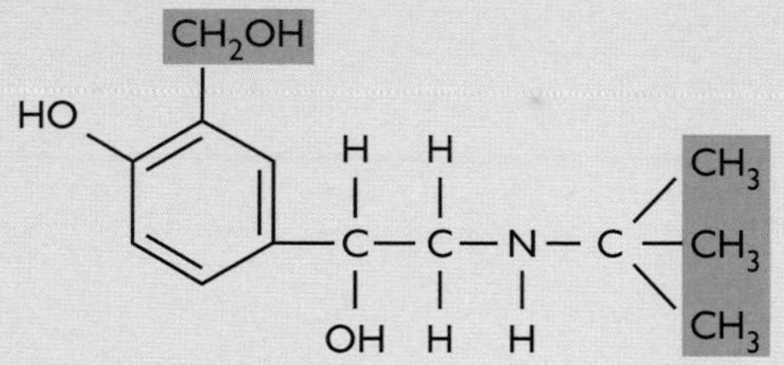

Terbutaline

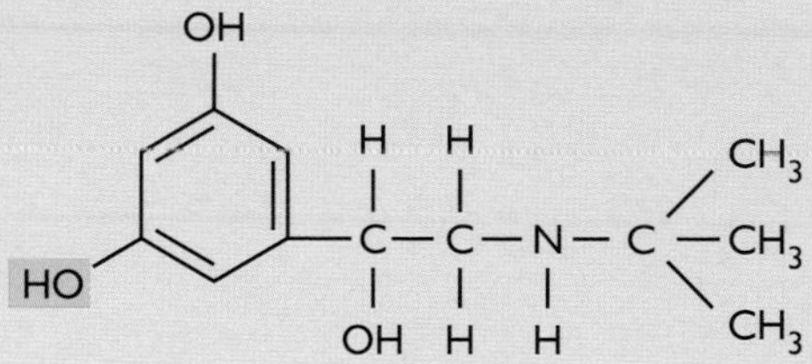

Fenoterol

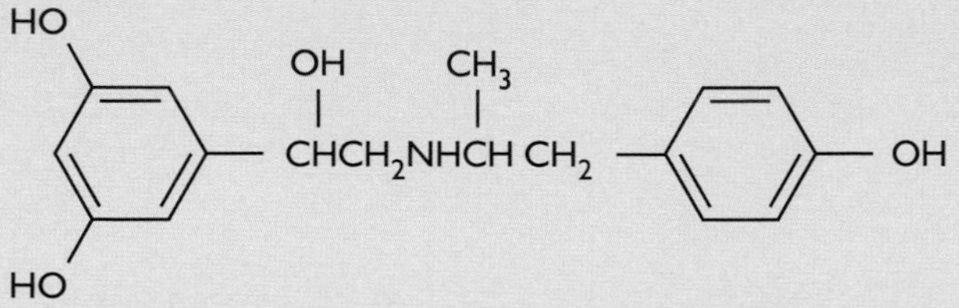

Salmeterol xinafoate

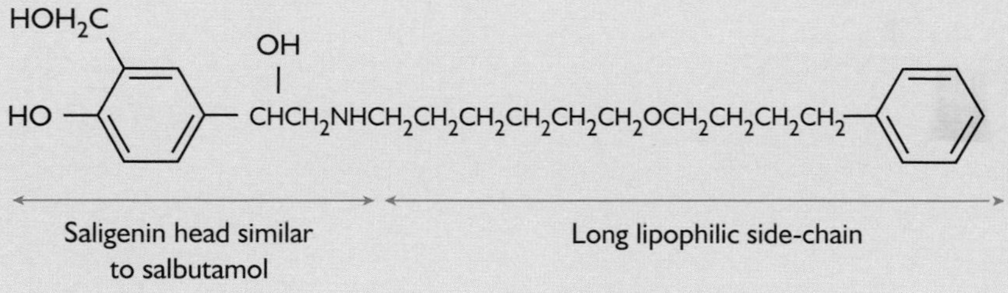

Saligenin head similar to salbutamol

Long lipophilic side-chain

Formoterol

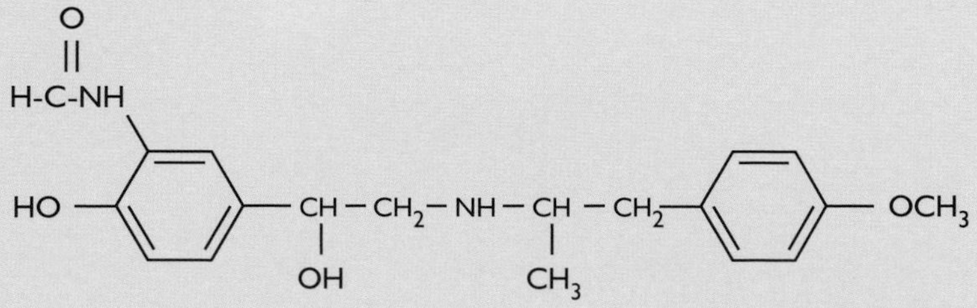

contrast, the parasympathetic system is finely regulated and controls day-to-day respiratory, cardiac, gastrointestinal and bladder functions.

Sympathetic nerve fibers arise from thoracolumbar portions of the spinal cord (Figures 5.11 and 5.12). There is a synapse within ganglia in the right and left sympathetic trunks that lie in a vertical row on the posterior thorax and abdominal walls. Long postganglionic sympathetic nerve fibers then mix with vagus nerve parasympathetic fibers to form the pulmonary autonomic nerve plexus. Rami from the autonomic plexus accompany the bronchi and bronchioles. The sympathetic neurotransmitter is noradrenaline (norepinephrine), whose effects can also be caused by release of adrenaline (epinephrine) into the circulation.

β₂-Adrenoceptor (Figure 5.28)

Bronchodilator therapy is based on the effects on the autonomic (involuntary) nervous system, and β₂-adrenoceptor agonists act on the sympathetic innervation of airway smooth muscle. β-Adrenoceptors have been divided into three subtypes based on drug selectivity but now confirmed by molecular cloning: β_1 on cardiac smooth muscle, β_2 on airway smooth muscle and β_3 on adipose tissue. β_2-Agonists cause bronchodilation by stimulation of β_2-adrenoceptors on the surface membrane of airway smooth muscle cells[28]. There are some 30–40 000 β_2-adrenoceptors on each smooth muscle cell, and the receptor is present on a variety of other cells, including lung epithelial and endothelial cells.

The β_2-adrenoceptor is a serpentine receptor and is a member of the seven-transmembrane family of receptors, with seven α-helices that cross the plasma membrane[91] (Figure 5.28). The β_2-adrenoceptor is composed of 413 amino acids[28]. The amino terminus is found outside the cell, while the carboxyl terminus is internal (cytoplasmic). A total of 17 single nucleotide polymorphisms (SNPs) have been described within the β_2-adrenoceptor gene and its

---

Figure 5.28   The human β₂-adrenoceptor on bronchial smooth muscle

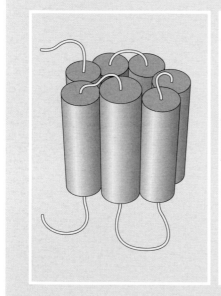
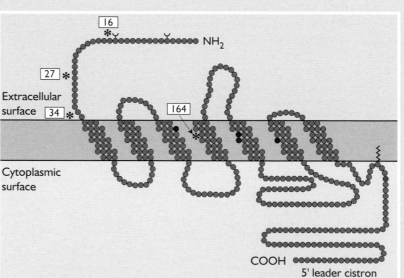

This is a serpentine receptor with seven transmembrane domains (TMD).
There are four amino acid polymorphisms (*) at positions 16, 27, 34, 164 from the amino (NH₂) terminal.
Important residues for binding to agonists (●)
Glycosylation sites (ⵧ)
The human receptor has 413 amino acids.

For details see Leggett SB. *J Allergy Clin Immunol* 2002;110:S223–8.

regulatory region[92]. Amino acid positions 16 (Arg or Gly), 27 (Gln or Glu), and 164 (Thr or Ile) are the most common SNPs.

Molecular action of β_2-agonists

Salbutamol is hydrophilic and interacts directly with the β_2-adrenoceptor receptor from the aqueous phase[93] (Figure 5.29). In contrast, salmeterol is lipophilic and associates predominantly initially with the lipid bilayer, followed by membrane translocation. For salmeterol, this indirect binding causes a delay in the onset of action[28]. Formoterol is partially lipophilic and forms a membrane depot; its action is more rapid in onset than that of salmeterol.

The molecular basis of the interaction between β_2-agonists and the active site has been determined[28,93] (Figure 5.30). The active site is located within hydrophilic amino acids of transmembrane domains 3, 5 and 6. Formoterol, salbutamol, and terbutaline bind to the active site but not to the exosite. The residues of critical importance for agonist binding to the active site are aspartate (Asp) at residue 113 of the transmembrane domain 3, two

serine (Ser) residues at 204 and 207 of the transmembrane domain 5, two phenylalanines (Phe) at 259 and 290 of transmembrane domain 6. Asp binds to nitrogen, while the two Ser residues interact with hydroxyl groups.

The molecular basis of the interaction of salmeterol with the active and exosite of the β_2-adrenoceptor is termed the salmeterol hinge (charniére) theory[28] (Figure 5.31):

- The lipophilic side-chain of salmeterol binds to the exosite (transmembrane domain 4) within a hydrophobic part of the β_2-adrenoceptor structure, and anchors salmeterol to the β_2-adrenoceptor. The molecular location of this exosite within the β_2-adrenoceptor has been identified by elegant site-directed mutagenesis studies[94].

- The oxygen 'O' within the lipophilic side-chain of salmeterol acts as a fulcrum or hinge.

- The saligenin head of salmeterol is involved in repeated engaging and disengaging with the active site (transmembrane domains 3, 5, 6) within the β_2-adrenoceptor.

Figure 5.29   Interaction of β_2-agonists with cell membrane

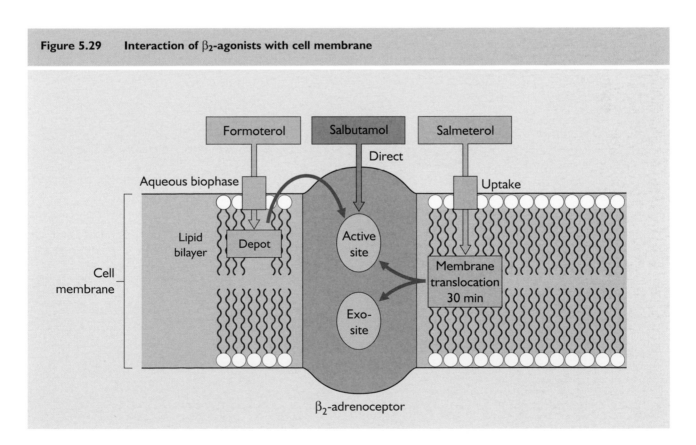

See text for details.

Figure 5.30   The β₂-adrenoceptor active site and exosite

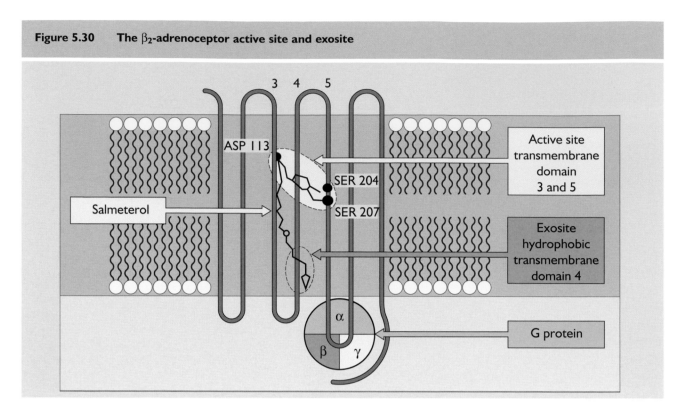

See text for details.

Figure 5.31   Mechanism of action of salmeterol

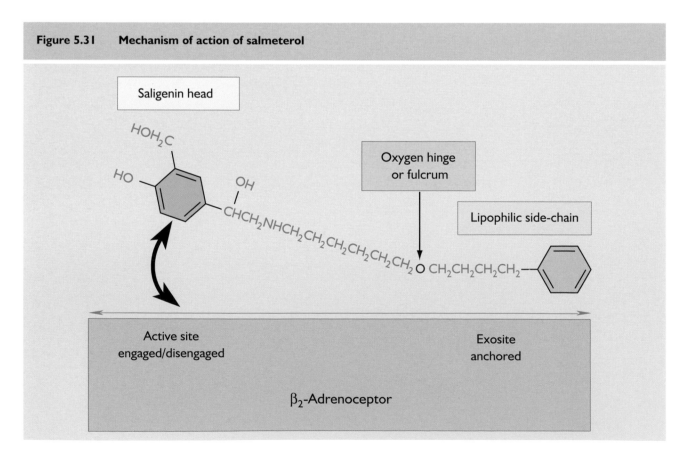

See text for details.

Comparison of formoterol and salmeterol (Figure 5.32)

Formoterol and salmeterol share the pharmacological property of being potent and selective for β_2-receptors, but they have major pharmacological differences. Both formoterol and salmeterol cause bronchodilation for at least 12 h after a single administration, but formoterol has almost immediate onset of action while that of salmeterol is delayed for approximately 15 min. Formoterol but not salmeterol can be used 'as required'[95], and the dose of formoterol is more flexible than that of salmeterol, which cannot be increased because of long-lasting systemic side-effects. Salmeterol is a partial agonist with lesser efficacy on isolated smooth muscle than the full agonist formoterol. However, while it has been speculated that full agonism may in certain cases lead to therapeutic advantages, there is also the theoretical possibility of increasing tolerance and adverse events[96].

β_2-Adrenoceptor signalling

G protein GTPase cycle (Figure 5.33)

The β_2-adrenoceptor is a G protein-coupled receptor (GPCR), the G protein being a heterotrimer, consisting of α, β and γ subunits[30,40]. There are four major families of α subunits: Gαs, GαI, Gαq11, and Gα12/13. In the basal state, the α subunit binds guanosine diphosphate (GDP), while, on receptor activation, GDP is replaced with GTP. GTP-bound Gα separates from the receptor and interacts with effector systems, in multiple cycles of GTP-binding and hydrolysis, within milliseconds. There is an expanding spectrum of G protein diseases[97].

Adenyl cyclase, cAMP, PKA, MLCK, relaxation

Gαs causes activation of membrane-bound adenyl cyclase, which catalyzes conversion of adenosine triphosphate (ATP) to cyclic adenosine monophosphate (cAMP)[30]. cAMP is a second messenger within the smooth muscle cell which can activate protein kinase A (PKA), which in turn phosphorylates many proteins. When PKA phosphorylates myosin regulatory light chain kinases (MLCK), affinity for calmodulin/calcium is decreased, and smooth muscle relaxation occurs.

Calcium, MLCK, contraction

Contraction of airway smooth muscle requires an increase in cytosolic calcium, generally through an influx of calcium from endoplasmic reticulum stores.

Figure 5.32   Comparative properties of β_2-agonists

	Salbutamol	Formoterol	Salmeterol
Potency	moderately potent	very potent	potent
Onset of action	rapid	rapid	delayed >10 min
Duration of action	4–6 h	> 12 h	> 12 h
β_2-receptor selectivity	very selective	selective	highly selective
Efficacy	partial agonist	full agonist	partial agonist
Mechanism of action	direct	membrane depot	exosite
Clinical role	rescue/acute use	rescue and maintenance	maintenance

Figure 5.33 β₂-adrenoceptor-mediated smooth muscle relaxation: cell signalling

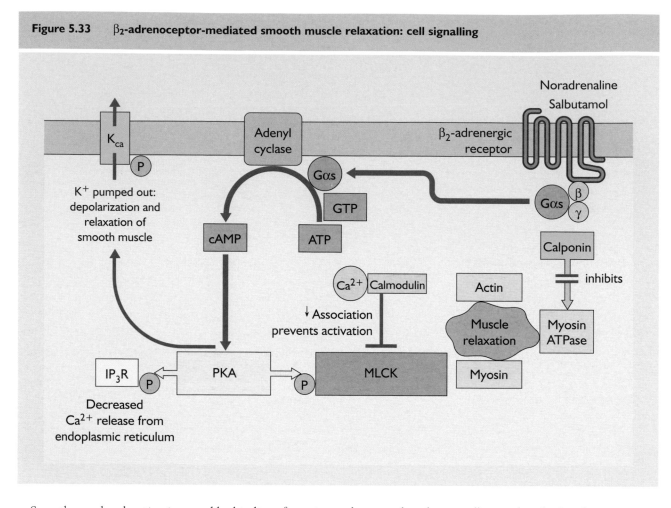

Smooth muscle relaxation is caused by binding of agonists such as noradrenaline or salbutamol to the β₂-adrenoceptor. This is a Gαs-coupled receptor that stimulates adenyl cyclase, resulting in the conversion of adenosine triphosphate (ATP) to cAMP. Increased cAMP levels activate protein kinase A (PKA) which phosphorylates myosin regulatory light chain kinase (MLCK). This decreases its association with calcium/calmodulin. In addition, inositol triphosphate receptors (IP₃R) on the endoplasmic reticulum (ER) are phosphorylated by PKA; this decreases Ca^{2+} release from the ER into the cytosol. The two pathways result in depolarization and relaxation of the smooth muscle. Adapted from Figure 4A of Johnson EN, Druey KM. *J Allergy Clin Immunol* 2002;109:592–602.

Calcium in smooth muscle cells binds calmodulin and activates MLCK, which, in turn, causes phosphorylation of myosin light chain 20 and facilitates actin–myosin interaction, cross-bridge cycling and smooth muscle contraction.

Clinical physiology (Figure 5.34)

β₂-Agonists are bronchodilators (or relievers) that lessen airway smooth muscle tone and reduce dynamic hyperinflation, thus causing relatively rapid relief of symptoms and improved exercise tolerance, but they do not alter the natural history of COPD. They have several actions[98]:

(1) *Bronchodilation* Relaxation of airway smooth muscle tone causes an increase in FEV₁, but, in COPD, these changes are generally small (< 10%). β₂-Agonists cause smooth muscle relaxation in large and small airways. They act as functional antagonists and reverse bronchoconstriction, irrespective of cause. Bronchodilator efficacy in COPD is generally assessed by the FEV₁, measured by spirometry, but this may not be useful[99]. Long-acting β₂-agonists cause bronchodilation for 12 h, and there is increasing evidence that these drugs are useful as additional bronchodilators in patients with COPD[100,101];

Figure 5.34   Actions of β₂-agonists in COPD

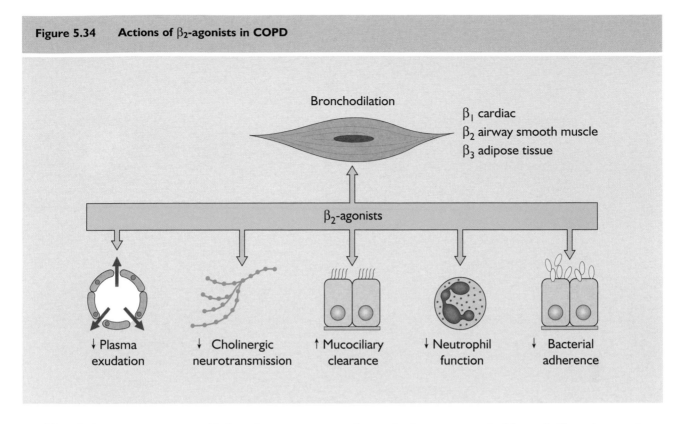

Although their primary action is likely to be on airway smooth muscle, there are several additional effects that may be beneficial. See text for details.

(2) *Decreased hyperinflation* Reduced dynamic hyperinflation with a reduction in residual volume and functional residual capacity may contribute to symptomatic benefits[36], since this makes breathing more comfortable and dyspnea is lessened[37,102];

(3) *Symptoms* Symptomatic improvement may be greater than indicated by changes in FEV₁, especially in moderate to severe COPD. Bronchodilator efficacy is often best judged by improvement in symptoms and improved exercise tolerance;

(4) *Exercise tolerance and health status* Improved exercise performance may be a conspicuous feature of bronchodilator usage in COPD[101], and can also be used to assess bronchodilator efficacy[99]. Salbutamol has been shown to increase exercise tolerance, but without necessarily having conspicuous effects on FEV₁[103]. Long-acting β₂-agonists cause improved symptoms, health-related quality of life and exercise performance[56,57,104];

(5) *Natural history* Usage of β₂-agonists does not modify the decline in lung function (FEV₁) in COPD[44];

(6) *Reduced plasma exudation* β₂-Agonists reduce plasma exudation in the airway by an action on the endothelial cells of post-capillary venules, thus closing the increased gaps between endothelial cells induced by inflammatory mediators[105–108];

(7) *Mucociliary clearance improvements* There is some evidence that β₂-agonists increase mucociliary clearance in patients with asthma and bronchitis[109,110];

(8) *Ventilatory drive* There is some evidence that β₂-agonists may increase the ventilatory drive to hypercapnia (but not to hypoxia)[111];

(9) *Inflammation* β₂-agonists have no obvious clinical effects on chronic inflammation, but may have increased activity in the presence of corticosteroids[112–114]. β₂-Agonists are potent mast cell stabilizing agents and have a variety of other potential anti-inflammatory actions;

169

(10) *Bacterial adherence*   Recent evidence suggests that β_2-agonists may reduce adherence of bacteria to airway epithelial cells and this may reduce the severity of infectious exacerbations[115];

(11) *Non-bronchodilator mechanisms*   Long-acting β_2-agonists have a range of alternative mechanisms other than as bronchodilators[83].

Clinical indications

* Salbutamol and terbutaline are indicated for relief symptoms on an 'as-required' basis for patients with COPD.

* Salmeterol and formoterol are selective long-acting β_2-agonists indicated for regular long-term chronic treatment of moderately severe COPD (GOLD Stage II), severe COPD (GOLD Stage III) and very severe (GOLD Stage IV).

* Salmeterol should not be taken for immediate relief (rescue) of acute symptoms of COPD or bronchospasm. This is because it has a relatively slow onset of some 10–20 min.

Dosage and administration

Inhalers for salbutamol (short-acting β_2-agonist), salmeterol (long-acting β_2-agonist), fluticasone propionate (corticosteroid) and fluticasone with salmeterol are shown in Figure 5.35.

Figure 5.35   A range of β_2-agonists and corticosteroid inhalers for the treatment of COPD

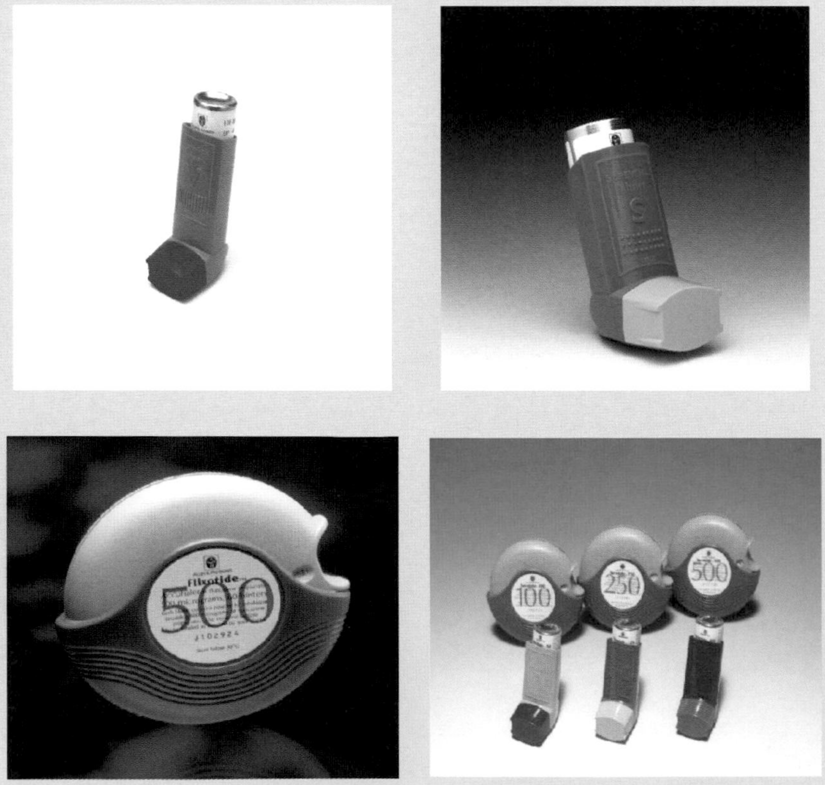

(a) Salbutamol (Ventolin®); (b) salmeterol (Serevent®); (c) fluticasone (Flixotide®); (d) salmeterol + fluticasone combined in a single dry powder inhaler (Discus® or Accuhaler®). Reproduced by courtesy of GlaxoSmithKline.

Salbutamol and terbutaline

These may be administered by dry powder inhaler or pressurized metered dose inhaler. A pressurized metered dose inhaler may be used in conjunction with a spacer. Salbutamol and terbutaline are generally given on an as-required basis.

- By pressurized metered dose inhaler, salbutamol is generally given as 100–200 µg (one to two puffs) up to four times daily, while, by dry powder inhaler, salbutamol may be given at 200–400 µg up to four times daily.

- By pressurized metered dose inhaler, terbutaline is generally given at 250–500 µg (one to two puffs) up to four times daily, while, by dry powder inhaler, terbutaline is usually given at 500 µg (one puff) up to four times daily.

Salmeterol

Salmeterol is generally given by inhalation at 50 µg (two puffs or one blister) twice daily for adults with COPD, although some patients may need 100 µg once or twice daily. Salmeterol (Serevent®, GlaxoSmithKline) is available as a dry powder inhaler in the Accuhaler® or Diskhaler®. Salmeterol is also available as a pressurized metered dose inhaler which is often best used in conjunction with a reservoir device such as a Volumatic spacer.

Formoterol

Formoterol is generally given by inhalation at 12 µg twice daily for adults with COPD, although some patients may need 24 µg once or twice daily. Foradil® (Novartis) is available as a dry powder inhaler, and Oxis Turbohaler® (AstraZeneca) is a dry powder inhaler.

Slow-release oral β₂-agonist preparations

Slow-release oral β_2-agonist preparations, such as bambuterol and slow-release salbutamol, are useful in some elderly patients who are unable to use inhalers. The advantage of these preparations is that they may treat peripheral airways more effectively, but the disadvantage is that side-effects are much more frequent than with inhaled preparations and they are slower in onset. Bambuterol is a prodrug which is slowly metabolized to terbutaline and is effective as a once-daily preparation in COPD[116]. In asthma at least, bambuterol appears to be as effective as inhaled salmeterol twice daily[117,118].

Efficacy

Salbutamol and terbutaline

Short-acting β_2-agonists have a relatively rapid onset of bronchodilator activity, although this is probably slower in COPD than in asthma. Salbutamol and terbutaline are partial agonists that act directly on the active site. The bronchodilator effects of salbutamol, terbutaline, and fenoterol usually wear off within 4–6 h[119]. When using the FEV_1 as the outcome, the dose–response relationship of salbutamol is relatively flat[120,121]. Following extended therapy, it has been demonstrated in a number of studies that ipratropium causes greater benefit than salbutamol[4]. In addition, salbutamol (albuterol) has less bronchodilator efficacy than Combivent® (ipratropium bromide combined with salbutamol in a single inhaler)[64].

Salmeterol

Onset and dose There is a delay of at least 10 min before onset of action of salmeterol in partially reversible COPD[122–124]. In a 16-week study, 50 µg of salmeterol twice-daily was found to be the optimal dose – it caused similar efficacy but less adverse events than with 100 µg twice daily.

Dyspnea Salmeterol reduces dyspnea and improves lung function in patients with COPD[56,98,125].

Exercise capacity Salmeterol increases the distance that patients with COPD can walk on a treadmill[126], and there is less perceived exertion on walking the same distance in 6 min[127]. Salmeterol and ipratropium have similar effects on dyspnea ratings during exercise[59].

Health-related quality of life Salmeterol at doses of 50 µg twice daily (but not for 100 µg twice daily) has been shown to have significant effects on health status[56,57,104,128]. The reduction in health status at higher doses is likely to be due to side-effects outweighing beneficial effects.

Additive effects Additive effects of salmeterol and theophylline have been described[129,130]. In addition, a study has found additive effects of salmeterol and ipratropium[101], although the combination has not been found to be more effective than salmeterol alone in patients with COPD[101,131].

Figure 5.36   Two studies comparing salmeterol with ipratropium bromide

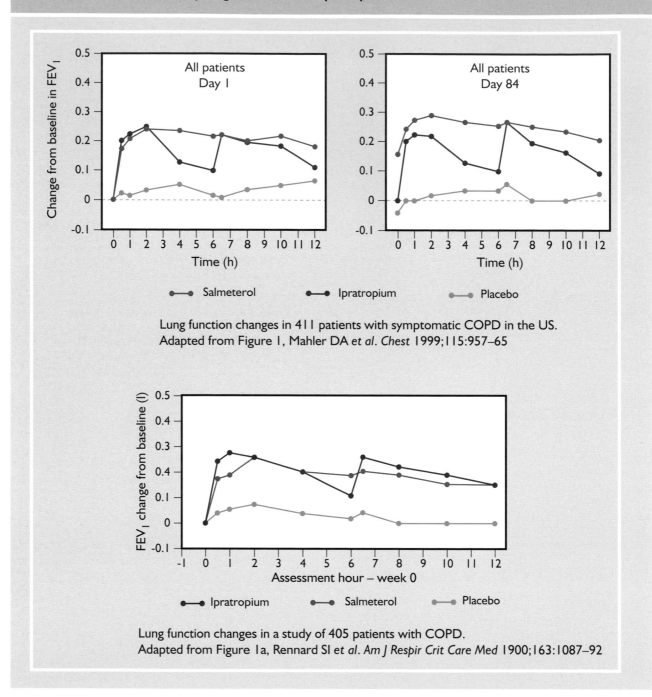

Lung function changes in 411 patients with symptomatic COPD in the US.
Adapted from Figure 1, Mahler DA *et al. Chest* 1999;115:957–65

Lung function changes in a study of 405 patients with COPD.
Adapted from Figure 1a, Rennard SI *et al. Am J Respir Crit Care Med* 1900;163:1087–92

Comparative studies   In one study, salmeterol has been demonstrated to cause superior bronchodilation to ipratropium in patients with COPD[57], while another study showed almost equivalent bronchodilation[56] (Figure 5.36). A recent 6-month large-scale study in patients with COPD has demonstrated that tiotropium once daily has superior effects than twice-daily salmeterol[33].

Formoterol

Onset, duration of action, dose response   Formoterol causes rapid bronchodilation, with onset as rapid as salbutamol, in patients with stable COPD[132,133], and faster onset of action than with salmeterol[134]. Formoterol has a duration of action of over 12 h in stable COPD[135], although salmeterol has a longer

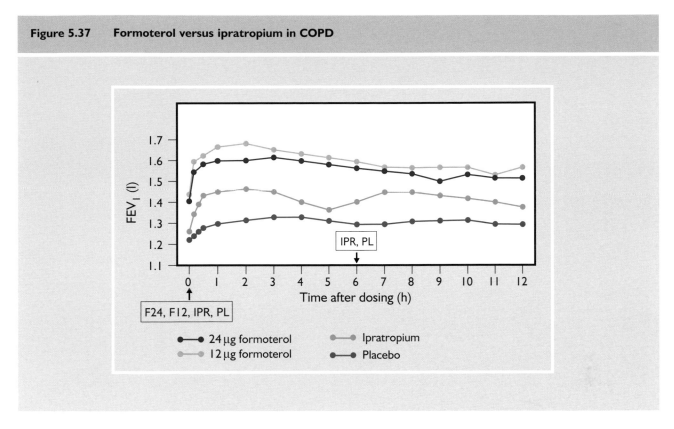

Figure 5.37 Formoterol versus ipratropium in COPD

12-h profile of mean FEV$_1$ measurements after 12 weeks dosing in the FICOPD I clinical study in 780 patients with COPD. Adapted from Figure 1B, Dahl R *et al. Am J Respir Crit Care Med* 2001;164:778–84.

duration[136]. Pretreatment with formoterol, salmeterol or oxitropium bromide still allows further bronchodilation with salbutamol[137]. A dose–response study with formoterol at 4.5, 9 or 18 µg versus placebo in 692 patients with COPD has been performed[138].

Pivotal studies An open, multicenter, 1-year trial in 242 patients with COPD demonstrated that formoterol 12 µg twice daily is effective[139]. In the FICOPD I Study in 780 patients with COPD, it was found that formoterol was superior to ipratropium bromide[60] (Figure 5.37). This was followed by the FICOPD II Study in 854 patients with COPD, which demonstrated that long-term treatment with inhaled formoterol is more effective and better tolerated than slow-release theophylline[140] (Figure 5.38).

Combination studies Effects of formoterol combined with ipratropium bromide[141] and formoterol with oxitropium bromide[142,143] are greater than with the two drugs alone. In addition, formoterol with ipratropium is more effective than salbutamol with ipratropium[144].

Contraindications and cautions

- *Hypersensitivity* Inhaled β$_2$-agonists are contraindicated in patients with a history of sensitivity to any of their constituents.

- *Hypertrophic cardiomyopathy* Avoid β$_2$-agonists because of their positive ionotropic effects. Extra care is required with myocardial insufficiency and hypokalemia.

- *Diabetes mellitus* Due to hyperglycemic effects of β$_2$-agonists, extra blood glucose measurements are initially recommended.

- *Thyrotoxicosis* Salmeterol should be administered with caution in patients with thyrotoxicosis.

Side-effects (Figure 5.39)

Following widespread clinical use of long-acting β$_2$-agonists, there is increasing reassurance on the safety of these agents when used within the context of

173

Figure 5.38   Comparison of the efficacy of formoterol with theophylline

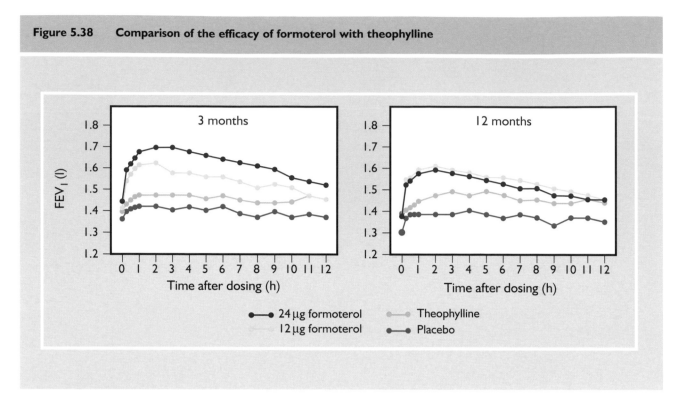

A study in 854 patients with symptomatic COPD from the FICOPD II Group. Adapted from Figure 1, Rossi A *et al.* *Chest* 2002;121:1058–69.

Figure 5.39   Side-effects of β_2-agonists

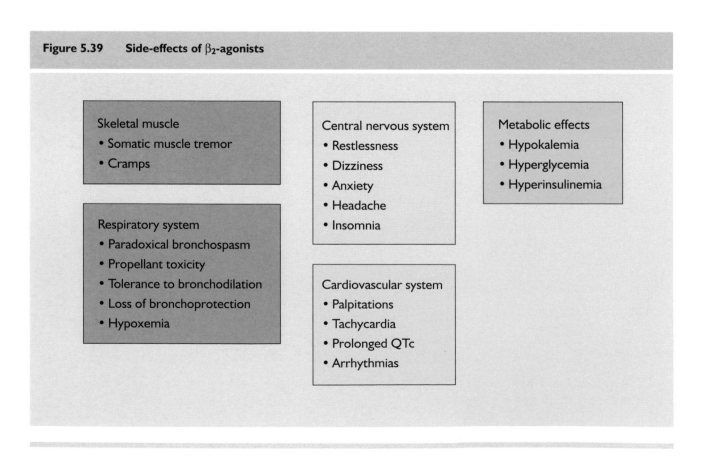

Skeletal muscle
- Somatic muscle tremor
- Cramps

Respiratory system
- Paradoxical bronchospasm
- Propellant toxicity
- Tolerance to bronchodilation
- Loss of bronchoprotection
- Hypoxemia

Central nervous system
- Restlessness
- Dizziness
- Anxiety
- Headache
- Insomnia

Cardiovascular system
- Palpitations
- Tachycardia
- Prolonged QTc
- Arrhythmias

Metabolic effects
- Hypokalemia
- Hyperglycemia
- Hyperinsulinemia

clinical guidelines for asthma and COPD. The pharmacological side-effects of β_2-agonist treatment, such as tremor, palpitations and headache, tend to be transient and reduce with regular therapy. In a study on healthy subjects, formoterol and salmeterol caused dose-related changes in systemic adverse events, with formoterol generally causing a more rapid onset of these adverse events[145]. The relative dose potencies for the systemic end-points were similar to the four-fold difference in recommended doses for salmeterol and formoterol, but a relatively modest therapeutic window was noted.

(1) *Skeletal muscle* Exaggerated somatic muscle tremor and cramps are troublesome in some elderly patients treated with high doses of β_2-agonists, due to a direct effect on skeletal muscle β_2-receptors;

(2) *Respiratory*

- *Paradoxical bronchospasm* has occurred on rare occasions and may be caused by propellants

- *Hypoxemia* can occur with mild falls in paO_2 after both short-acting and long-acting β_2-agonists. The clinical significance of this hypoxemia is doubtful, and may be caused by increased V/Q mismatch due to pulmonary vasodilatation. Oxygen consumption can be increased under resting conditions

- *Tolerance to bronchodilation* and *loss of bronchoprotection* have been described in asthma

(3) *Cardiovascular system* Sinus tachycardia, palpitations, prolonged QTc interval, vasodilation, and precipitation of cardiac rhythm disturbances in susceptible patients are relatively rare events. The mechanism may be caused by a direct effect on atrial β_2-receptors, combined with a reflex effect from increased peripheral vasodilatation via β_2-receptors. Short-acting inhaled β_2-agonists do not increase the risk of acute myocardial infarction in patients with COPD[146];

(4) *Central nervous system* Headache, restlessness, tension, dizziness and nervousness, and insomnia may occur;

(5) *Metabolic effects*

- *Hypokalemia* is caused by a direct effect on skeletal muscle uptake of potassium via β_2-receptors, and is usually a small effect and of no clinical significance, but it can be serious. In severe asthma, serum potassium levels should be monitored. Hypokalemia can occur, especially when treatment is combined with thiazide diuretics

- *Hyperglycemia* Increased blood glucose and insulin levels have also been reported, and are more relevant in diabetic patients

- *Tachyphylaxis* to metabolic effects occurs, unlike with the actions of bronchodilators.

THEOPHYLLINE

Summary

Reserve bronchodilator Theophylline slow-release (SR) is a reserve bronchodilator in patients with chronic stable COPD in the recent GOLD guidelines[1,147].

Oral The oral administration of theophylline (SR) has the advantage of treating small airways[148], and may be useful because many patients with COPD do not use their inhalers properly[149].

Biochemical actions Phosphodiesterase type 4 (PDE4) inhibition, adenosine antagonism and induction of histone deacetylase (HDAC) may be responsible for some of the actions of theophylline.

Physiological properties Beneficial properties of theophylline in stable COPD include bronchodilation, with improved respiratory drive and diaphragmatic strength, as well as increased mucociliary clearance, improved inspiratory muscle function, and anti-inflammatory effects.

Clinical benefits Clinically, there are improvements in lung function, with less dyspnea, and benefits during exercise and sleep, with improved quality of life.

Adverse events The major limitations to the use of theophylline are the variable hepatic metabolism and the tendency to side-effects, so that therapeutic monitoring of plasma levels is mandatory.

History

Caffeine is a plant alkaloid found in coffee beans, kola nuts (coca cola) and tea leaves (Figure 5.40), and caffeinated drinks have activities as central nervous system and cardiac stimulants, diuretics and bronchodilators. Henry Hyde Salter, a physician in Charing Cross Hospital in Victorian England, recognized the clinical benefits for asthma sufferers in drinking strong black coffee[11,150]. In the early 1970s, there were reports of theophylline slow-release being a useful monotherapy in asthma[151]. By 1980, theophylline had become a leading medication for asthma[151,152]. Following this, theophylline has been used alone and in combination with other bronchodilators for COPD[153–155]. Theophylline is off patent, and is a cheap and readily available medication.

Molecular structure

The natural metabolite xanthine is a precursor of uric acid, and theophylline and caffeine are methylated xanthine derivatives (Figure 5.41). Methyl attachments at nitrogen-1 (possibly) and nitrogen-3 enhance the bronchodilator properties of xanthine, and 1,3 dimethyl xanthine comprises theophylline.

Mode of action

The mode of action of methylxanthines remains controversial.

- *PDE inhibition* Phosphodiesterase (PDE) inhibition increases cyclic AMP and cyclic GMP levels, and is probably important for bronchodilator action[156]. This weak and non-selective PDE inhibition may also be important in reducing neutrophilic inflammation and levels of tumor necrosis factor-α (TNF-α)[157,158]. Non-specific inhibition of different subtypes of PDE4 inhibitors may explain the large variety of toxic side-effects.

- *HDAC induction* Induction of histone deacetylase (HDAC) activity by theophylline has recently been shown to decrease inflammatory gene expression[159]. This occurs at therapeutic concentrations of theophylline and is independent of other known pharmacological actions. It predicts a potentiation of the anti-inflammatory action of corticosteroids, which work through a similar mechanism.

- *A_1 and A_2 receptor antagonism* Adenosine receptor antagonism accounts for some of the

Figure 5.40   Botanical origin of methylxanthines

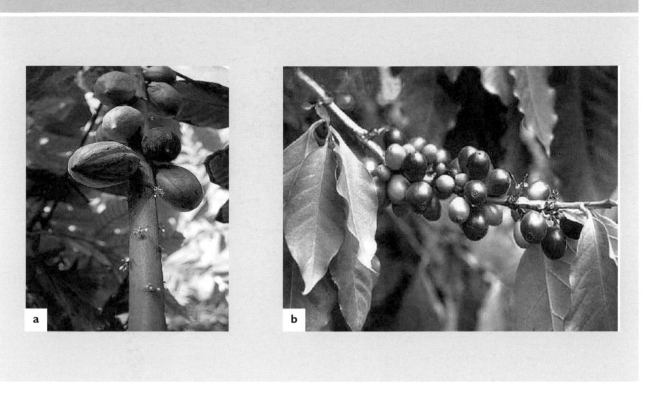

(a) Theobromine pods (cocoa); (b) coffee arabica beans. Reproduced by permission of Henriette Kress (www.iblio.org/herbmed).

Figure 5.41   Structures of xanthine derivatives

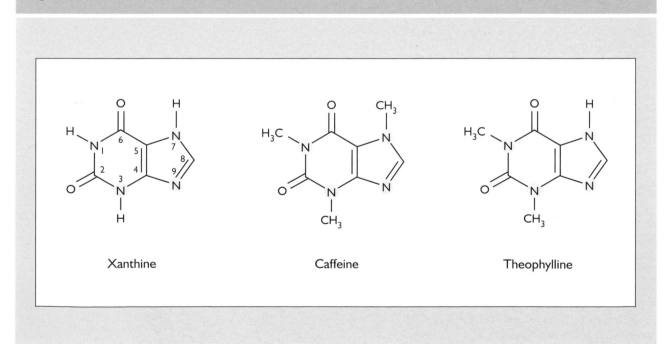

Xanthine   Caffeine   Theophylline

side-effects, but there is little evidence that this is relevant for bronchodilator effects. Theophylline inhibits both A_1 and A_2 receptors.

Physiological mode of action (Figure 5.42)

- *Bronchodilation* Theophylline is a useful additional second-line bronchodilator in patients with COPD, and oral administration has the advantage of treating small airways[148]. While not as effective a bronchodilator as salmeterol, theophylline has an additive effect when the two drugs are used together[130]. Theophylline has effects on lung function, dyspnea, and exercise tolerance[154]. Theophylline also has an additive effect when combined with ipratropium bromide and salbutamol[160]. Withdrawal of theophylline in patients with severe COPD results in significant deterioration, despite the continuation of other bronchodilator therapy[161].

- *Respiratory muscles* Changes in diaphragmatic and respiratory muscle function have been reported[162,163], but it is unknown whether this translates into effects on dynamic lung volumes.

Theophylline may give good symptomatic improvement without any change in spirometry (FEV_1); this may be due to lung deflation and a reduction in residual volume[148,164].

- Mucociliary clearance is increased[165].

- *Anti-inflammatory effects* These may be important in COPD, with an inhibitory effect on neutrophilic inflammation[157]. Induced sputum neutrophils, IL-8 and myeloperoxidase are reduced by theophylline, and there is decreased neutrophil chemotactic activity[158].

Clinical indications

- Theophylline is a reserve bronchodilator for patients with Stage II (moderate), Stage III (severe) and Stage IV (very severe) stable COPD not controlled by either regular inhaled anticholinergics nor short- and long-acting β_2-agonists[1].

- Theophylline is effective in stable COPD, but, due to its narrow therapeutic : toxic ratio, inhaled bronchodilators (anticholinergics and β_2-agonists) are generally preferred. Theo-

Figure 5.42   Actions of theophylline in COPD

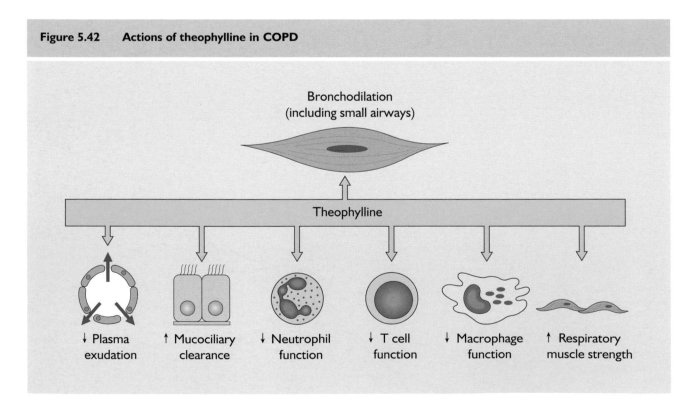

There may be several mechanisms of action of this drug.

phylline may be especially useful in patients who have symptoms at night[166].

Dosage and administration

- A slow-release (SR) preparation of theophylline should be given orally twice daily in COPD; slow absorption causes less adverse effects.

- For chronic use, initial slow increments in the dose of theophylline in a slow upward titration must be employed. For example,

  200 mg every 12 h, increased after 1 week to 300 mg every 12 h

  300 mg every 12 h, increased after 1 week to 400 mg every 12 h

  Every week the dose can be adjusted by 100–150 mg steps, as required.

- Depending on the formulation and manufacturer's recommendations, theophylline may eventually be given at up to 1000 mg daily, usually comprising up to 500 mg every 12 h.

- A larger evening or morning dose may be used to give effects when symptoms are most severe.

- For chronic COPD, theophylline doses should generally be titrated to give steady-state serum concentrations of 10–12 mg/l (µg/ml) (55–66 µmol/l), although sometimes a wider serum range of 10–20 mg/l (µg/ml) (55–110 µmol/l) is used.

Serum theophylline levels (Figure 5.43)

- Measurement of serum theophylline levels is useful in all patients given theophylline, with particular levels loosely corresponding to effects[151].

- Serum theophylline levels are best taken at the time of peak absorption of the drug, this being 5–9 h after the morning dose of theophylline sustained release (SR).

- Serum theophylline levels for optimal responses in COPD are 10–12 mg/l (55–66 µmol/l)[167].

- The toxic : therapeutic ratio is small, and most of the benefit occurs when near toxic doses are

Figure 5.43   Serum theophylline levels

Theophylline serum level (µg/ml)	Clinical effect
> 30	seizures
> 25	cardiac arrhythmias
> 20	nausea and vomiting
10–20	therapeutic range
10–12	optimal range
< 5	no bronchodilator effects seen

given[167]. Toxic effects may occur within the therapeutic range of theophylline[168].

Factors affecting theophylline blood levels (Figure 5.44)

Theophylline does not distribute into fatty tissues; hence lean body weight should be used in calculating theophylline doses. Data on duration of action for slow-release theophylline in COPD are not available. The therapeutic effect of theophylline is related to serum concentration, which is affected by several factors that alter clearance. Theophylline is largely metabolized by the liver – especially by hepatic cytochrome P450 mixed function oxidases (in particular, CYP1A2). Not surprisingly, an increased dose may be required for the heavy-drinking and -smoking, protein-eating, younger male. A decreased dose is required in older females, with a high carbohydrate diet and heart, respiratory and liver disease[169]. If in doubt as to whether therapeutic or toxic levels are present, always repeat measurements of theophylline serum concentration. Theophylline is largely eliminated by the kidneys.

Efficacy

- Improved respiratory function and reduced dyspnea have been reported[163,164,170,171] with increased respiratory drive[172].

- Dose responses are relatively flat for low, medium and high doses[148].

- Improved cardiorespiratory exercise performance[173–176], sleep[177] and nocturnal oxygen saturation[178] have been reported.

- Quality of life is improved[170].

- Diaphragmatic strength is increased[162].

- Theophylline withdrawal results in deterioration in 72% of patients[161].

Comparative clinical studies

The addition of theophylline to salbutamol in patients with COPD results in improvement compared with using the drugs alone[171]. However, another study concluded that adding theophylline to

---

Figure 5.44   Factors affecting theophylline blood levels

Increased clearance (increased dose)	Decreased clearance (decreased dose)
1. Enzyme induction: rifampicin anticonvulsants phenobarbitone	1. Enzyme inhibition: cimetidine (not ranitidine) erythromycin, ciprofloxacin, allopurinol, ketoconazole, zafirlukast
2. Ethanol	2. Old age
3. Cigarette smoking: tobacco, marijuana	3. Congestive heart failure
4. Childhood	4. Respiratory acidosis and pneumonia
5. High-protein, low-carbohydrate diet	5. Liver cirrhosis
6. Barbecued meat	6. Viral hepatitis
	7. High-carbohydrate diet

ipratropium bromide and salbutamol may be of little value[160]. It is noteworthy that, in a major recent study, theophylline was found to be inferior to formoterol in stable COPD[140] (Figure 5.38).

Cautions

Slow-release theophylline has a narrow toxic : therapeutic ratio, and monitoring of serum theophylline levels is mandatory. Factors that increase or decrease the clearance of theophylline must be considered, and the potential for drug interactions is large. In addition, caution must be employed in patients with heart, respiratory and liver disease.

Side-effects (Figure 5.45)

Side-effects are generally related to serum concentration, although some patients may be particularly susceptible. Side-effects may be reduced by slowly increasing the dose of theophylline in an initial gradual-dose titration when theophylline is introduced. The following side-effects may occur:

* Nausea and vomiting, appetite loss, gastric upset, abdominal discomfort, heartburn, gastroesophageal reflux, diarrhea and hematemesis

* Headache, anxiety, restlessness, insomnia and tremor

* Epileptic seizures include full-blown grand mal episodes, irrespective of past epileptic history

* Diuresis

* Cardiac arrhythmias: palpitations, atrial and ventricular arrhythmias, supraventricular tachycardia, ventricular tachycardia, hypotension

* Risk of overdose, unlike with other bronchodilators

Figure 5.45   Side-effects of theophylline

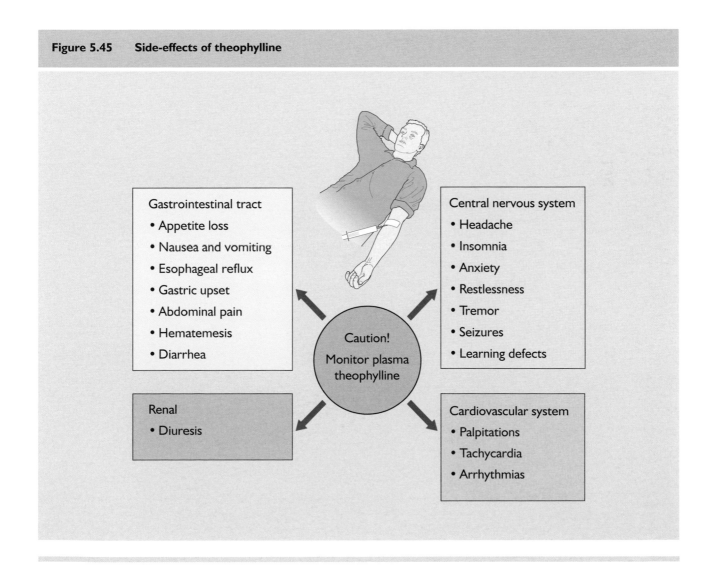

Gastrointestinal tract
• Appetite loss
• Nausea and vomiting
• Esophageal reflux
• Gastric upset
• Abdominal pain
• Hematemesis
• Diarrhea

Renal
• Diuresis

Caution!
Monitor plasma theophylline

Central nervous system
• Headache
• Insomnia
• Anxiety
• Restlessness
• Tremor
• Seizures
• Learning defects

Cardiovascular system
• Palpitations
• Tachycardia
• Arrhythmias

INHALED CORTICOSTEROIDS

Summary

The role of inhaled steroids in COPD patients is currently controversial[179,180]. The cumulative experience from four 3-year large-scale studies is that inhaled corticosteroids do not alter the rate of loss of lung function (FEV_1) in COPD, and thus they do not affect the natural history of COPD. However, there is evidence that inhaled corticosteroids may improve quality of life, decrease exacerbations and improve survival. In some studies, improvement in exercise tolerance has been demonstrated. A proportion of patients with COPD have coexisting asthma and show a pronounced corticosteroid response; these patients should be labelled as having combined COPD with asthma and treated with long-term inhaled corticosteroids[181]. It should be noted that there are significant adverse events from use of long-term, high-dose, inhaled corticosteroids in some elderly patients with COPD[182].

Figure 5.46   Structure of hydrocortisone and inhaled corticosteroids

Hydrocortisone

Budesonide

Beclomethasone dipropionate

Fluticasone propionate

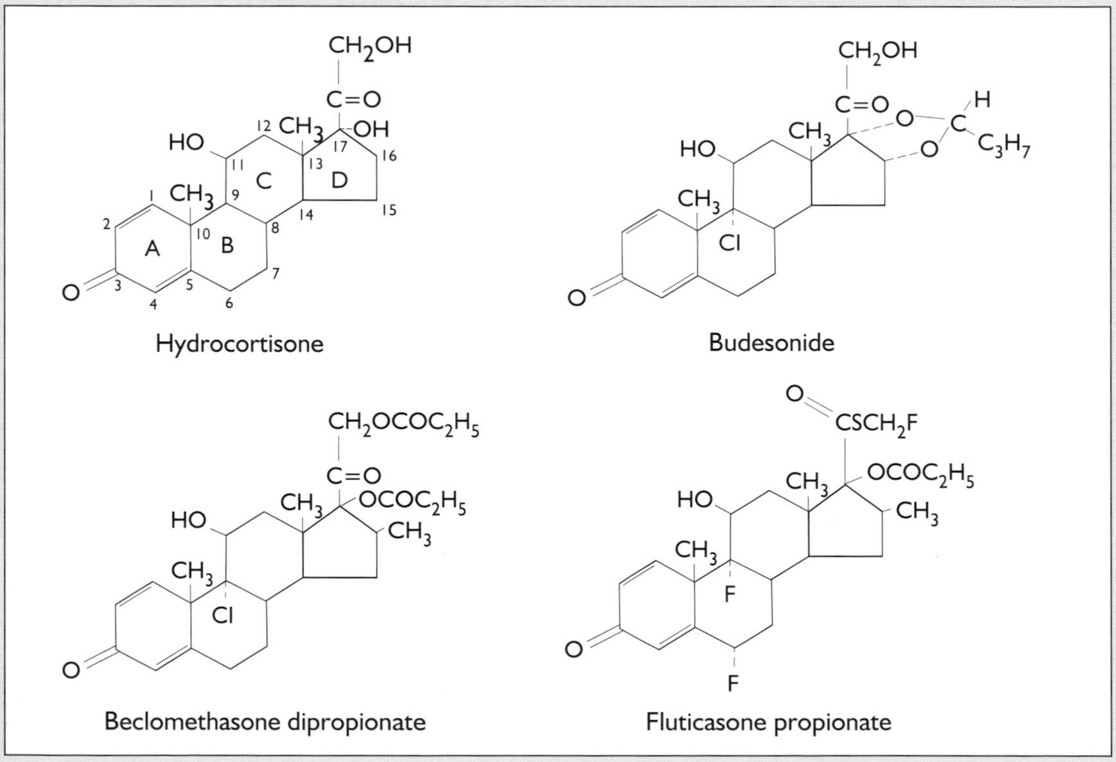

Molecular structures

Natural hormones with glucocorticoid action include hydrocortisone (cortisol), corticosterone and cortisone; these compounds regulate metabolism and provide resistance to stress. Corticosteroids such as hydrocortisone and synthetic dexamethasone were given by inhalation for asthma in the 1950s, but caused prominent side-effects due to systemic absorption.

Hydrocortisone contains the characteristic steroid nucleus, consisting of three 6-carbon rings (ABC), and a single 5-carbon ring (D) (Figure 5.46). Hydrocortisone is the major glucocorticoid

Figure 5.47   Corticosteroid GR dimer transactivation

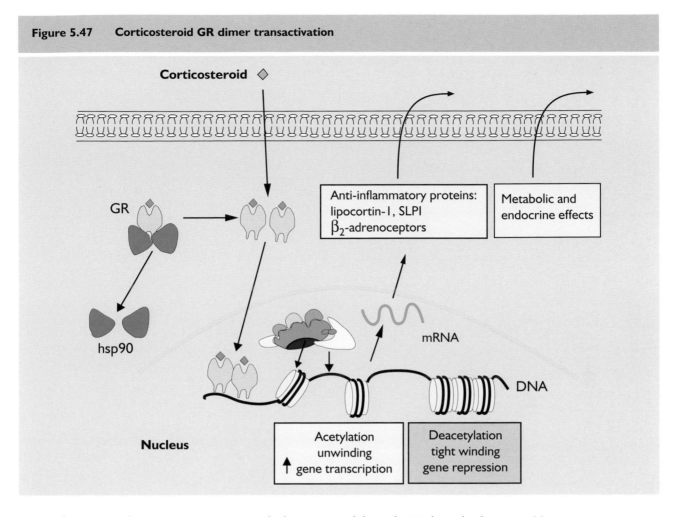

GR, glucocorticoid receptor; SLPI, secretory leukoprotease inhibitor; hsp90, heat shock protein 90.

produced by the adrenal cortex, while cortisone differs from hydrocortisone by having a ketone group at C11.

Beclomethasone dipropionate, budesonide and fluticasone propionate are synthetic analogs of hydrocortisone and have a high topical anti-inflammatory activity. Among the synthetic corticosteroids, modifications at C16 and C17 positions have significantly topical anti-inflammatory potency:

- *Beclomethasone dipropionate* (BDP) has two propionate groups at C17, and the active metabolite is beclomethasone monopropionate (17-BMP).

- *Budesonide* is a non-halogenated corticosteroid with high topical anti-inflammatory potency and low systemic bioavailability.

- *Fluticasone propionate* is a trifluorinated glucocorticoid that is derived from the 17 carbothioate (sulfur-containing) series.

Mechanism of action

Corticosteroids freely diffuse from the circulation across cell membrane where they interact with cytoplasmic glucocorticoid receptors (GR) in almost all nucleated cells[183] (Figure 5.47). Following steroid binding, the receptor is activated and discards heat shock protein 90 (hsp90) fragments; these 'molecular chaperones' previously prevented unoccupied GR localizing to the nuclear compartment.

Transcription of anti-inflammatory protein (transactivation by GR dimer)

The activated GR-steroid dimerizes and translocates to the nucleus, where it binds to specific DNA sequences, glucocorticoid response elements (GRE) within the promoter region of genes. Binding of GR homodimers via zinc fingers to the GRE causes unfolding of DNA. This permits access of the cAMP

Figure 5.48   **The transcription factor–CREB binding protein–RNA polymerase II complex**

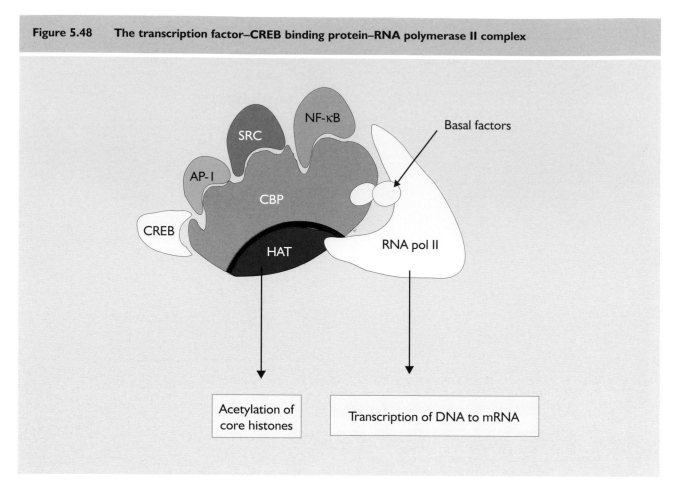

CREB, cAMP response element binding protein; CBP, CREB binding protein; NF-κB, nuclear factor-κB; SRC, steroid receptor coactivator – glucocorticoid activated glucocorticoid receptors (GR) bind to SRC; AP-1, activator protein-1; HAT, histone acetylase; RNA pol II, RNA polymerase II.

Figure 5.49   **Corticosteroid GR dimer transactivation**

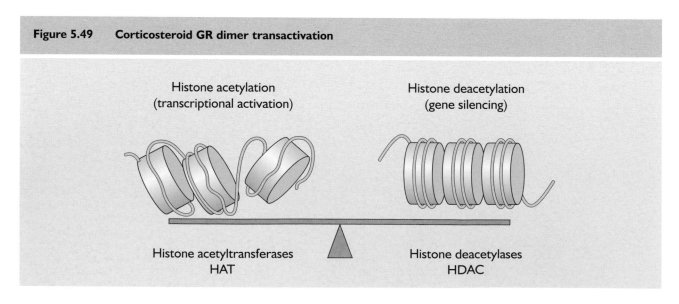

Histone acetylation (HAT) causes unwinding of DNA and permits transcriptional activation through access to RNA polymerase. Conversely, histone deacetylation (HDAC) causes tight winding of DNA and gene silencing.

response element binding protein (CREB)-binding protein (CBP), which forms a scaffold for attached transcription factors, and has histone acetyl transferase (HAT) activity (Figure 5.48). Acetylation of histones permits unwinding of the local DNA and permits the RNA polymerase II (RNA pol II) to transcribe messenger RNA (Figure 5.49). Anti-inflammatory proteins that are transcribed through corticosteroid action include secretory leukoprotease inhibitor (SLPI). The endocrine and metabolic effects of corticosteroids are thought to be mediated via GRE binding.

Repression of transcription factors (transrepression by GR monomer)

Most of the anti-inflammatory effects of corticosteroids are thought to be mediated by the repression of transcription factors (Figure 5.50). GR acting as a monomer interacts with CBP, causing an inhibition of CBP-mediated HAT activity. In addition, GR may also recruit histone deacetylases (HDACs) to the CBP complex; this deacetylation leads to tight nucleosome compaction and repression of transcription.

Effects in COPD

Theoretically, it might be expected that inhaled steroids would be beneficial in the long term if they suppress the inflammatory response in the airways. In COPD, anti-inflammatory drugs are required to reduce neutrophil and macrophage inflammation. However, these effects have not been demonstrated in COPD with even high doses of oral or inhaled corticosteroids, with no changes in neutrophil

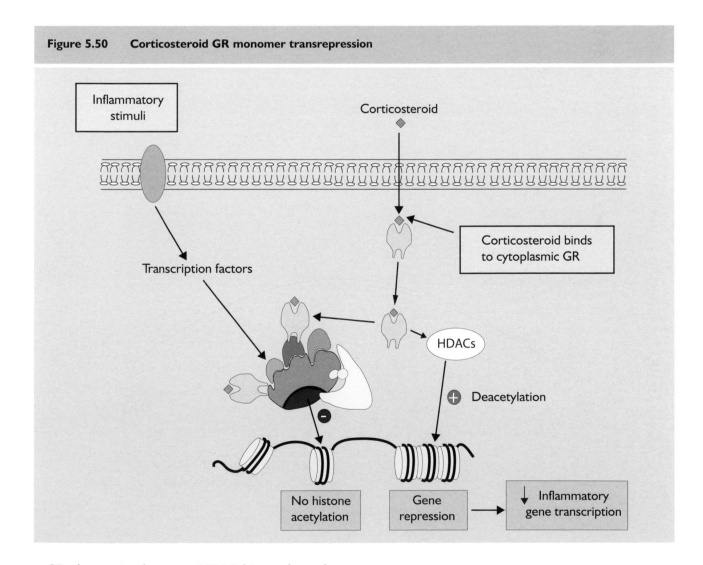

Figure 5.50   Corticosteroid GR monomer transrepression

GR, glucocorticoid receptor; HDAC, histone deacetylase.

counts, neutrophil activation markers, inflammatory cytokines or proteases[184–186]. This may be because neutrophilic inflammation in humans is not suppressible, since neutrophil survival is prolonged by steroids[187,188]. Indeed, there may be a resistance to the anti-inflammatory effects of corticosteroids in COPD, as corticosteroids inhibit, in normal subjects and asthmatic patients, the expression of cytokines which are not inhibited in patients with COPD. Cigarette smoke and oxidative stress appear to interfere with the molecular mechanism of corticosteroid action[189].

Corticosteroid resistance

There may be an active resistance to corticosteroids in COPD, since high doses of steroids fail to reduce levels of cytokines and chemokines[184,185]. The molecular mechanisms of steroid resistance remain obscure, but could be the same as those that result in amplification of inflammatory responses. Thus, a reduction in HDAC in macrophages[189] may prevent the anti-inflammatory action of steroids through failure of HDAC recruitment to the inflammatory gene complex[190]. Similarly, latent adenovirus induces corticosteroid resistance in animal experiments[191].

Clinical studies

Effects on natural history of FEV₁

Four long-term studies have examined the use of long-term inhaled corticosteroids on the progression of COPD (Figure 5.51). The place of inhaled corticosteroids in the management of COPD remains uncertain after these studies, which failed to report a statistically significant effect on the rate of decline of FEV_1.

- The Copenhagen Lung Study investigated a similar group of patients with mild asthma from a single population and found no benefit of inhaled budesonide (800 µg daily) compared with placebo over 3 years[192].

- The EuroSCOP study investigated patients with mild COPD and compared budesonide 800 µg daily with placebo over 3 years of therapy. There was no significant change in the rate of decline in FEV_1[193]. Note that there was some effect of budesonide in the first 3 months, before the fall in FEV_1 seemed to continue at the same rate as with placebo (Figure 5.52).

- The ISOLDE study investigated a more severe group of patients and demonstrated no effect of fluticasone propionate (1000 µg daily) on the rate of decline in lung function over 3 years, although there was some improvement in the quality of life and a small reduction in exacerbations[194].

- The Lung Health Study II showed that triamcinolone 600 µg twice daily had no effect on the decline in lung function over 3.5 years in patients with moderate COPD[195].

Effects on survival and exacerbations

Recently, in a study in general practice, it has been found that regular use of inhaled fluticasone propionate, alone or in combination with salmeterol, causes increased survival in COPD patients[196]. In a population-based study in Ontario, Canada ($n = 22\,620$), it was found that inhaled corticosteroid therapy was associated with decreased COPD-related morbidity and mortality in elderly patients[197] (Figure 5.53). In a group of patients who had suffered from repeated exacerbations, inhaled fluticasone propionate for 6 months was found to have some clinical benefits in the prevention of exacerbations[198]. Furthermore, prevention of exacerbations is a feature of the ISOLDE study[194], and this effect is seen predominantly in patients with a post-bronchodilator FEV_1 of < 50% predicted[199]. On discontinuation of inhaled fluticasone in patients with COPD, there is a more rapid onset of exacerbations[200]. In 24 elderly men with severe irreversible airway obstruction, withdrawal of inhaled beclomethasone dipropionate led to a deterioration in ventilatory function and increased exercise-induced dyspnea[201].

Combined inhaled corticosteroids and long-acting β₂-agonists

The combination of fluticasone (F) and salmeterol (S) in a single inhaler (Seretide®, GlaxoSmithKline) improves pre-dose lung function and severity of dyspnea in patients with COPD[202–204]. In particular, the TRISTAN study (TRial of Inhaled STeroids ANd long-acting β₂-agonist) demonstrated that the combination (F + S) at 52 weeks improved pre-treatment (also without bronchodilator) FEV_1 over a 1-year period compared with placebo by 133 ml, when salmeterol alone caused a 73 ml improvement

Figure 5.51   Long-term studies of inhaled corticosteroids (ICS) in COPD

Study	Copenhagen	EuroSCOP[a]	ISOLDE[b]	Lung Health Study II
References	*Lancet* 1999; 353:1819–23	*N Engl J Med* 1999; 340:1948–53	*BMJ* 2000; 320:1297–303	*N Engl J Med* 2000; 343:1902–9
Recruitment	from Copenhagen Heart Study: epidemiological study	mass media advertisements	from UK hospital clinics	from LHS I in USA
Reversibility assessment	< 15% increase over pre-bronchodilator FEV_1 after β_2-agonist < 15% increase over post-bronchodilator FEV_1 with prednisolone	< 10% predicted FEV_1 increase after β_2-agonist	< 10% predicted FEV_1 increase after β_2-agonist	no limit averaged 3.7% predicted FEV_1
Mean age (years)	59	52	64	56
Mean post-bronchodilator FEV_1 (l)	2.38	2.65	1.40	2.28
Mean post-bronchodilator FEV_1 (% predicted)	86	79	50	68
Randomized (n)	290	1277	751	1116
Current smoking (%)	76	100 continue smoking	48	
Completed (%)	70	71	53	>90
Therapy (daily dose)	budesonide 120 µg for 6 months 800 µg for 30 months	budesonide 800 µg for 36 months	fluticasone 1000 µg for 36 months	triamcinolone 1200 µg for 36 months
Primary end-point	All four studies assessed effects of inhaled corticosteroids in subjects with: • smoking-related airways obstruction • poor reversibility to inhaled β_2-agonists Slope of change in post-bronchodilator FEV_1 was main outcome			
Slope change in FEV_1 (% predicted), ml/year	ICS 46 placebo 49	57 69	50 59	44 47
Total change in FEV_1 (% predicted) ml over 0–36 mths	ICS – placebo –	140 180	133 197	– –
Health status			fluticasone deterioration by 2 U/year placebo deterioration by 3.2 U/year	
Exacerbations (number/subject/year)	0.36	<0.20	fluticasone 1.32 placebo 0.99 25% decrease	
Adverse events				

[a] EuroSCOP, European Respiratory Society study on Chronic Obstructive Pulmonary Disease
[b] ISOLDE, the Inhaled Steroids in Obstructive Lung Disease in Europe study

187

Figure 5.52   EuroSCOP: effects of budesonide on FEV₁

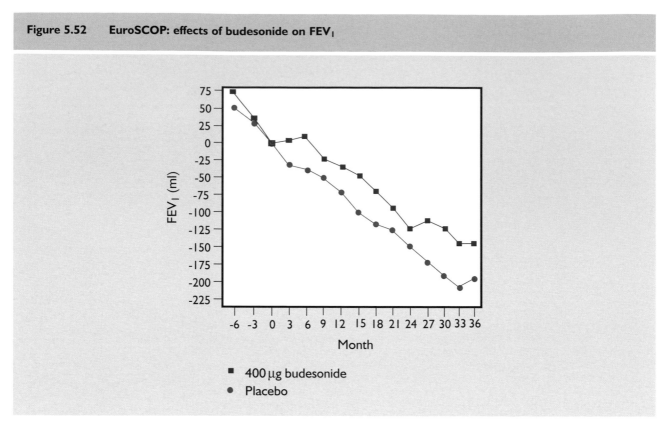

Adapted from Figure 1, Pauwels *et al.* *N Engl J Med* 1999;340:1948–53. EuroSCOP: European Respiratory Society Study on COPD

Figure 5.53   Hospitalization-free survival after inhaled corticosteroids

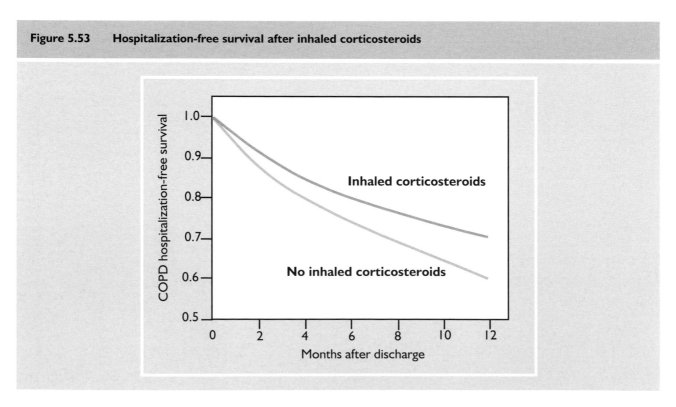

Adjusted probability of hospitalization-free survival in COPD patients who did and did not receive inhaled corticosteroids post-discharge from hospital. Adapted from Sin DD, Tu JB. *Am J Respir Crit Care Med* 2001;164:S80–4

and fluticasone caused a 95 ml improvement[203,204] (Figure 5.54). The TRISTAN study demonstrated reduced frequency of exacerbations with Seretide®, while combined budesonide and formoterol (Symbicort®, Astra-Zeneca) has been found to decrease the number of severe exacerbations of COPD when compared with placebo and formoterol[205] (Figure 5.54).

Side-effects

It is important to consider the risk of side-effects of inhaled corticosteroids (Figure 5.55). Patients with COPD are at particular risk of systemic effects of inhaled corticosteroids (osteoporosis, cataracts, skin bruising, glaucoma) as they are elderly, immobile and often have a poor diet[179]. The Lung Health II Study showed a reduction in bone density in the lumbar spine and femur in the triamcinolone-treated group[195]. Furthermore, in a population-based case–control study, inhaled corticosteroids were associated with a dose-related increase in hip fracture[206].

Corticosteroid trial

Inhaled corticosteroids are recommended in those patients who have concomitant asthma, as demonstrated by a bronchodilator response, or a clear improvement on oral corticosteroids[179]. However, the GOLD guidelines note that a short course of oral corticosteroids is a poor predictor of long-term response to inhaled corticosteroids[194,207]. A formal trial of 2 weeks of oral or 4–6 weeks of inhaled corticosteroids may be used to exclude chronic asthma, and these patients may have increased numbers of eosinophils in the sputum and an increase in exhaled nitric oxide[181,208].

Clinical indications

The updated GOLD guidelines of 2003 recommend inhaled corticosteroids for the treatment of symptomatic patients with severe (stage III) and very severe (stage IV) COPD with frequent exacerbations (Figure 5.1):

Figure 5.54 Effect of combined inhaled corticosteroid and long-acting β₂-agonist on FEV₁ in COPD

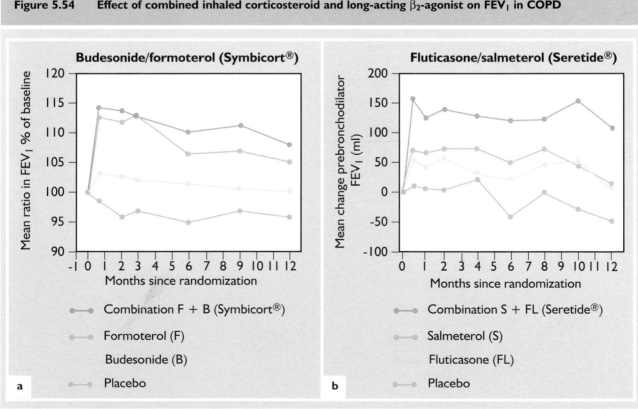

(a) Adapted from Fig 2, Szafranski W, *et al. Eur Respir J* 2003;21:74–81; (b) Adapted from Fig 2A, Calverley P, *et al. Lancet* 2003;361:449–56

Figure 5.55   Potential adverse effects of inhaled corticosteroids

Local	Systemic
• Oropharyngeal fungal infections: *Candida albicans* or *Aspergillus niger* • Dysphonia due to adductor vocal cord myopathy and paresis • Cough and bronchoconstriction	• Suppression of hypothalamic–pituitary–adrenal axis • Osteoporosis and decreased bone mineral density • Growth abnormalities • Spontaneous and easy bruising • Cataracts • Glaucoma

- Symptomatic COPD with a pre-bronchodilator FEV$_1$ of < 50%

- Repeated exacerbations, e.g. three in the past 3 years

GOLD (2003) notes that corticosteroids combined with long-acting β$_2$-agonists are more effective than the components alone.

MISCELLANEOUS COPD THERAPY

Vaccination

- Influenza vaccine is recommended for all patients with COPD, since they are subject to severe exacerbations with this infection, and there is evidence for a reduction in acute exacerbations and hospital admissions[209]. There is now convincing evidence that influenza vaccination is cost-effective in elderly people and should be more so in patients with COPD[210]. Influenza vaccination should be given every autumn.

- Polyvalent pneumococcal vaccine is used in many countries to protect against the development of pneumococcal lung infections[211]. Pneumococcal vaccination is cost-effective in reducing infective exacerbations in COPD, but there is insufficient evidence to support general use in COPD patients.

- OM85-BV (Broncho-vaxom®) is a mixture of bacterial products that activate macrophage function. There is some evidence that it may reduce the severity of acute exacerbations, but it cannot be recommended as a routine treatment[212].

Mucolytics

Because mucus hypersecretion is a prominent feature of chronic bronchitis, various mucolytic therapies have been used to increase the ease of mucus expectoration, in the belief that this will improve lung function[213].

- *Smoking cessation* is the most effective way to reduce mucus hypersecretion.

- *Anticholinergics* may decrease mucus hypersecretion.

- β$_2$-*Agonists and theophylline* may improve mucus clearance.

- *Steam inhalation* (with or without aromatics) may provide symptomatic relief, but there is no evidence that it improves lung function or long-term symptom control.

- Several drugs, such as *carbocisteine, bromhexol and ambroxol*, reduce mucus viscosity *in vitro*, but there is little evidence from controlled trials that they improve lung function in patients with COPD, and they cannot be recommended as routine therapy.

- Expectorants, such as *guaiphenesin* and *potassium iodide*, similarly have no proven beneficial effects.

- *Recombinant human DNAse* (alfadornase, Pulmozyme®) has beneficial effects in some patients with cystic fibrosis, but was unsuccessful in the treatment of exacerbations in patients with COPD[214].

Antioxidants

Since oxidant damage may be critical in the pathophysiology of COPD, antioxidant therapy is logical, but the GOLD guidelines do not recommend use of antioxidants[215]. *N*-acetyl-cysteine (NAC) was originally developed as a mucolytic, but has well-documented antioxidant effects. Controlled trials have demonstrated that it reduces the frequency and severity of acute exacerbations of COPD[216] and, in an open study, significantly reduces the rate of decline in lung function[217]. NAC may therefore be useful in long-term management of COPD, but is not currently available on prescription in the UK. A recent meta-analysis has demonstrated a beneficial effect of NAC in reducing exacerbations of COPD by approximately 25%[216,218].

Neuraminidase inhibitors

Inhibitors of neuraminidase, such as zanamivir (inhaled) and oseltamivir (oral) speed the recovery from influenza and may protect against its development[219,220]. However, there are no specific trials in patients with COPD and it is not yet certain whether this treatment is cost-effective.

Antitussives

Cough is often a troublesome symptom of COPD, but may have a protective effect in clearing secretions. The regular use of antitussives is therefore not recommended in COPD[221].

REFERENCES

1. National Institutes of Health (NIH), National Heart Lung and Blood Institute (NHLBI), World Health Organisation (WHO). Global Initiative for Chronic Obstructive Lung Disease (GOLD) : Global Strategy for the Diagnosis, Management, and Prevention of Chronic Obstructive Pulmonary Disease NHLBI/WHO Workshop Report.www.goldcopd.com/workshop/index.html. 2001

2. MacNee W, Calverley PM. Chronic obstructive pulmonary disease. 7. Management of COPD. *Thorax* 2003;58:261–5

3. British Thoracic Society. BTS guidelines for the management of chronic obstructive pulmonary disease. *Thorax* 1997;52(Suppl 5):S1–28

4. Rennard SI, Serby CW, Ghafouri M, Johnson PA, Friedman M. Extended therapy with ipratropium is associated with improved lung function in patients with COPD. A retrospective analysis of data from seven clinical trials. *Chest* 1996;110:62–70

5. Vincken W, van Noord JA, Greefhorst AP, Bantje TA, Kesten S, Korducki L, *et al.* Improved health outcomes in patients with COPD during 1 yr's treatment with tiotropium. *Eur Respir J* 2002;19:209–16

6. Hansel TT, Barnes PJ. Tiotropium bromide: a novel once-daily anticholinergic bronchodilator for the treatment of COPD. *Drugs Today* 2002;38:585–600

7. van Noord JA. Tiotropium: a new once-daily inhaled M3-receptor blocker for the treatment of COPD. *Essentials* COPD 2002;Issue 3:1–19

8. Van Noord JA, Aumann J, Janssens E, *et al.* Tiotropium maintenance therapy in patients with COPD and the 24-h spirometric benefit of adding once or twice daily formoterol during 2-week treatment periods. *Am J Respir Crit Care Med* 2003;167(7):A95

9. Van Noord JA, Aumann J, Janssens E, *et al.* Comparison of once daily tiotropium, twice daily formoterol and the free combination, once daily, in patients with COPD. *Am J Respir Crit Care Med* 2003;167(7):A320

10. Vanden Burgt JA, Busse WW, Martin RJ, Szefler SJ, Donnell D. Efficacy and safety overview of a new inhaled corticosteroid, QVAR (hydrofluoroalkane-beclomethasone extrafine inhalation aerosol), in asthma. *J Allergy Clin Immunol* 2000;106:1209–26

11. Sakula A. A history of asthma. The FitzPatrick lecture 1987. *J R Coll Physicians Lond* 1988;22:36–44

12. Rau JL Jr. *Respiratory Care Pharmacology*, 6th edn. St Louis, MO: Mosby, 2002

13. Gross NJ. Ipratropium bromide. *N Engl J Med* 1988;319:486–94

14. Chapman KR. History of anticholinergic treatment in airways disease. In Gross NJ, ed. *Anticholinergic Therapy in Obstructive Airways Disease*. London: Franklin Scientific Publications, 1993:9–17

15. Herxheimer H. Atropine cigarettes in asthma emphysema. *Br Med J* 1959;2:167

16. Gandevia B. Historical review of the use of parasympatholytic agents in the treatment of respiratory disorders. *Postgrad Med J* 1975;51:S13–20

17. Barnes PJ. Tiotropium bromide. *Expert Opin Investig Drugs* 2001;10:733–40

18. Hvizdos KM, Goa KL. Tiotropium bromide. *Drugs* 2002;62:1195–203

19. Barnes PJ. Muscarinic receptor subtypes in airways. *Life Sci* 1993;52:521–8

20. Eglen RM, Choppin A, Watson N. Therapeutic opportunities from muscarinic receptor research. *Trends Pharmacol Sci* 2001;22:409–14

21. Disse B. Antimuscarinic treatment for lung diseases from research to clinical practice. *Life Sci* 2001;68:2557–64

22. Witek TJ Jr, Disse B. Inhaled anticholinergic therapy: applied pharmacology and interesting developments. *Curr Opin Invest Drugs* 2001;2:53–8

23. Disse B, Speck GA, Rominger KL, Witek TJ, Hammer R. Tiotropium (Spiriva) mechanistical considerations and clinical profile in obstructive lung disease. *Life Sci* 1999;64:457–64

24. Barnes PJ. The pharmacological properties of tiotropium. *Chest* 2000;117(Suppl 2):63–6S

25. Disse B, Reichl R, Speck G, Traunecker W, Rominger KL, Hammer R. A novel long-acting anticholinergic bronchodilator. *Life Sci* 1993;52:537–44

26. Haddad EB, Mak JC, Barnes PJ. Characterization of [3H]Ba 679 BR, a slowly dissociating muscarinic antagonist, in human lung: radioligand binding and autoradiographic mapping. *Mol Pharmacol* 1994;45:899–907

27. Takaisha T, Belvisi MG, Patel H, Ward JK, Tadjkarimi S, Yacoub MH, *et al*. Effect of BA 679 Br, a novel long-acting anticholonergic agent, on cholinergic neurotransmission in guinea pig and human airways. *Am J Respir Crit Care Med* 1994;150:1640–5

28. Johnson M. Beta2-adrenoceptors: mechanisms of action of beta2-agonists. *Paediatr Respir Rev* 2001;2:57–62

29. Billington CK, Penn RB. M3 muscarinic acetylcholine receptor regulation in the airway. *Am J Respir Cell Mol Biol* 2002;26:269–72

30. Johnson EN, Druey KM. Heterotrimeric G protein signaling: role in asthma and allergic inflammation. *J Allergy Clin Immunol* 2002;109:592–602

31. Anderson GP, Rabe KF. Bronchodilators: an overview. In Hansel TT, Barnes PJ, eds. *New Drugs for Asthma, Allergy and COPD*, 1st edn. Basel, Switzerland: Karger, 2001:54–9

32. Tashkin D, Kesten S. Long-term treatment benefits with tiotropium in COPD patients with and without short-term bronchodilator responses. *Chest* 2003;123:1441–9

33. Donohue JF, van Noord JA, Bateman ED, Langley SJ, Lee A, Witek TJ Jr, *et al*. A 6-month, placebo-controlled study comparing lung function and health status changes in COPD patients treated with tiotropium or salmeterol. *Chest* 2002;122:47–55

34. Donohue JF, Menjoge S, Kesten S. Tolerance to bronchodilating effects in salmeterol in COPD. *Respir Med* 2003;97:1014–20

35. Brusasco V, Hodder R, Miravitlles M, Korducki L, Towse L, Kesten S. Health outcomes following treatment for six months with once daily tiotropium compared with twice daily salmeterol in patients with COPD. *Thorax* 2003;58:399–404

36. Nisar M, Earis JE, Pearson MG, Calverley PMA. Acute bronchodilator trials in chronic obstructive pulmonary disease. *Am Rev Respir Dis* 1992;146:555–9

37. O'Donnell DE, Lam M, Webb KA. Measurement of symptoms, lung hyperinflation, and endurance during exercise in chronic obstructive pulmonary disease. *Am J Respir Crit Care Med* 1998;158:1557–6

38. Magnussen H, O'Donnell DE, Casaburi R, *et al*. Spiriva® (tiotropium) reduces lung hyperinflation in COPD. *Am J Respir Crit Care Med* 2002;165(8): A227 (abstr)

39. Celli BR, ZuWallack RL, Wang S, Kesten S. Improvement in resting inspiratory capacity and hyperinflation with tiotropium in COPD patients with increased static lung volumes. *Chest* 2003, in press

40. Casaburi R, Mahler DA, Jones PW, Wanner A, San PG, ZuWallack RL, *et al*. A long-term evaluation of once-daily inhaled tiotropium in chronic obstructive pulmonary disease. *Eur Respir J* 2002;19:217–24

41. O'Donnell DE, Lam M, Webb KA. Spirometric correlates of improvement in exercise performance after anticholinergic therapy in chronic obstructive pulmonary disease. *Am J Respir Crit Care Med* 1999;160:542–9

42. Huchon G, Verkindre C, Bart F, *et al*. Improvements with tiotropium on endurance measured by the shuttle walking test (SWT) and on health related quality of life (HRQoL) in COPD patients. *Eur Respir J* 2002;20(Suppl 38):287s (abstr)

43. O'Donnell DE, Magnussen H, Aguilaniu B, *et al*. Spiriva® (tiotropium) improves exercise tolerance in COPD. *Am J Respir Crit Care Med* 2002;165(8): A227 (abstr)

44. Anthonisen NR, Connett JE, Kiley JP, Altose MD, Bailey WC, Buist AS, et al. Effects of smoking intervention and the use of an inhaled anticholinergic bronchodilator on the rate of decline of FEV1. The Lung Health Study. J Am Med Assoc 1994;272:1497–505

45. Campbell S. For COPD a combination of ipratropium bromide and albuterol sulfate is more effective than albuterol base. Arch Intern Med 1999;159:156–60

46. Chodosh S, Flanders JS, Kesten S, Serby CW, Hochrainer D, Witek TJ Jr. Effective delivery of particles with the HandiHaler dry powder inhalation system over a range of chronic obstructive pulmonary disease severity. J Aerosol Med 2001;14:309–15

47. Leusch A, Eichhorn B, Muller G, Rominger KL. Pharmacokinetics and tissue distribution of the anticholinergics tiotropium and ipratropium in the rat and dog. Biopharm Drug Dispos 2001;22:199–212

48. Skorodin MS, Gross NJ, Moritz T, King FW, Armstrong W, Wells D, et al. Oxitropium bromide, a new anticholinergic bronchodilator. Ann Allergy 1986;56:229–32

49. Teramota S, Ouchi Y. Inhaled oxitropium is currently used as the first-line therapy of patients with chronic pulmonary disease in Japan. Eur Respir J 1999;13:473–5

50. Gross NJ, Petty TL, Friedman M, Skorodin MS, Silvers GW, Donohue JF. Dose response to ipratropium as a nebulized solution in patients with chronic obstructive pulmonary disease. A three-center study. Am Rev Respir Dis 1989;139:1188–91

51. Frith PA, Jenner B, Dangerfield R, Atkinson J, Drennan C. Oxitropium bromide. Dose-response and time-response study of a new anticholinergic bronchodilator drug. Chest 1986;89:249–53

52. Flohr E, Bischoff KO. Oxitropium bromide, a new anticholinergic drug, in a dose-response and placebo comparison in obstructive airway diseases. Respiration 1979;38:98–104

53. Braun SR, Levy SF. Comparison of ipratropium bromide and albuterol in chronic obstructive pulmonary disease: a three-center study. Am J Med 2002;91(Suppl 4A):28–32S

54. COMBIVENT Inhalation Solution Study Group. Routine nebulized ipratropium and albuterol together are better than either alone in COPD. Chest 1997;112:1514–21

55. Gross N, Tashkin D, Miller R, Oren J, Coleman W, Linberg S, et al. Inhalation by nebulisation of albuterol-ipratropium combination (Dey Combination) is superior to either agent alone in the treatment of chronic obstructive pulmonary disease. Respiration 2002;65:354–62

56. Rennard SI, Anderson W, ZuWallack R, Broughton J, Bailey W, Friedman M, et al. Use of a long-acting inhaled beta2-adrenergic agonist, salmeterol xinafoate, in patients with chronic obstructive pulmonary disease. Am J Respir Crit Care Med 2001;163:1087–92

57. Mahler DA, Donohue JF, Barbee RA, Goldman MD, Gross NJ, Wisniewski ME, et al. Efficacy of salmeterol xinafoate in the treatment of COPD. Chest 1999;115:957–65

58. Khoukaz G, Gross NJ. Effects of salmeterol on arterial blood gases in patients with stable chronic obstructive pulmonary disease. Comparison with albuterol and ipratropium. Am J Respir Crit Care Med 1999;160:1028–30

59. Ayers ML, Mejia R, Ward J, Lentine T, Mahler DA. Effectiveness of salmeterol versus ipratropium bromide on exertional dyspnoea in COPD. Eur Respir J 2001;17:1132–7

60. Dahl R, Greefhorst LA, Nowak D, Nonikov V, Byrne AM, Thomson MH, et al. Inhaled formoterol dry powder versus ipratropium bromide in chronic obstructive pulmonary disease. Am J Respir Crit Care Med 2001;164:778–84

61. Bleecker ER, Britt EJ. Acute bronchodilating effects of iprotropium bromide and theophylline in chronic obstructive pulomonary disease. Am J Med 1991;91(Suppl 4A):24S–7S

62. Karpel JP, Kotch A, Zinny M, Pesin J, Alleyne W. A comparison of inhaled ipratropium, oral theophylline plus inhaled β-agonist, and the combination of all three in patients with COPD. Chest 1994;105:1089–94

63. COMBIVENT Inhalation Aerosol Study Group. In chronic obstructive pulmonary disease, a combination of ipratropium and albuterol is more effective than either agent alone. An 85-day multicentre trial. Chest 1994;105:1411–19

64. Wilson JD, Serby CW, Menjoge SS, Witek TJ. The efficacy and safety of combination bronchodilator therapy. Eur Respir Rev 1996;6:286–9

65. Hughes JA, Tobin MJ, Bellamy D, Hutchison DC. Effects of ipratropium bromide and fenoterol aerosols in pulmonary emphysema. Thorax 1982;37:667–70

66. Morton O. Response to Duovent of chronic reversible airways obstruction – a controlled trial in general practice. Postgrad Med J 1984;60(Suppl 1):32–5

67. Serra C, Giacopelli A. Controlled clinical study of a long-term treatment of chronic obstructive lung disease using a combination of fenoterol and ipratropium bromide in aerosol form. *Respiration* 1986;50(Suppl 2):249–53

68. Marlin GE. Studies of ipratropium bromide and fenoterol administered by metered-dose inhaler and aerosolized solution. *Respiration* 1986;50(Suppl 2):290–3

69. Wesseling G, Mostert R, Wouters EEM. A comparison of the effects of anticholinergic and beta2-agonist and combination therapy on respiratory impedence in COPD. *Chest* 1992;101:166–73

70. Imhof E, Elsasser S, Karrer W, Grossenbacher M, Emmons R, Perruchoud AP. Comparison of bronchodilator effects of fenoterol/ipratropium bromide and salbutamol in patients with chronic obstructive lung disease. *Respiration* 1993;60:84–8

71. Fernandez A, Munoz J, de la Calle B, Alia I, Ezpeleta A, de la Cal MA, *et al.* Comparison of one versus two bronchodilators in ventilated COPD patients. *Intensive Care Med* 1994;20:199–202

72. Guerin C, Chevre A, Dessirier P, Poncet T, Becquemin MH, Dequin PF, *et al.* Inhaled fenoterol-ipratropium bromide in mechanically ventilated patients with chronic obstructive pulmonary disease. *Am J Respir Crit Care Med* 1999;159:1036–42

73. Maesen FPV, Smeets JJ, Costongs MAL, Wald FDM, Comelissen PJG. Ba 679 Br, a new long-acting antimuscarinic bronchodilator:a pilot dose-escalation study in COPD. *Eur Respir J* 1993;6:1031–6

74. Maesen FPV, Smeets JJ, Sledsens TJH, Wald FDM, Cornelissen PJG. Tiotropium bromide, a new long-acting antimuscarinic bronchodilator:a pharmacodynamic study in patients with chronic obstructive disease (COPD). *Eur Respir J* 1995;8:1506–13

75. O'Connor BJ, Towse LJ, Barnes PJ. Prolonged effect of tiotropium bromide on methacholine-induced bronchoconstriction in asthma. *Am J Respir Crit Care Med* 1996;154:876–80

76. van Noord JA, Smeets JJ, Custers FL, Korducki L, Cornelissen PJ. Pharmacodynamic steady state of tiotropium in patients with chronic obstructive pulmonary disease. *Eur Respir J* 2002;19:639–44

77. Littner MR, Ilowite JS, Tashkin DP, Friedman M, Serby CW, Menjoge SS, *et al.* Long-acting bronchodilation with once-daily dosing of tiotropium (Spiriva) in stable chronic obstructive pulmonary disease. *Am J Respir Crit Care Med* 2000;161:1136–42

78. van Noord JA, Bantje TA, Eland ME, Korducki L, Cornelissen PJ. A randomised controlled comparison of tiotropium and ipratropium in the treatment of chronic obstructive pulmonary disease. The Dutch Tiotropium Study Group. *Thorax* 2000;55:289–94

79. Casaburi R, Briggs DD Jr, Donohue JF, Serby CW, Menjoge SS, Witek TJ Jr. The spirometric efficacy of once-daily dosing with tiotropium in stable COPD: a 13-week multicenter trial. The US Tiotropium Study Group. *Chest* 2000;118:1294–302

80. Rees PJ. Tiotropium in the management of chronic obstructive pulmonary disease. *Eur Respir J* 2002;19:205–6

81. Calverley PM. The future for tiotropium. *Chest* 2000;117(Suppl 2):67–9S

82. Jarvis B, Markham A. Inhaled salmeterol: a review of its efficacy in chronic obstructive pulmonary disease. *Drugs Aging* 2001;18:441–72

83. Johnson M, Rennard S. Alternative mechanisms for long-acting beta(2)-adrenergic agonists in COPD. *Chest* 2001;120:258–70

84. Cazzola M, Donner CF. Long-acting beta2 agonists in the management of stable chronic obstructive pulmonary disease. *Drugs* 2000;60:307–20

85. Kips J. The clinical role of long-acting beta2-agonists in COPD. *Respir Med* 2000;94(Suppl E):S1–5

86. van Schayck CP. Do long-acting beta2-adrenergic agonists deserve a different place in guidelines for the treatment of asthma and COPD? *Eur Respir J* 2000;15:631–4

87. Lotvall J. Pharmacology of bronchodilators used in the treatment of COPD. *Respir Med* 2000;94(Suppl E):S6–10

88. Chapman KR. Seretide for obstructive lung disease. *Expert Opin Pharmacother* 2002;3:341–50

89. Bielory L, Lupoli K. Herbal interventions in asthma and allergy. *J Asthma* 1999;36:1–65

90. Aranson R, Rau JL Jr. The evolution of beta-agonists. *Respir Care Clin N Am* 1999;5:479–519

91. Liggett SB. Update on current concepts of the molecular basis of beta2-adrenergic receptor signaling. *J Allergy Clin Immunol* 2002;110:S223–8

92. Liggett SB. The pharmacogenetics of beta 2-adrenergic receptors: relevance to asthma. *J Allergy Clin Immunol* 2000;105:S487–92

93. Anderson GP, Linden A, Rabe KF. Why are long-acting beta-adrenoceptor agonists long-acting? *Eur Respir J* 1994;7:569–78

94. Green SA, Spasoff AP, Coleman RA, Johnson M, Liggett SB. Sustained activation of a G protein-coupled receptor via 'anchored' agonist binding. Molecular localization of the salmeterol exosite

within the 2-adrenergic receptor. *J Biol Chem* 1996;271:24029–35

95. Tattersfield AE, Lofdahl CG, Postma DS, Eivindson A, Schreurs AG, Rasidakis A, *et al*. Comparison of formoterol and terbutaline for as-needed treatment of asthma: a randomised trial. *Lancet* 2001;357:257–61

96. Bremner P, Siebers R, Crane J, Beasley R, Burgess C. Partial vs full β-receptor agonist. A clinical study of inhaled albuterol and fenoterol. *Chest* 1996;109:957–62

97. Farfel Z, Bourne HR, Iiri T. The expanding spectrum of G protein diseases. *N Engl J Med* 1999;340:1012–20

98. Mahler DA. The effect of inhaled beta2-agonists on clinical outcomes in chronic obstructive pulmonary disease. *J Allergy Clin Immunol* 2002;110(Suppl 6):S298–303

99. O'Donnell DE. Assessment of bronchodilator efficacy in symptomatic COPD: is spirometry useful? *Chest* 2000;117(Suppl 2):42–7S

100. Appleton S, Smith B, Veale A, Bara A. Long-acting beta2-agonists for chronic obstructive pulmonary disease. *Cochrane Database Syst Rev* 2000;issue 2:CD001104

101. van Noord JA, de Munck DR, Bantje TA, Hop WC, Akveld ML, Bommer AM. Long-term treatment of chronic obstructive pulmonary disease with salmeterol and the additive effect of ipratropium. *Eur Respir J* 2000;15:878–85

102. Belman MJ, Botnick WC, Shin JW. Inhaled bronchodilators reduce dynamic hyperinflation during exercise in patients with chronic obstructive pulmonary disease. *Am J Respir Crit Care Med* 1996;153:967–75

103. Jenkins SC, Heaton RW, Fulton TJ, Moxham J. Comparison of domiciliary nebulized salbutamol and salbutamol from a metered-dose inhaler in stable chronic airflow limitation. *Chest* 1987;91:804–7

104. Boyd G, Morice AH, Pounsford JC, Siebert M, Peslis N, Crawford C. An evaluation of salmeterol in the treatment of chronic obstructive pulmonary disease (COPD). *Eur Respir J* 1997;10:815–21

105. Erjefalt I, Persson CG. Pharmacologic control of plasma exudation into tracheobronchial airways. *Am Rev Respir Dis* 1991;143:1008–14

106. Tokuyama K, Kuo HP, Rohde JA, Barnes PJ, Rogers DF. Neural control of goblet cell secretion in guinea pig airways. *Am J Physiol* 1990;259:L108–15

107. Hui KP, Ventresca P, Brown AC, Barnes PJ, Chung KF. Modulation of neurally mediated airway microvascular leak in guinea pig airways by beta2 adrenoceptor agonists. *Agents Actions* 1992;32:29–33

108. Proud D, Reynolds CJ, Lichtenstein LM, Kagey-Sobotka A, Togias A. Intranasal salmeterol inhibits allergen-induced vascular permeability but not mast cell activation or cellular infiltration. *Clin Exp Allergy* 1998;28:868–75

109. Devalia JL, Sapsford RJ, Rusznak C, Toumbis MJ, Davies RJ. The effects of salmeterol and salbutamol on ciliary beat frequency of cultured human bronchial epithelial cells, *in vitro*. *Pulm Pharmacol* 1992;5:257–63

110. Melloni B, Germouty J. The influence of a new beta agonist: formoterol on mucociliary function. *Rev Mal Respir* 1992;9:503–7

111. Suzuki S, Watanuki Y, Yoshiike Y, Okubo T. Effects of fenoterol on ventilatory response to hypercapnia and hypoxia in patients with chronic obstructive pulmonary disease. *Thorax* 1997;52:125–9

112. Johnson M. Effects of beta2-agonists on resident and infiltrating inflammatory cells. *J Allergy Clin Immunol* 2002;110(Suppl 6):S282–90

113. Adcock IM, Maneechotesuwan K, Usmani O. Molecular interactions between glucocorticoids and long-acting beta2-agonists. *J Allergy Clin Immunol* 2002;110(Suppl 6):S261–8

114. Jeffery PK, Venge P, Gizycki MJ, Egerod I, Dahl R, Faurschou P. Effects of salmeterol on mucosal inflammation in asthma: a placebo-controlled study. *Eur Respir J* 2002;20:1378–85

115. Dowling RB, Johnson M, Cole PJ, Wilson R. Effect of salmeterol on *Haemophilus influenzae* infection of respiratory mucosa *in vitro*. *Eur Respir J* 1998;11:86–90

116. McDonald CF, Pierce RJ, Thompson PJ, Allen D, Bowler S, Breslin AB, *et al*. Comparison of oral bambuterol and terbutaline in elderly patients with chronic reversible airflow obstruction. *J Asthma* 1997;34:53–9

117. Crompton GK, Ayres JG, Basran G, Schiraldi G, Brusasco V, Eivindson A, *et al*. Comparison of oral bambuterol and inhaled salmeterol in patients with symptomatic asthma and using inhaled corticosteroids. *Am J Respir Crit Care Med* 1999;159:824–8

118. Wallaert B, Brun P, Ostinelli J, Murciano D, Champel F, Blaive B, *et al*. A comparison of two long-acting beta-agonists, oral bambuterol and inhaled salmeterol, in the treatment of moderate to severe asthmatic patients with nocturnal symptoms. The French Bambuterol Study Group. *Respir Med* 1999;93:33–8

119. van Schayck CP, Folgering H, Harbers H, Maas KL, van Weel C. Effects of allergy and age on responses

to salbutamol and ipratropium bromide in moderate asthma and chronic bronchitis. *Thorax* 1991;46:355–9

120. Vathenen AS, Britton JR, Ebden P, Cookson JB, Wharrad HJ, Tattersfield AE. High-dose inhaled albuterol in severe chronic airflow limitation. *Am Rev Respir Dis* 1988;138:850–5

121. Higgins BG, Powell RM, Cooper S, Tattersfield AE. Effect of salbutamol and ipratropium bromide on airway calibre and brochial reactivity in asthma and chronic bronchitis. *Eur Respir J* 1991;4:415–20

122. Celik G, Kayacan O, Beder S, Durmaz G. Formoterol and salmeterol in partially reversible chronic obstructive pulmonary disease: a crossover, placebo-controlled comparison of onset and duration of action. *Respiration* 1999;66:434–9

123. Cazzola M, Santangelo G, Piccolo A, Salzillo A, Matera MG, D'Amato G, *et al.* Effect of salmeterol and formoterol in patients with chronic obstructive pulmonary disease. *Pulm Pharmacol* 1994;7:103–7

124. Matera MG, Cazzola M, Vinciguerra A, Di Perna F, Calderaro F, Caputi M, *et al.* A comparison of the bronchodilating effects of salmeterol, salbutamol and ipratropium bromide in patients with chronic obstructive pulmonary disease. *Pulm Pharmacol* 1995;8:267–71

125. Ramirez-Venegas A, Ward J, Lentine T, Mahler DA. Salmeterol reduces dyspnea and improves lung function in patients with COPD. *Chest* 1997;112:336–40

126. Patakas D, Andreadis D, Mavrofridis E, Argyropoulou P. Comparison of the effects of salmeterol and ipratropium bromide on exercise performance and breathlessness in patients with stable chronic obstructive pulmonary disease. *Respir Med* 1998;92:1116–21

127. Grove A, Lipworth BJ, Reid P, Smith RP, Ramage L, Ingram CG, *et al.* Effects of regular salmeterol on lung function and exercise capacity in patients with chronic obstructive airways disease. *Thorax* 1996;51:689–93

128. Di Lorenzo G, Morici G, Drago A, Pellitteri ME, Mansueto P, Melluso M, *et al.* Efficacy, tolerability, and effects on quality of life of inhaled salmeterol and oral theophylline in patients with mild-to-moderate chronic obstructive pulmonary disease. SLMT02 Italian Study Group. *Clin Ther* 1998;20:1130–48

129. Cazzola M, Di Lorenzo G, Di Perna F, Calderaro F, Testi R, Centanni S. Additive effects of salmeterol and fluticasone or theophylline in COPD. *Chest* 2000;118:1576–81

130. ZuWallack RL, Mahler DA, Reilly D, Church N, Emmett A, Rickard K, *et al.* Salmeterol plus theophylline combination therapy in the treatment of COPD. *Chest* 2001;119:1661–70

131. Matera MG, Caputi M, Cazzola M. A combination with clinical recommended dosages of salmeterol and ipratropium is not more effective than salmeterol alone in patients with chronic obstructive pulmonary disease. *Respir Med* 1996;90:497–9

132. Cazzola M, Centanni S, Regorda C, di Marco F, Di Perna F, Carlucci P, *et al.* Onset of action of single doses of formoterol administered via Turbuhaler in patients with stable COPD. *Pulm Pharmacol Ther* 2001;14:41–5

133. Benhamou D, Cuvelier A, Muir JF, Leclerc V, Le G, V, Kottakis J, *et al.* Rapid onset of bronchodilation in COPD: a placebo-controlled study comparing formoterol (Foradil Aerolizer) with salbutamol (Ventodisk). *Respir Med* 2001;95:817–21

134. Kottakis J, Cioppa GD, Creemers J, Greefhorst L, Lecler V, Pistelli R, *et al.* Faster onset of bronchodilation with formoterol than with salmeterol in patients with stable, moderate to severe COPD: results of a randomized, double-blind clinical study. *Can Respir J* 2002;9:107–15

135. Maesen BL, Westermann CJ, Duurkens VA, van den Bosch JM. Effects of formoterol in apparently poorly reversible chronic obstructive pulmonary disease. *Eur Respir J* 1999;13:1103–8

136. Cazzola M, Matera MG, Santangelo G, Vinciguerra A, Rossi F, D'Amato G. Salmeterol and formoterol in partially reversible severe chronic obstructive pulmonary disease: a dose-response study. *Respir Med* 1995;89:357–62

137. Cazzola M, Di Perna F, Noschese P, Vinciguerra A, Calderaro F, Girbino G, *et al.* Effects of formoterol, salmeterol or oxitropium bromide on airway responses to salbutamol in COPD. *Eur Respir J* 1998;11:1337–41

138. Aalbers R, Ayres J, Backer V, Decramer M, Lier PA, Magyar P, *et al.* Formoterol in patients with chronic obstructive pulmonary disease: a randomized, controlled, 3-month trial. *Eur Respir J* 2002;19:936–43

139. Schultze-Werninghaus G. Multicenter 1-year trial on formoterol, a new long-acting beta 2-agonist, in chronic obstructive airway disease. *Lung* 1990;168 (Suppl):83–9

140. Rossi A, Kristufek P, Levine BE, Thomson MH, Till D, Kottakis J, *et al.* Comparison of the efficacy, tolerability, and safety of formoterol dry powder and oral, slow-release theophylline in the treatment of COPD. *Chest* 2002;121:1058–69

141. Sichletidis L, Kottakis J, Marcou S, Constantinidis TC, Antoniades A. Bronchodilatory responses to formoterol, ipratropium, and their combination in patients with stable COPD. *Int J Clin Pract* 1999;53:185–8

142. Cazzola M, Di Perna F, Califano C, Vinciguerra A, D'Amato M. Incremental benefit of adding oxitropium bromide to formoterol in patients with stable COPD. *Pulm Pharmacol Ther* 1999;12:267–71

143. Cazzola M, Matera MG, Di Perna E, Califano C, D'Amato M, Mazzarella G. Influence of higher than conventional doses of oxitropium bromide on formoterol-induced bronchodilation in COPD. *Respir Med* 1999;93:909–11

144. D'Urzo AD, De Salvo MC, Ramirez-Rivera A, Almeida J, Sichletidis L, Rapatz G, *et al*. In patients with COPD, treatment with a combination of formoterol and ipratropium is more effective than a combination of salbutamol and ipratropium. *Chest* 2001;119:1347–56

145. Guhan AR, Cooper S, Oborne J, Lewis S, Bennett A, Tattersfield AE. Systemic effects of formoterol and salmeterol: a dose-response comparison in healthy subjects. *Thorax* 2000;55:650–6

146. Suissa S, Assimes T, Ernst P. Inhaled short acting beta agonist use in COPD and the risk of acute myocardial infarction. *Thorax* 2003;58:43–6

147. Barnes PJ. Theophylline. New perspectives for an old drug. *Am J Respir Crit Care Med* 2003;167:813–18

148. Chrystyn H, Mulley BA, Peake MD. Dose response relation to oral theophylline in severe chronic obstructive airways disease. *Br Med J* 1988;297:1506–10

149. van der Palen J, Klein JJ, Kerkhoff AH, van Herwaarden CL. Evaluation of the effectiveness of four different inhalers in patients with chronic obstructive pulmonary disease. *Thorax* 1995;50:1183–7

150. Persson CG. On the medical history of xanthines and other remedies for asthma: a tribute to HH Salter. *Thorax* 1985;40:881–6

151. Weinberger M, Hendeles L. Theophylline in asthma. *N Engl J Med* 1996;334:1380–8

152. Weinberger M, Hendeles L, Bighley L. The relation of product formulation to absorption of oral theophylline. *N Engl J Med* 1978;299:852–7

153. Rennard SI. Combination bronchodilator therapy in COPD. *Chest* 1995;107(Suppl 5):171S–5S

154. Pauwels R. The use of theophylline in chronic obstructive pulmonary disease. *Clin Exp Allergy* 1996;26(Suppl 2):55–9

155. Cazzola M, Donner CF, Matera MG. Long acting beta(2) agonists and theophylline in stable chronic obstructive pulmonary disease. *Thorax* 1999;54:730–6

156. Rabe KF, Magnussen H, Dent G. Theophylline and selective PDE inhibitors as bronchodilators and smooth muscle relaxants. *Eur Respir J* 1999;8:637–42

157. Culpitt S, Maziak W, Loukides S, Keller A, Barnes P.J. Effects of theophylline on induced sputum inflammatory indices in COPD patients. *Am J Respir Crit Care Med* 1997;157:A797

158. Culpitt SV, De Matos C, Russell RE, Donnelly LE, Rogers DF, Barnes PJ. Effect of theophylline on induced sputum inflammatory indices and neutrophil chemotaxis in chronic obstructive pulmonary disease. *Am J Respir Crit Care Med* 2002;165:1371–6

159. Ito K, Lim S, Caramori G, Cosio B, Chung F, Adcock IM, *et al*. A molecular mechanism of action of theophylline: induction of histone deacetylase activity to decrease inflammatory gene expression. *Proc Natl Acad Sci USA* 2002;99:8921–6

160. Nishimura K, Koyama H, Ikeda A, Izumi T. Is oral theophylline effective in combination with both inhaled anticholinergic agent and inhaled beta 2-agonist in the treatment of stable COPD? *Chest* 1993;104:179–84

161. Kirsten DK, Wegner RE, Jorres RA, Magnussen H. Effects of theophylline withdrawal in severe chronic obstructive pulmonary disease. *Chest* 1993;104:1101–7

162. Murciano D, Aubier M, Lecocguic Y, Pariente R. Effects of theophylline on diaphragmatic strength and fatigue in patients with chronic obstructive pulmonary disease. *N Engl J Med* 1984;311:349–53

163. Murciano D, Auclair MH, Pariente R, Aubier M. A randomized, controlled trial of theophylline in patients with severe chronic obstructive pulmonary disease. *N Engl J Med* 1989;320:1521–5

164. Mahler DA, Matthay RA, Snyder PE, Wells CK, Loke J. Sustained-release theophylline reduces dyspnea in nonreversible obstructive airway disease. *Am Rev Respir Dis* 1985;131:22–5

165. Ziment I. Theophylline and mucociliary clearance. *Chest* 1987;92(Suppl 1):38–43S

166. Martin RJ, Pak J. Overnight theophylline concentrations and effects on sleep and lung function in

chronic obstructive pulmonary disease. *Am Rev Respir Dis* 1992;145:540–4

167. Holford N, Black P, Couch R, Kennedy J, Briant R. Theophylline target concentration in severe airways obstruction – 10 or 20 mg/L? A randomised concentration-controlled trial. *Clin Pharmacokinet* 1993;25:495–505

168. Johnston ID. Theophylline in the management of airflow obstruction. 2. Difficult drugs to use, few clinical indications. *Br Med J* 1990;300:929–31

169. Powell JR, Vozeh S, Hopewell P, Costello J, Sheiner LB, Riegelman S. Theophylline disposition in acutely ill hospitalized patients. The effect of smoking, heart failure, severe airway obstruction, and pneumonia. *Am Rev Respir Dis* 1978;118:229–38

170. Guyatt GH, Townsend M, Pugsley SO, Keller JL, Short HD, Taylor DW, *et al.* Bronchodilators in chronic air-flow limitation. Effects on airway function, exercise capacity, and quality of life. *Am Rev Respir Dis* 1987;135:1069–74

171. Thomas P, Pugsley JA, Stewart JH. Theophylline and salbutamol improve pulmonary function in patients with irreversible chronic obstructive pulmonary disease. *Chest* 1992;101:160–5

172. Ashutosh K, Sedat M, Fragale-Jackson J. Effects of theophylline on respiratory drive in patients with chronic obstructive pulmonary disease. *J Clin Pharmacol* 1997;37:1100–7

173. Fink G, Kaye C, Sulkes J, Gabbay U, Spitzer SA. Effect of theophylline on exercise performance in patients with severe chronic obstructive pulmonary disease. *Thorax* 1994;49:332–4

174. Tsukino M, Nishimura K, Ikeda A, Hajiro T, Koyama H, Izumi T. Effects of theophylline and ipratropium bromide on exercise performance in patients with stable chronic obstructive pulmonary disease. *Thorax* 1998;53:269–73

175. Mulloy E, McNicholas WT. Theophylline improves gas exchange during rest, exercise, and sleep in severe chronic obstructive pulmonary disease. *Am Rev Respir Dis* 1993;148:1030–6

176. Melani AS, Pirrelli M, Di Gregorio A. Effects of inhaled salmeterol and orally dose-titrated theophylline on exercise capacity of stable COPD patients. *Eur Respir J* 1996;9(Suppl 23):391s

177. Berry RB, Desa MM, Branum JP, Light RW. Effect of theophylline on sleep and sleep-disordered breathing in patients with chronic obstructive pulmonary disease. *Am Rev Respir Dis* 1991;143:245–50

178. Man GC, Champman KR, Ali SH, Darke AC. Sleep quality and nocturnal respiratory function with once-daily theophylline (Uniphyl) and inhaled

salbutamol in patients with COPD. *Chest* 1996;110:648–53

179. Barnes PJ. Inhaled corticosteroids are not beneficial in chronic obstructive pulmonary disease. *Am J Respir Crit Care Med* 2000;161:342–4

180. Calverley PM. Inhaled corticosteroids are beneficial in chronic obstructive pulmonary disease. *Am J Respir Crit Care Med* 2000;161:341–2

181. Papi A, Romagnoli M, Baraldo S, Braccioni F, Guzzinati I, Saetta M, *et al.* Partial reversibility of airflow limitation and increased exhaled NO and sputum eosinophilia in chronic obstructive pulmonary disease. *Am J Respir Crit Care Med* 2000;162:1773–7

182. McEvoy CE. Adverse effects of corticosteroid therapy for COPD A critical review. *Chest* 1997; 111:732–43

183. Adcock IM. Glucocorticoid-regulated transcription factors. *Pulm Pharmacol Ther* 2001;14:211–19

184. Keatings VM, Jatakanon A, Worsdell YM, Barnes PJ. Effects of inhaled and oral glucocorticoids on inflammatory indices in asthma and COPD. *Am J Respir Crit Care Med* 1997;155:542–8

185. Culpitt SV, Maziak W, Loukidis S, Nightingale JA, Matthews JL, Barnes PJ. Effect of high dose inhaled steroid on cells, cytokines, and proteases in induced sputum in chronic obstructive pulmonary disease. *Am J Respir Crit Care Med* 1999;160:1635–9

186. Loppow D, Schleiss MB, Kanniess F, Taube C, Jorres RA, Magnussen H. In patients with chronic bronchitis a four week trial with inhaled steroids does not attenuate airway inflammation. *Respir Med* 2001;95:115–21

187. Meagher LC, Cousin JM, Seckl JR, Haslett C. Opposing effects of glucocorticoids on the rate of apoptosis in neutrophilic and eosinophilic granulocytes. *J Immunol* 1996;156:4422–8

188. Nightingale JA, Rogers DF, Fan CK, Barnes PJ. No effect of inhaled budesonide on the response to inhaled ozone in normal subjects. *Am J Respir Crit Care Med* 2000;161:479–86

189. Ito K, Lim S, Caramori G, Chung KF, Barnes PJ, Adcock IM. Cigarette smoking reduces histone deacetylase 2 expression, enhances cytokine expression and inhibits glucocorticoid actions in alveolar macrophages. *FASEB J* 2001;15:1100–2

190. Ito K, Barnes PJ, Adcock IM. Glucocorticoid receptor recruitment of histone deacetylase 2 inhibits interleukin-1beta-induced histone H4 acetylation on lysines 8 and 12. *Mol Cell Biol* 2000;20:6891–903

191. Yamada K, Elliott WM, Brattsand R, Valeur A, Hogg JC, Hayashi S. Molecular mechanisms of decreased steroid responsiveness induced by latent adenoviral infection in allergic lung inflammation. *J Allergy Clin Immunol* 2002;109:35–42

192. Vestbo J, Sorensen T, Lange P, Brix A, Torre P, Viskum K. Long-term effect of inhaled budesonide in mild and moderate chronic obstructive pulmonary disease: a randomised controlled trial. *Lancet* 1999;353:1819–23

193. Pauwels RA, Lofdahl CG, Laitinen LA, Schouten JP, Postma DS, Pride NB, *et al*. Long-term treatment with inhaled budesonide in persons with mild chronic obstructive pulmonary disease who continue smoking. European Respiratory Society Study on Chronic Obstructive Pulmonary Disease. *N Engl J Med* 1999;340:1948–53

194. Burge PS, Calverley PM, Jones PW, Spencer S, Anderson JA, Maslen TK. Randomised, double blind, placebo controlled study of fluticasone propionate in patients with moderate to severe chronic obstructive pulmonary disease: the ISOLDE trial. *Br Med J* 2000;320:1297–303

195. Lung Health Study Research Group. Effect of inhaled triamcinolone on the decline in pulmonary function in chronic obstructive pulmonary disease. *N Engl J Med* 2000;343:1902–9

196. Soriano JB, Vestbo J, Pride NB, Kiri V, Maden C, Maier WC. Survival in COPD patients after regular use of fluticasone propionate and salmeterol in general practice. *Eur Respir J* 2002;20:819–25

197. Sin DD, Tu JV. Inhaled corticosteroids and the risk of mortality and readmission in elderly patients with chronic obstructive pulmonary disease. *Am J Respir Crit Care Med* 2001;164:580–84

198. Paggiaro PL, Dahle R, Bakran I, Frith L, Hollingworth K, Efthimiou J. Multicentre randomised in placebo-controlled trial of inhaled fluticasone propionate in patients with chronic obstructive pulmonary disease. *Lancet* 1998;351:773–80

199. Jones PW, Willits LR, Burge PS, Calverley PMA on behalf of the ISOLDE investigators. Disease severity and the effect of fluticasone propionate on chronic obstructive pulmonary disease exacerbations. *Eur Repir J* 2003;21:68–73

200. van der Valk P, Monninkhof E, van der Palen J, Zielhuis G, van Herwaarden C. Effect of discontinuation of inhaled corticosteroids in patients with chronic obstructive pulmonary disease: the COPE study. *Am J Respir Crit Care Med* 2002;166:1358–63

201. O'Brien A, Russo-Magno P, Karki A, Hiranniramol S, Hardin M, Kaszuba M, Sherman C, Rounds S. Effects of withdrawal of inhaled steroids in men with severe irreversible airflow obstruction. *Am J Respir Crit Care Med* 2001;164:365–71

202. Mahler DA, Wire P, Horstman D, Chang CN, Yates J, Fischer T, *et al*. Effectiveness of fluticasone propionate and salmeterol combination delivered via the Diskus device in the treatment of chronic obstructive pulmonary disease. *Am J Respir Crit Care Med* 2002;166:1084–91

203. Calverley PMA, Pauwels R, Vestbo J, Jones P, Pride NB, Gulsvik A, *et al*. Combined salmeterol and fluticasone in the treatment of chronic obstructive pulmonary disease: a randomised controlled trial. *Lancet* 2003;361:449–56

204. Rennard SI. COPD: treatments benefit patients. *Lancet* 2003;361:444–5

205. Szafranski W, Cukier A, Ramirez A, Menga G, Sansores R, Nahabedian S, *et al*. Efficacy and safety of budesonide/formoterol in the management of chronic obstructive pulmonary disease. *Eur Respir J* 2003;21:74–81

206. Hubbard RB, Smith CJ, Smeeth L, Harrison TW, Tattersfield AE. Inhaled corticosteroids and hip fracture: a population-based case-control study. *Am J Respir Crit Care Med* 2002;166:1563–6

207. Senderovitz T, Vestbo J, Frandsen J, Maltbaek N, Norgaard M, Nielsen C, *et al*. Steroid reversibility test followed by inhaled budesonide or placebo in outpatients with stable chronic obstructive pulmonary disease. The Danish Society of Respiratory Medicine. *Respir Med* 1999;93:715–18

208. Brightling CE, Monteiro W, Ward R, Parker D, Morgan MD, Wardlaw AJ, *et al*. Sputum eosinophilia and short-term response to prednisolone in chronic obstructive pulmonary disease: a randomised controlled trial. *Lancet* 2000;356:1480–5

209. Poole PJ, Chacko E, Wood-Baker RW, Cates CJ. Influenza vaccine for patients with chronic obstructive pulmonary disease. *Cochrane Database Syst Rev* 2000;issue 4:CD002733

210. Nichol KL, Baken L, Wuorenma J, Nelson A. The health and economic benefits associated with pneumococcal vaccination of elderly persons with chronic lung disease. *Arch Intern Med* 1999;159:2437–42

211. Fedson DS, Shapiro ED, LaForce FM, Mufson MA, Musher DM, Spika JS, *et al*. Pneumococcal vaccine after 15 years of use. Another view. *Arch Intern Med* 1994;154:2531–5

212. Collet JP, Shapiro P, Ernst P, Renzi T, Ducruet T, Robinson A. Effects of an immunostimulating agent on acute exacerbations and hospitalizations in patients with chronic obstructive pulmonary disease.

The PARI-IS Study Steering Committee and Research Group. Prevention of Acute Respiratory Infection by an Immunostimulant. *Am J Respir Crit Care Med* 1997;156:1719–24

213. Poole PJ, Black PN. Oral mucolytic drugs for exacerbations of chronic obstructive pulmonary disease: systematic review. *Br Med J* 2001;322:1271–4

214. Hudson TJ. Dornase in treatment of chronic bronchitis. *Ann Pharmacother* 1996;30:674–5

215. Wedzicha JA, Cotes PM, Empey DW, *et al.* Serum immunoreactive erythropoietin in hypoxic lung disease with and without polycythemia. *Clin Sci* 1985;69:413–22

216. Grandjean EM, Berthet P, Ruffmann R, Leuenberger P. Efficacy of oral long-term N-acetylcysteine in chronic bronchopulmonary disease: a meta-analysis of published double-blind, placebo-controlled clinical trials. *Clin Ther* 2000;22:209–21

217. Lundback B, Lindstrom M, Jonsson E, Anderson S, van Herwaarden CL. Effect of N-acetylcysteine on the decline in lung function in patients with COPD. *Eur Respir J* 1995;5(Suppl 15):895

218. Poole PJ, Black PN. Oral mucolytic drugs for exacerbations of chronic obstructive pulmonary disease: systematic review. *Br Med J* 2001;322:1271–4

219. Dunn CJ, Goa KL. Zanamivir: A review of its use in influenza. *Drugs* 1999;58:761–84

220. Bardsley-Elliot A, Noble S. Oseltamivir. *Drugs* 1999;58:851–60

221. Irwin RS, Boulet LP, Cloutier MM, Fuller R, Gold PM, Hoffstein V, *et al.* Managing cough as a defense mechanism and as a symptom. A consensus panel report of the American College of Chest Physicians. *Chest* 1998;114:133–81S

6

Management of exacerbations of COPD

CONTENTS

SUMMARY

Extent of the problem

Exacerbations of symptoms requiring medical intervention are a major clinical event in COPD; they carry a high morbidity and mortality, profoundly affect health-related quality of life for the individual patient, and frequently require intensive and costly clinical therapy.

Definition based on clinical features

Although there is no widely accepted definition of an acute exacerbation of COPD, a commonly used definition encompasses the three major clinical findings of increasing dyspnea, increasing sputum volume, and increasing sputum purulence. The clinical features, arterial blood gas profile, and causes of type 1 and type 2 respiratory failure are compared.

Causes

The most common causes of an exacerbation of COPD are viral and bacterial infection of the tracheobronchial tree and air pollution, but the cause of approximately one-third of exacerbations cannot be identified.

Investigations

- *Spirometry* An initial test of lung function may be useful for comparison with values prior to the exacerbation. However, spirometry to measure FEV_1 is *not* useful to diagnose an exacerbation nor judge the severity of an exacerbation, and FEV_1 is a poor predictor of outcome.
- *Arterial blood gases* This is the major monitoring test and, following admission to a hospital, arterial blood gases are required for diagnosis and monitoring. In severe exacerbations, it is generally useful to establish a radial arterial line.
- *Chest X-ray (CXR)* This is an important test for patients admitted for acute exacerbation of COPD, and assists in the differential diagnosis and monitoring. Electrocardiogram (ECG), echocardiography and CT scan may be required to detect cardiac disease and pulmonary embolism.

Four management steps

(1) Bronchodilators/systemic steroids/antibiotics   Home management
(2) Controlled oxygen (FiO_2 24–28%) therapy   ER/hospital management
(3) Non-invasive intermittent positive pressure ventilation   High dependency area
(4) Invasive mechanical ventilation   Intensive care unit

Treatment modalities

- *Bronchodilation* Inhaled anticholinergic bronchodilators (ipratropium bromide) and/or short-acting β_2-agonists are mandatory. Since the inhaled anticholinergic bronchodilators have fewer and more benign side-effects, they are generally considered first. Methylxanthines (theophylline or aminothylline) are not of proven efficacy, are not supported by some guidelines, and should only be used with caution in relation to monitoring of blood therapeutic levels.

- *Systemic corticosteroids* Intravenous and oral steroids given for up to 2 weeks are of proven efficacy in patients not previously given long-term oral steroid therapy.

- *Antibiotics* In severe exacerbations of COPD, initial narrow-spectrum antibiotics are reasonable first choices, since the superiority of newer broad-spectrum antibiotics has not been established. Antibiotics should only be given if patients have worsening dyspnea and cough, with increasing sputum volume and purulence.

- *Controlled oxygen therapy* Oxygen (fractional concentration in dry inspired gas, FiO_2 of 24–28%) is mandatory when used with caution and arterial blood gas monitoring in hypoxemic patients.

- *NIPPV and invasive mechanical ventilation* Non-invasive positive pressure ventilation (NIPPV) may be indicated for the treatment of respiratory acidosis and should be given in a high dependency area. Invasive mechanical ventilation (IMV) is reserved for the most serious exacerbations and should be administered under the care of a specialist physician in the intensive care unit (ICU).

INTRODUCTION

There are more than 16 million adults with COPD in the United States, and exacerbations of COPD have been estimated to account for 500 000 hospitalizations a year, with 110 000 deaths a year, at a cost of $18 billion in direct health-care costs[1]. Exacerbations of COPD cause considerable morbidity and mortality, with a recent study noting an in-hospital mortality rate of 11%, with a 50% rate of rehospitalization within 6 months of discharge[2–4]. The Lung Health Study recently noted that active smokers have more frequent exacerbations than non-smokers[5]. The American College of Chest Physicians (ACCP) and the American College of Physicians–American Society of Internal Medicine (ACP–ASIM) have recently issued evidence-based guidelines on the management of acute exacerbations of COPD[1,6]. This chapter attempts to integrate the recommendations of GOLD and ACCP and ACP–ASIM on the care of patients with acute exacerbations of COPD[7].

DEFINITION OF AN EXACERBATION OF COPD (Figure 6.1)

Anthonisen and colleagues defined exacerbations in terms of three main features: increased dyspnea, sputum production and sputum purulence. These signs are indicative or suggestive of an infectious etiology, and this is a somewhat restricted definition[8]. Mild exacerbations can be defined on the basis of the presence of one out of these three features, moderate exacerbations with two out of three

| Figure 6.1 | Definition of an exacerbation of COPD |

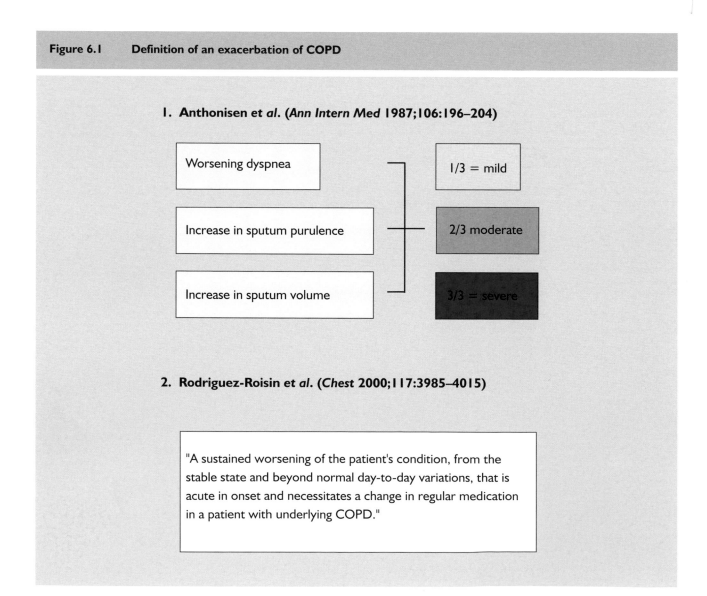

1. Anthonisen et al. (*Ann Intern Med* 1987;106:196–204)

Worsening dyspnea

Increase in sputum purulence

Increase in sputum volume

1/3 = mild

2/3 moderate

3/3 = severe

2. Rodriguez-Roisin et al. (*Chest* 2000;117:3985–4015)

"A sustained worsening of the patient's condition, from the stable state and beyond normal day-to-day variations, that is acute in onset and necessitates a change in regular medication in a patient with underlying COPD."

features, and severe exacerbations with all three features. This division of exacerbations into mild, moderate and severe categories is the basis of the ACCP and ACP–ASIM guidelines for the treatment of exacerbations of COPD[1,6]. However, the grading of severity is best made through the gold standard of arterial blood gas analysis.

An international workshop has given a broader definition of COPD exacerbation[9]:

'A sustained worsening of the patient's condition, from the stable state and beyond normal day-to-day variations, that is acute in onset and necessitates a change in regular medication in a patient with underlying COPD.'

CLINICAL FEATURES OF AN ACUTE EXACERBATION (Figure 6.2)

Acute exacerbations of COPD present as a worsening of the previously stable situation. The three cardinal features from the history used to classify severity in the ACCP and ACP–ASIM guidelines are[1,6,8]:

- Increase in dyspnea (measure rate of breathing)
- Increase in sputum purulence
- Increase in sputum volume

Important clinical signs are (Figure 6.3):

- CO_2 *retention* This can occur in conjunction with hypoxia and respiratory acidosis. The most important sign of a severe exacerbation with type 2 respiratory failure and CO_2 narcosis may be a change in the alertness and mental state of the patient, when immediate hospital evaluation is required. Other clinical features of CO_2 retention are warm flushed peripheries due to vasodilation, a bounding pulse, and CO_2 retention flap (asterixis).

- *Hypoxia* Tachypnea and tachycardia occur with use of accessory respiratory muscles and pursed lip breathing. Cyanosis occurs when there is an

---

Figure 6.2   Clinical features of an acute exacerbation of COPD

History	General signs
Three clinical features to classify severity: • Increase in dyspnea • Increase in sputum purulence • Increase in sputum volume	• Reduced alertness • Central cyanosis

Respiratory signs	Cardiovascular signs

• Tachypnea
• Use of accessory muscles of respiration
• Paradoxical chest wall movements
• Hyperinflation
• Pursed lip breathing
	• Tachycardia
	• Hemodynamic instability
	• Right heart failure
	  - raised jugular venous pressure
	  - pulsatile liver edge
	  - ankle and sacral edema

increased amount of reduced hemoglobin, and central cyanosis occurs on the lips and within the mouth.

- *Cardiovascular signs* relate to hemodynamic instability and right-sided congestive cardiac failure.

TYPES OF RESPIRATORY FAILURE IN COPD (Figure 6.3)

Either type 1 respiratory failure, or type 2 respiratory failure, or, more frequently, a mixture of both can occur in an exacerbation of COPD.

- Type 1 respiratory failure in COPD patients is hypoxia due to factors affecting function of the alveolar-capillary membrane leading to inadequate gas exchange. Ventilation perfusion defects as well as an increase in intrapulmonary shunt may be present. Emphysema with destruction of the capillary bed can itself cause type 1 respiratory failure, or an exacerbation

can increase intrapulmonary blood shunt through atelectasis, consolidation, and pulmonary edema. In most cases, type 1 respiratory failure will respond to controlled oxygen therapy. In a minority of cases, continuous positive airways pressure (CPAP) may be beneficial in type 1 respiratory failure, since it splints open small airways and leads to recruitment of non-ventilated areas of lung.

- Type 2 respiratory failure in COPD patients occurs due to a ventilatory defect that causes hypoxia with a respiratory acidosis. This commonly occurs in exacerbations of COPD when patients are put on controlled oxygen therapy and have reduced ventilatory drive. Type 2 respiratory failure is caused by decreased ventilatory drive (oxygen therapy and opiates), neuromuscular weakness as occurs in COPD, and increased impedance to ventilation, as with changes in elastic recoil in emphysema. Type 2 respiratory failure is

Figure 6.3   Respiratory failure in COPD exacerbations

	Type 1 Hypoxic respiratory failure	Type 2 Ventilatory respiratory failure
Arterial blood gases	Hypoxia	• Hypoxia • Hypercapnia • Respiratory acidosis
Causes	Impaired gas exchange at alveolar-capillary membrane 1. Ventilation–perfusion inequality emphysema 2. Increased intrapulmonary shunt • atelectasis • consolidation • pulmonary edema	Decreased central ventilatory drive: • oxygen therapy • opiates Neuromuscular weakness Increased impedence to ventilation • loss of elastic recoil in emphysema
Clinical features	Features of hypoxia • tachypnea and tachycardia • use of accessory respiratory muscles • pursed lip breathing • cyanosis	Features of hypoxia (see left) Features of hypercapnia: • peripheral vasodilation – pink hands and faces • bounding pulse • CO_2 retention flap • CO_2 narcosis – drowsiness

generally first treated by non-invasive positive pressure ventilation (NIPPV), but in extreme cases may require invasive mechanical ventilation (IMV).

Figure 6.4	External causes of acute exacerbations of COPD

Viruses
Rhinovirus, influenza,
Parainfluenza, coronavirus

Bacteria
Haemophilus influenzae
Streptococcus pneumoniae
Pseudomonas aeruginosa
Moraxella catarrhalis
Mycoplasma pneumoniae
Chlamydia pneumoniae

Air pollutants and irritants

CAUSES AND DIFFERENTIAL DIAGNOSIS
(Figures 6.4 and 6.5)

Acute exacerbations of COPD may be due to viral and, less commonly, bacterial infections, or to non-infective causes[10,11]. It is often stated that the cause of about one-third of exacerbations cannot be identified. Note that, in the course of an exacerbation of COPD, secondary pathophysiology may frequently occur, especially in more severe exacerbations when pulmonary and cardiovascular pathology can be complex.

INVESTIGATIONS

Lung function: spirometry

When a patient with COPD is suffering an acute exacerbation, it is frequently difficult for them to carry out lung function tests properly. Except in patients with very severe baseline airflow obstruction, a PEF of < 100 l/min or an $FEV_1 < 1.0$ liter indicates a severe exacerbation. An initial test of lung function may be useful for comparison with values prior to the exacerbation. However, spirometry to measure FEV_1 is *not* useful to diagnose an

Figure 6.5	Differential diagnosis of an acute exacerbation of COPD

Pulmonary
Pneumonia
Pulmonary embolism
Pneumothorax
Pleural effusion
Lung cancer
Upper airway obstruction

Cardiac
Right and/or left congestive
   heart failure
Cardiac arrhythmias

Skeletal
Rib fractures
Chest trauma

Drug-related
Adverse events of sedatives,
   narcotics, β-blockers

exacerbation nor judge the severity of an exacerbation, and FEV_1 is a poor predictor of outcome.

Arterial blood gases (Figure 6.6)

Arterial blood samples are generally taken from the radial artery into a heparinized syringe, and are important in the monitoring of blood gases and acid–base status. For hospitalized patients, it is mandatory to monitor arterial blood gases, and, in some cases, repeat arterial blood gas stabs can be performed. However, it is generally more convenient for a severe exacerbation of COPD in hospital to introduce a radial arterial line, so that, in the acute phase, arterial blood gases can be measured every 30 min.

Following administration of controlled oxygen (FiO_2 at 24–28%), attempts are made to restore arterial O_2 to > 8.0 kPa. While on controlled O_2, there is a danger of CO_2 retention (hypercapnia) with respiratory acidosis; hence it is important to repeat arterial blood gas evaluation, especially in the initial phases of oxygen therapy.

Chest X-ray

A posterior/anterior plus lateral chest X-ray is an important test for patients admitted for acute exacerbation of COPD, and assists in the differential diagnosis and monitoring. Electrocardiogram (ECG), echocardiography and CT scan may be required to detect cardiac disease and pulmonary embolism.

Electrocardiogram

This is also an important test for patients in hospital with an exacerbation of COPD. An ECG is useful in the diagnosis of right heart hypertrophy, cardiac arrhythmias, and myocardial ischemic episodes.

Spiral CT scan

A spiral CT scan may be useful to identify a pulmonary embolism, which can be very difficult to distinguish from a severe exacerbation with right ventricular hypertrophy and large pulmonary arteries. A low systolic blood pressure with an inability to increase PaO_2 above 8.0 kPa (60 mmHg) while on oxygen is suspicious for a pulmonary embolism.

When there is a strong suspicion that a pulmonary embolism is present, it is best to commence treatment of the embolism along with the exacerbation.

Venous blood tests

- Hemoglobin and hematocrit to identify polycythemia (hematocrit > 55%) or anemia

- The white cell count is not generally informative

- Biochemical tests are important to identify electrolyte disturbances (especially hyponatremia and hypokalemia), elevated blood glucose or hypoalbuminemia

- C-reactive protein (CRP) is increased in infective exacerbations

Sputum examination

The presence of increased volumes of purulent sputum with an increase in dyspnea is sufficient to justify commencing antibiotics. If there is no response to initial antibiotics, a sputum culture and antibiogram should be performed.

STEPS IN MANAGEMENT OF AN EXACERBATION

The ACCP and ACP–ASIM guidelines provide an algorithm for the care of acute exacerbation of COPD[1,6]. Figure 6.7 illustrates the way that management of COPD exacerbations can be based on the presence of symptoms that comprise up to three diagnostic criteria; one diagnostic criterion signifies a mild exacerbation, two diagnostic criteria a moderate exacerbation, and three diagnostic criteria a severe exacerbation. Based on additional input from the GOLD strategy[7], four steps in the management of COPD exacerbations are proposed:

(1) Bronchodilators/systemic steroids/antibiotics in management at home;

(2) Controlled oxygen (FiO_2 24–28%) therapy in management in the emergency room/hospital;

(3) Non-invasive intermittent positive pressure ventilation in hospital;

(4) Invasive mechanical ventilation in the intensive care unit.

Figure 6.6   Arterial blood gases and acute exacerbations of COPD

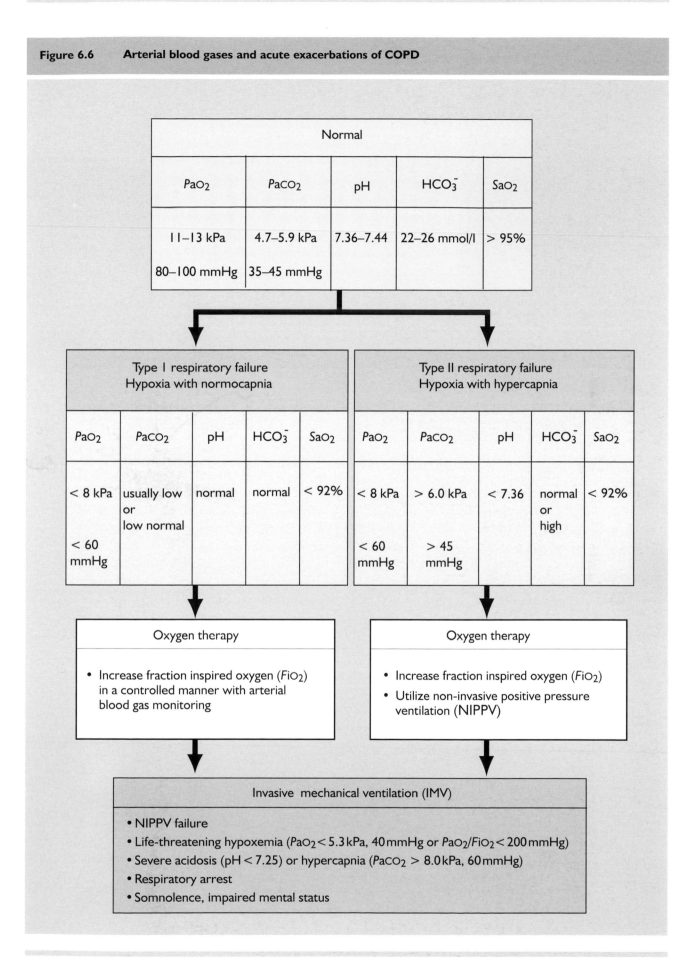

Figure 6.7 Algorithm for management of COPD exacerbations

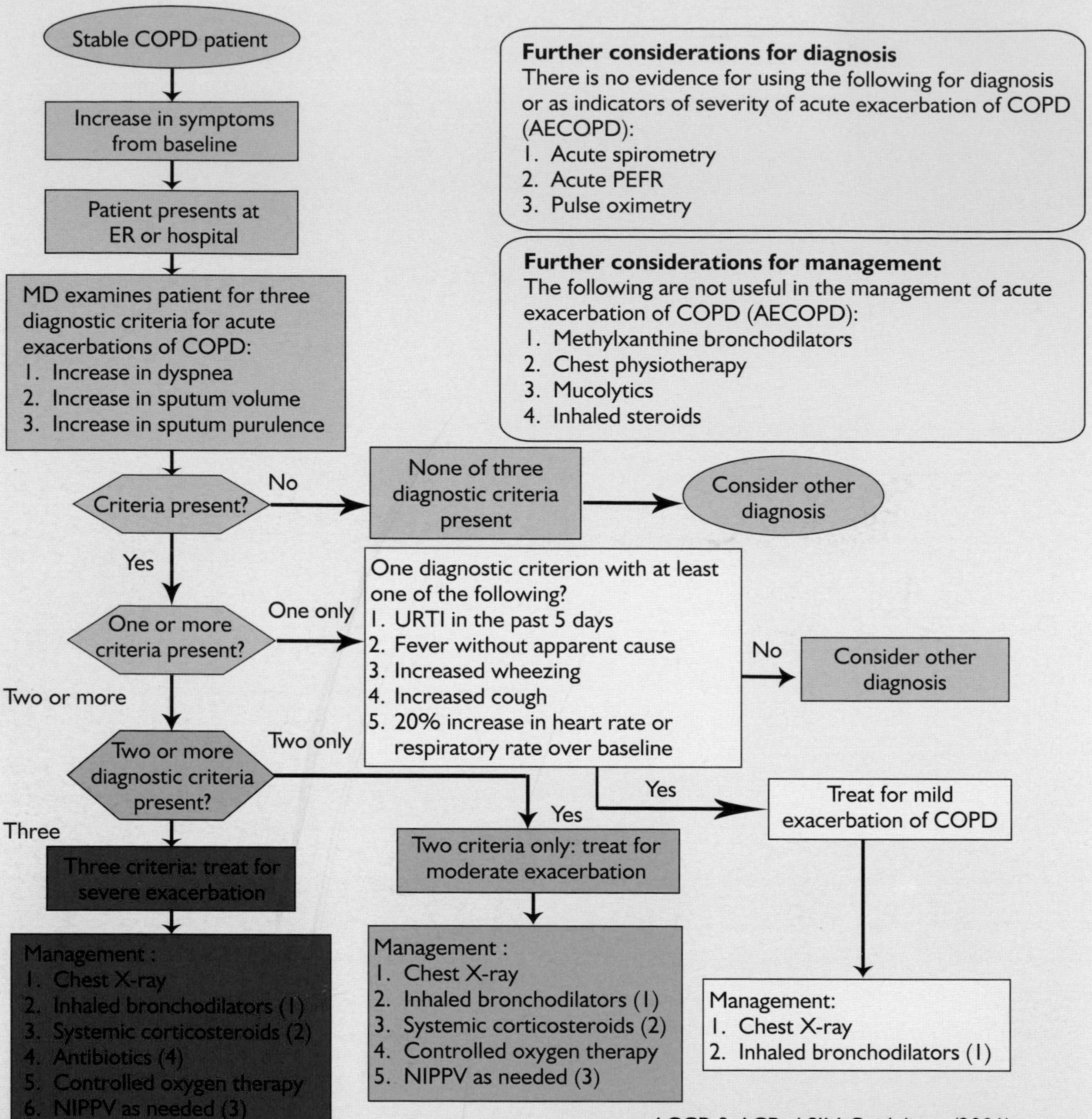
Stable COPD patient
Increase in symptoms from baseline
Patient presents at ER or hospital
MD examines patient for three diagnostic criteria for acute exacerbations of COPD:
1. Increase in dyspnea
2. Increase in sputum volume
3. Increase in sputum purulence
Criteria present?
No
None of three diagnostic criteria present
Consider other diagnosis
Yes
One or more criteria present?
One only
One diagnostic criterion with at least one of the following?
1. URTI in the past 5 days
2. Fever without apparent cause
3. Increased wheezing
4. Increased cough
5. 20% increase in heart rate or respiratory rate over baseline
No
Consider other diagnosis
Two or more
Two or more diagnostic criteria present?
Two only
Yes
Yes
Treat for mild exacerbation of COPD
Three
Three criteria: treat for severe exacerbation
Two criteria only: treat for moderate exacerbation
Management :
1. Chest X-ray
2. Inhaled bronchodilators (1)
3. Systemic corticosteroids (2)
4. Antibiotics (4)
5. Controlled oxygen therapy
6. NIPPV as needed (3)
Management :
1. Chest X-ray
2. Inhaled bronchodilators (1)
3. Systemic corticosteroids (2)
4. Controlled oxygen therapy
5. NIPPV as needed (3)
Management:
1. Chest X-ray
2. Inhaled bronchodilators (1)
Further considerations for diagnosis
There is no evidence for using the following for diagnosis or as indicators of severity of acute exacerbation of COPD (AECOPD):
1. Acute spirometry
2. Acute PEFR
3. Pulse oximetry
Further considerations for management
The following are not useful in the management of acute exacerbation of COPD (AECOPD):
1. Methylxanthine bronchodilators
2. Chest physiotherapy
3. Mucolytics
4. Inhaled steroids

ACCP & ACP–ASIM Guidelines (2001)

Glossary

ACCP and ACP–ASIM: American College of Chest Physicians and the American College of Physicians–American Society of Internal Medicine
PEFR: Peak expiratory flow rate
URTI: Upper respiratory tract infection
NIPPV: Non-invasive positive pressure ventilation
COPD: Chronic obstructive pulmonary disease
ER: Emergency room

Footnotes

1. Use anticholinergic bronchodilators first, once at maximum dose, then add β_2-agonist bronchodilators
2. Dosing regimen used in the SCOPE trial: 3 days intravenous methylprednisolone, 125 mg every 6 h followed by oral prednisolone, taper to complete the 2-week course (60 mg/day on days 4–7, 40 mg/day on days 8–11, and 20 mg/day on days 12–15)
3. Non-invasive positive pressure ventilation should be administered under the supervision of a trained physician
4. Use narrow-spectrum antibiotics; the agents favored in the trials were amoxicillin, trimethoprim-sulfamethoxazole, and tetracycline

Step 1: bronchodilators, systemic steroids, antibiotics (Figure 6.8)

Bronchodilators

Short-acting inhaled bronchodilators are the preferred bronchodilators for treating acute exacer-

bations of COPD[12–23]. Inhaled anticholinergics and β_2-agonists have equivalent efficacy for treatment of an exacerbation of COPD, but anticholinergics are generally preferred because they cause less adverse events.

(1) *Inhaled anticholinergic bronchodilators (ipratropium bromide)* Ipratropium bromide

Figure 6.8   Step 1: Home management with bronchodilators, systemic corticosteroids and antibiotics

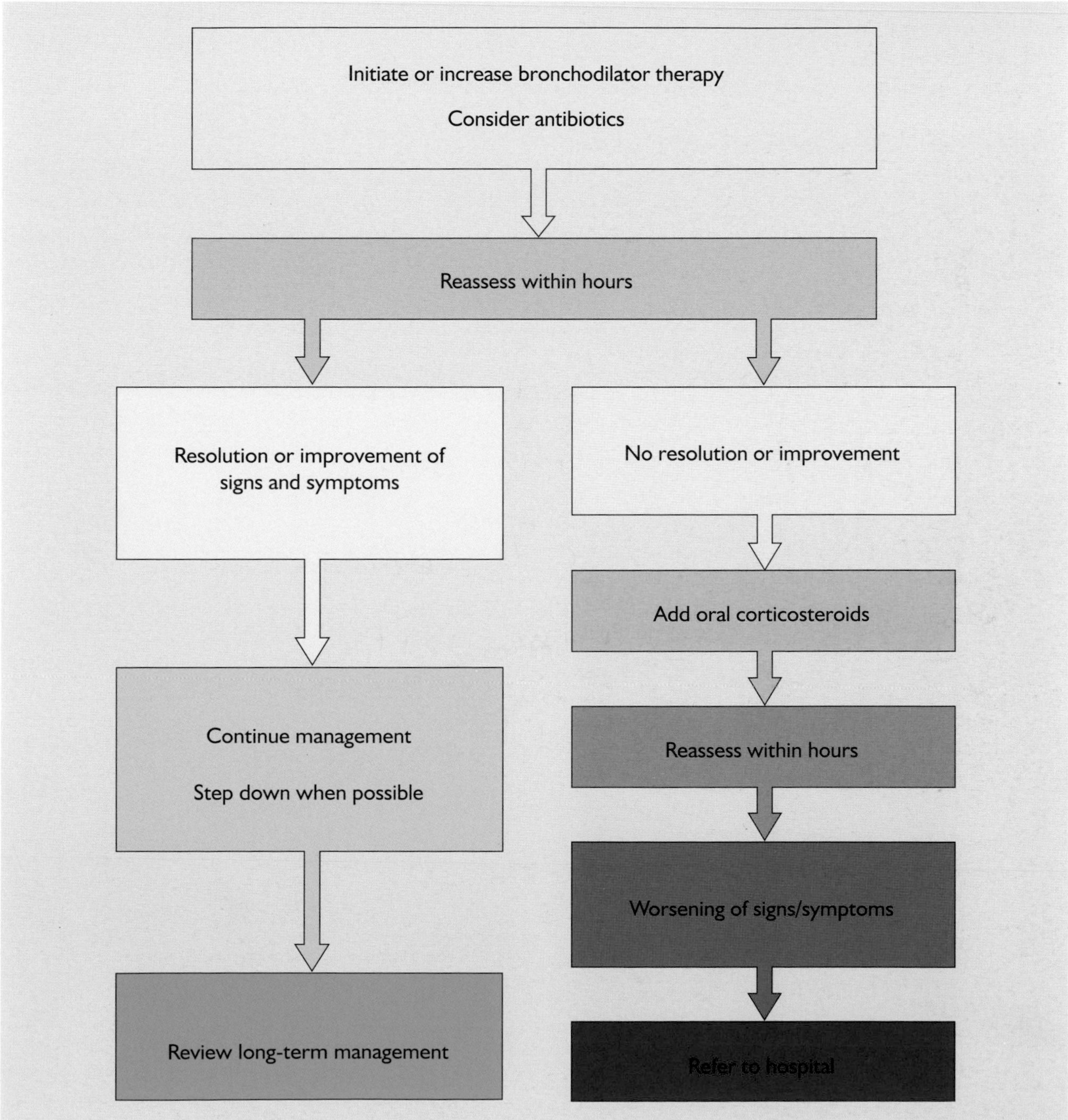

Initiate or increase bronchodilator therapy

Consider antibiotics

Reassess within hours

Resolution or improvement of signs and symptoms

No resolution or improvement

Add oral corticosteroids

Continue management

Step down when possible

Reassess within hours

Worsening of signs/symptoms

Review long-term management

Refer to hospital

Adapted from GOLD strategy (2003)

211

(40–80 µg 4 times daily) by pressurized metered dose inhaler (pMDI) with a spacer, or 250–500 µg 4 times daily with a jet nebulizer.

(2) *Inhaled short-acting β2-agonists (salbutamol)* Salbutamol 100–200 µg by pMDI with spacer, 4 times daily or salbutamol 2.5–5 mg by nebulization, 4 times daily and continued for 24–48 h.

(3) *Combined anticholinergic and short-acting β2-agonists* may be given if there is a poor response to a single bronchodilator.

(4) *Methylxanthines* are controversial because current evidence does not support the use of methylxanthines for acute COPD[24–27]. If there is no response to ipratropium bromide with salbutamol, oral theophylline or intravenous aminophylline can be added in hospital[28]. If the patient has not previously been taking methylxanthines, then a loading dose of 250–500 mg intravenous aminophylline is given over 30 min, followed by 250–500 mg over 24 h, adjusted according to plasma theophylline. Note that close monitoring of serum theophyllines and electrolyte balance is required to avoid the common side-effects of these drugs.

Systemic steroids

There is clear evidence that systemic corticosteroids are useful in acute exacerbations of COPD and improve the rate of recovery, although this effect is relatively small[29–33]. Their mechanism of action in acute exacerbations is unexplained. It is possible that corticosteroids reduce airway edema or that there is a different pattern of inflammation in exacerbations which is corticosteroid-sensitive. Thus, in acute exacerbations, an increase in the number of eosinophils has been reported and these cells are potently suppressed by corticosteroids[34].

Because corticosteroids are useful in the acute management of exacerbations of COPD, inhaled corticosteroids have been assessed in the prevention of acute exacerbations. High-dose fluticasone propionate has a small protective effect against severe exacerbations[35], so inhaled steroids are not indicated in the treatment of acute exacerbations of COPD.

Oral corticosteroids are indicated for a severe exacerbation (prednisolone 30–40 mg daily for 7–14 days). A course of oral steroids in the first 72 h speeds recovery and reduces hospital stay. However,

side-effects may be a problem and there is no evidence that there is any long-term benefit[30,31,36].

Oral steroids (prednisolone 40 mg daily on days 1–7, then 20 mg daily on days 8–10) are indicated if this has previously been shown to improve lung function or if airflow obstruction has not responded to increased bronchodilator doses. Outpatient treatment with oral prednisone (40 mg once daily for 10 days) following emergency treatment of COPD was found to offer a small advantage over placebo in preventing relapse[37].

In a large study (Systemic Corticosteroids in COPD Exacerbations), the following schedule was utilized:

Days 1–3   intravenous methylprednisolone (125 mg every 6 h)
Days 4–7   oral prednisone (60 mg/day)
Days 8–11   oral prednisone (40 mg/day)
Days 12–15   oral prednisone (20 mg/day)

The most common adverse event associated with systemic corticosteroids is hyperglycemia, although most cases occur in patients with known diabetes mellitus.

Antibiotics

The American guidelines on treatment of exacerbations of COPD found evidence that antibiotics are effective only if sputum is purulent, with an increase in sputum volume, and there is increased breathlessness[1,6]. Not all infective exacerbations are due to bacteria. There has been a considerable literature on antibiotics for the treatment of exacerbations of COPD, for which a useful meta-analysis was published in 1995[38].

Since infection is often the cause of progression or acute deterioration in patients with COPD, the combatting of infection by the appropriate use of antibiotics is an important part of therapy. In fact, the organisms causing pulmonary infections are often the same as those found normally in the upper respiratory tract, and it may be difficult to know if a pathogen isolated from the sputum is responsible for the exacerbation. For most of the time, the sputum in COPD is mucoid, but becomes yellow or green with exacerbations of infection. When this occurs, it is usual to begin empirical antibiotic therapy. Purulence of sputum is due to an increase in degranulating neutrophils and may not necessarily imply bacterial infection. Indeed, many exacerbations of COPD are likely to be due to upper respiratory tract virus infections, such as rhinovirus, corona virus and parainfluenza virus[39] (Figure 6.9). This means that antibiotics are often used inappropriately, but it is difficult to tell clinically whether an infection is viral or bacterial in origin. In a meta-analysis of placebo-controlled trials of antibiotics for COPD, there was a small but significant difference in peak expiratory flow between patients treated with antibiotics and placebo[38].

The common bacterial organisms responsible for exacerbations of COPD include *Streptococcus pneumoniae*, *Haemophilus influenzae*, *Moraxella catarrhalis*, and *Mycoplasma pneumoniae* (less common) (Figure 6.9). The choice of antibiotic depends upon the likely organisms, the likely sensitivity of the organisms in the community, the tolerance of the patient for the drug, and the response to treatment.

The treatment of choice in the community will often be either amoxicillin or co-trimoxazole (Septrin®). Co-trimoxazole is not recommended as development of resistance is common and side-effects due to the sulphonamide component are relatively common. However, because many strains of *H. influenzae* are now β-lactamase producers and hence resistant to ampicillin/amoxicillin, the treatment for initial therapy commonly lies between:

- Amoxicillin/clavulanic acid (Augmentin®)

Figure 6.9   Viruses and bacteria than can cause exacerbations of COPD

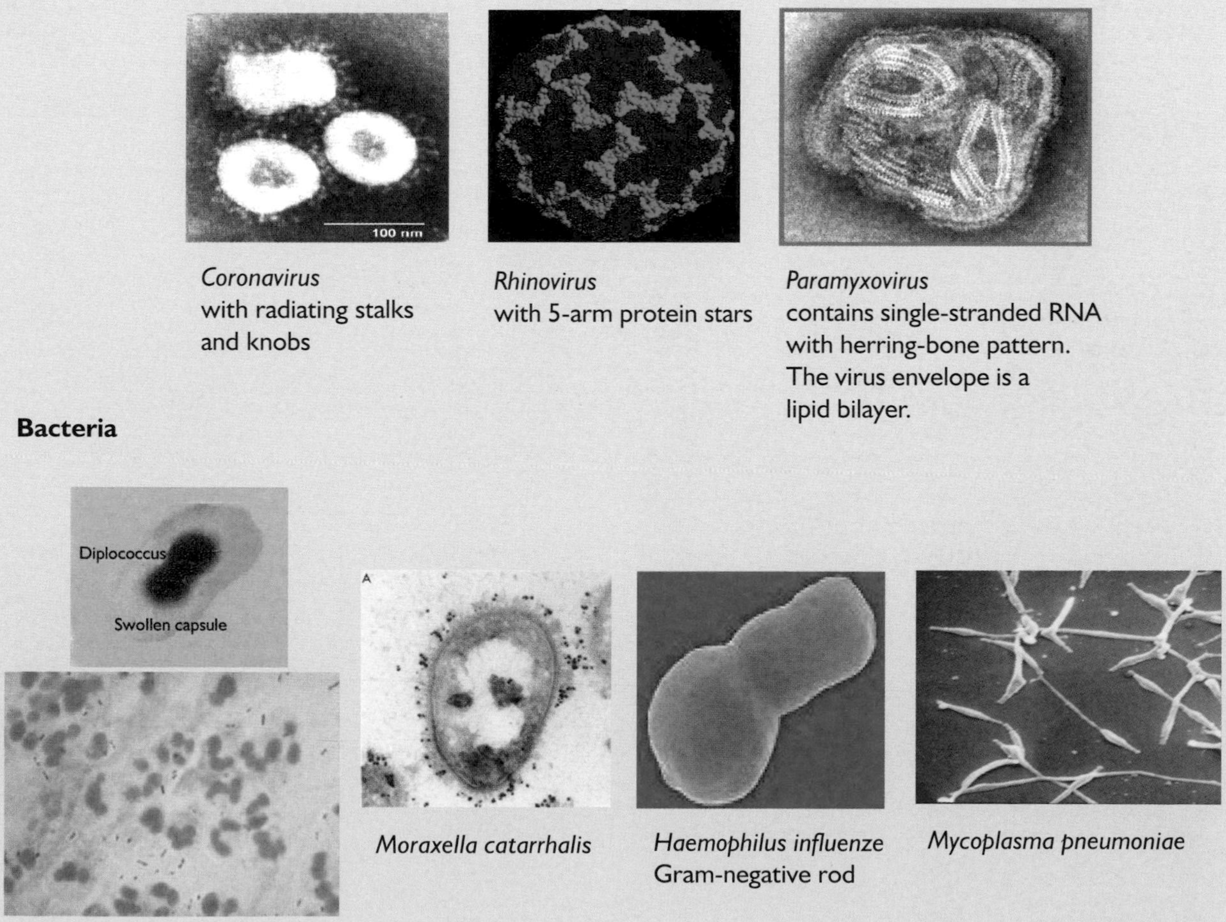

Viruses

Coronavirus with radiating stalks and knobs

Rhinovirus with 5-arm protein stars

Paramyxovirus contains single-stranded RNA with herring-bone pattern. The virus envelope is a lipid bilayer.

Bacteria

Diplococcus

Swollen capsule

Moraxella catarrhalis

Haemophilus influenze Gram-negative rod

Mycoplasma pneumoniae

Streptococcus pneumoniae Gram-positive spheres in pairs (bluish diplococci)

- Erythromycin or other macrolides (clarithromycin, azithromycin)
- A cephalosporin, e.g. cefaclor
- A tetracycline, e.g. doxycycline

There are advantages and disadvantages to each drug and the choice may finally be based on finding out which drug works for a given patient. Cost is also a factor and there is no justification for using an expensive drug when a cheaper one works just as well. In most cases, the choice usually falls between amoxicillin, amoxicillin/clavulanic acid or doxycycline for the typical ambulatory patient.

The antibiotic should be given in full therapeutic doses for a course lasting about 10–14 days, except for clarithromycin and azithromycin, which are given for shorter periods (3 days). Treatment is then stopped, provided the patient has responded. If there has been a poor response, a change of antibiotic may be indicated, usually to one of the newer broad-spectrum agents such as clarithromycin if this has

not already been tried. Continuous antibiotic administration is not recommended in COPD, as this has not been shown to alter the course of the disease and is likely to lead to an increase in resistant organisms.

Step 2: controlled oxygen therapy
(Figure 6.10)

Most patients can be managed at home, but hospital management should be considered if the features in Figure 6.8 are present. Controlled oxygen therapy is the cornerstone of hospital treatment of COPD exacerbations, and has obvious benefit to hypoxemic patients[40]. A major concern when administering oxygen is that hypercapnia will result in respiratory failure[41–44].

- Arterial blood gas assessment is mandatory before and after oxygen therapy, and a chest X-ray should be performed.

Figure 6.10   Step 2: Hospital management and controlled oxygen therapy

Indications for admission	Investigations and treatment

• Marked increase in intensity of symptoms, such as sudden development of resting dyspnea
• Severe background COPD
• Onset of new physical signs (e.g. cyanosis, peripheral edema)
• Failure of exacerbation to respond to initial medical management
• Significant co-morbidities
• Newly occurring arrhythmias
• Diagnostic uncertainty
• Older age
• Insufficient home support
	• Assess severity of symptoms, blood gases, chest X-ray
	• Administer controlled oxygen therapy and repeat arterial blood gas measurements after 30 min
	• Bronchodilators:
	  - Increase doses or frequency
	  - Combined β_2-agonists and anticholinergics
	  - Use spacers or air-driven nebulizers
	  - Consider adding intravenous aminophylline, if needed
	• Add oral or intravenous glucocorticosteroids
	• Consider antibiotics:
	  - When signs of bacteria infection, oral or occasionally intravenous
	• Consider non-invasive mechanical ventilation
	• At all times:
	  - Monitor fluid balance and nutrition
	  - Identify and treat associated conditions (e.g. heart failure, arrhythmias)
	  - Closely monitor condition of the patient

Adapted from GOLD strategy (2003)

- Oxygen (FiO_2 generally commencing at 24% and moving as required up to 28%) is generally given initially via a Venturi mask. Nasal prongs (*see* Figure 7.9) are more comfortable but less accurate for oxygen administration. The major mechanism of hypoxemia in an acute exacerbation of COPD is ventilation–perfusion inequality, and this is generally correctable with a relatively small increase in the percentage of inspired oxygen.

- Once oxygen is started, arterial blood gas estimation should be performed within 30 min. Depending on the clinical response, periodic assessment of arterial blood gases is performed. Aim to initially achieve a PaO_2 of at least 6.6 kPa (50 mmHg) without a fall in pH to < 7.35, thus avoiding a respiratory acidosis. Subsequently, oxygen therapy should be adjusted to permit a PaO_2 of > 8.0 kPa (60 mmHg), or saturation of > 90%, again without an increase in $PaCO_2$ or reduction in pH.

- Failure to restore arterial blood oxygenation with 24% oxygen raises the possibility of pneumonia, pulmonary embolism or a pneumothorax being present.

- Caution is required because CO_2 retention (hypercapnia) and respiratory acidosis can arise insidiously with little change in symptoms. The important clinical features of CO_2 retention are warm flushed peripheries due to vasodilation, a bounding pulse, CO_2 retention flap (asterixis), and CO_2 narcosis manifested as drowsiness. Arterial blood gas estimation is used to assess the degree of respiratory acidosis.

- Oxygen saturation by pulse oximetry may be used to monitor response, providing $PaCO_2$ and pH are normal.

- Bronchodilators (ipratropium bromide nebulized at 0.25–0.5 mg plus salbutamol 2.5–5 mg) should be given by nebulization every 4–6 h and continued for 24–48 h. If there is no response, intravenous aminophylline may be added with caution, as stated previously[28].

- Systemic corticosteroids should be given as stated above.

- Antibiotics should be started if indicated (as stated previously). In severe exacerbations, sputum culture and an antibiogram should be performed for antibiotic sensitivity.

- Manage complications: diuretics are indicated if there is peripheral edema, and fluid replacement may be required.

Step 3: non-invasive positive pressure ventilation (NIPPV)

Non-invasive positive pressure ventilation (NIPPV) has been a major advance in the treatment of patients with exacerbations of COPD, and has been studied in randomized controlled trials in acute respiratory failure[45–52]. The British Thoracic Society has recently issued a guideline on non-invasive ventilation in acute respiratory failure[53]. Further research is required to further define selection criteria for NIPPV, and identify patients most likely to benefit from NIPPV (Figure 6.11).

NIPPV has the following properties:

- Improves ventilation
- Increases pH to correct respiratory acidosis
- Reduces $PaCO_2$
- Reduces the severity of breathlessness in the first 4 h
- Decreases the length of hospital stay
- Avoids the need for intubation and invasive mechanical ventilation
- Decreases mortality

Step 4: invasive mechanical ventilation

Conventional invasive mechanical ventilation (IMV) is reserved for more severe indications (Figures 6.12 and 6.13). It is important to consider whether weaning from IMV will be possible, and whether IMV will benefit the individual patient.

Dynamic hyperinflation is caused by the lungs being prevented from reaching their passive functional residual capacity. Dynamic hyperinflation occurs during exacerbations of COPD and is caused by:

- Bronchoconstriction
- Airway inflammation
- Increased mucous secretion
- Loss of elastic recoil

An elastic threshold load, the intrinsic or auto-positive end-expiratory pressure is imposed on the inspiratory muscles at the beginning of inspiration, and increases the work of breathing.

Figure 6.11   Step 3: Selection and exclusion criteria for NIPPV

Selection criteria (at least two should be present)

- Moderate to severe dyspnea with use of accessory muscles and paradoxical abdominal motion

- Moderate to severe acidosis (pH < 7.35) and hypercapnia ($PaCO_2$ > 6.0 kPa, > 45 mmHg)

- Respiratory frequency > 25 breaths per min

Exclusion criteria (any may be present)

- Respiratory arrest

- Cardiovascular instability (hypotension, arrhythmias, myocardial infarction)

- Somnolence, impaired mental status, uncooperative patient

- High aspiration risk; viscous or copious secretions

- Recent facial or gastroesophageal surgery

- Craniofacial trauma, fixed nasopharyngeal abnormalities

- Burns

- Extreme obesity

Adapted from GOLD strategy (2003)

Figure 6.12   Step 4: Indications for admission to intensive care unit and invasive mechanical ventilation

Admission to intensive care unit	Invasive mechanical ventilation
• Severe dyspnea that responds inadequately to initial emergency therapy • Confusion, lethargy, coma • Persistent or worsening hypoxia ($PaO_2 < 6.7$ kPa, 50 mmHg), and/or severe/worsening hypercapnia ($PaCO_2 > 9.3$ kPa, 70 mmHg), and/or severe/worsening respiratory acidosis (pH < 7.30) despite supplemental oxygen and NIPPV	• NIPPV failure (or exclusion criteria) • Severe dyspnea with use of accessory muscles and paradoxical abdominal motion • Respiratory frequency > 35 breaths per min • Life-threatening hypoxia ($PaO_2 < 5.3$ kPa, 40 mmHg or $PaO_2/FiO_2 < 200$ mmHg) • Severe acidosis (pH < 7.25) and hypercapnia ($PaCO_2 > 8.0$ kPa, 60 mmHg) • Respiratory arrest • Somnolence, impaired mental status • Cardiovascular complications (hypotension, shock, heart failure) • Other complications (metabolic abnormalities, sepsis, pneumonia, pulmonary embolism, barotrauma, massive pleural effusion)

Adapted from GOLD strategy (2003)

Figure 6.13   Invasive mechanical ventilation (IMV)

Indication	**Acute respiratory failure due to an exacerbation of COPD with the following features:** • Remediable cause, e.g. pneumonia • First episode of respiratory failure • Acceptable quality of life and a reasonable level of activity could be restored	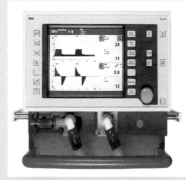
Delivery	Invasive mechanical ventilator with delivery via: • Endotracheal intubation • Tracheostomy	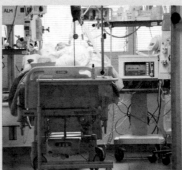
Oxygen source	Hospital oxygen supply	
Delivery regimen	Generally, intermittent positive pressure ventilation (IPPV)	
Monitoring	Closely monitor arterial blood gases	

The EVITA 4 system is shown by courtesy of Draeger Medical, Luebeck, Germany

OTHER TREATMENTS

Fluid and electrolyte administration

In the context of an acute exacerbation of COPD, it is important to carefully monitor and treat fluid and electrolyte abnormalities.

Nutrition

Supplementary nutrition is required when the patient is too breathless to eat.

Low-molecular-weight heparin

This should be considered in immobilized, polycythemic and dehydrated patients regardless of a past history of thromboembolic disease. Low-molecular-weight heparin is mandatory in those with a past history of thromboembolic disease.

Sputum clearance

Mucus clearance strategies using physiotherapy have not been convincingly demonstrated to be effective.

Mucolytics

DNAse (Pulmozyme®) was ineffective when used in the treatment of acute exacerbations of COPD.

Respiratory stimulants

Doxapram may be indicated in the management of an acute exacerbation of COPD if there is hypercapnia and hypoventilation, in order to tide the patient over 24–36 h until the underlying cause (e.g. infection) is controlled. However, it is likely that the use of doxapram in this situation will decline as nasal intermittent positive pressure ventilation becomes more widely available. There is no role for respiratory stimulants, such as doxapram or almitrine, in the long-term management of COPD, since there is no evidence that central ventilatory drive is impaired, ventilation being limited by mechanical rather than neurophysiological factors.

Neuraminidase inhibitors

Inhibitors of neuraminidase, such as zanamivir (inhaled) and oseltamivir (oral) speed the recovery from influenza and may protect against its development[54,55]. However, there are no specific trials in patients with exacerbations of COPD, and it is not yet certain whether this treatment is cost-effective.

Opiates

Breathlessness is a problem in many patients, particularly 'pink puffers'. Several drugs, including nebulized opiates, slow-release morphine, dihydrocodeine and benzodiazepines, may reduce the sensation of dyspnea. However, the reduction in ventilatory drive is potentially dangerous and these drugs should *not* be given during exacerbations[56].

Figure 6.14 Resolution of an exacerbation of COPD

Discharge criteria

- Inhaled β_2-agonist therapy is required no more frequently than every 4 h
- Patient, if previously ambulatory, is able to walk across room
- Patient is able to eat and sleep without frequent awakening by dyspnea
- Patient has been clinically stable for 12–24 h
- Arterial blood gases have been stable for 12–24 h
- Patient (or home care-giver) fully understands correct use of medications
- Follow-up and home care arrangements have been completed (e.g. visiting nurse, oxygen delivery, meal provisions)
- Patient, family and physician are confident that patient can manage successfully

Follow-up

- Ability to cope in usual environment
- Measurement of FEV_1
- Reassessment of inhaler technique
- Understanding of recommended treatment regimen
- Need for long-term oxygen therapy and/or home nebulizer (for patients with severe COPD)

Adapted from GOLD strategy (2003)

DISCHARGE FROM HOSPITAL (Figure 6.14)

- Record FEV$_1$ before discharge

- Check arterial blood gases in patients with a low PaO_2 on admission or with respiratory failure

- Switch nebulized bronchodilators to pressurized metered dose inhaler or dry powder inhaler at least 24 h before discharge

- Check inhaler technique

- Review all medication

- Check that patient understands how to use medication

- Assess home needs. Consider stair lifts, bathing aids, wheelchairs, home help with physiotherapist, occupational therapists and social services

- Consider smoking cessation, influenza vaccination, pulmonary rehabilitation

- Give follow-up appointment 4–6 weeks after discharge

REFERENCES

1. Bach PB, Brown C, Gelfand SE, McCrory DC. Management of acute exacerbations of chronic obstructive pulmonary disease: a summary and appraisal of published evidence. *Ann Intern Med* 2001;134:600–20

2. Connors AF, Jr, Dawson NV, Thomas C, Harrell FE, Jr, Desbiens N, Fulkerson WJ, *et al*. Outcomes following acute exacerbation of severe chronic obstructive lung disease. The SUPPORT investigators (Study to Understand Prognoses and Preferences for Outcomes and Risks of Treatments). *Am J Respir Crit Care Med* 1996;154:959–67

3. Stoller JK. Clinical practice. Acute exacerbations of chronic obstructive pulmonary disease. *N Engl J Med* 2002;346:988–94

4. Sherk PA, Grossman RF. The chronic obstructive pulmonary disease exacerbation. *Clin Chest Med* 2000;21:705–21

5. Kanner RE, Anthonisen NR, Connett JE. Lower respiratory illnesses promote FEV(1) decline in current smokers but not ex-smokers with mild chronic obstructive pulmonary disease: results from the lung health study. *Am J Respir Crit Care Med* 2001;164:358–64

6. Snow V, Lascher S, Mottur-Pilson C. Evidence base for management of acute exacerbations of chronic obstructive pulmonary disease. *Ann Intern Med* 2001;134:595–9

7. National Institutes of Health (NIH), National Heart Lung and Blood Institute (NHLBI), World Health Organisation (WHO). Global Initiative for Chronic Obstructive Lung Disease (GOLD): Global Strategy for the Diagnosis, Management, and Prevention of Chronic Obstructive Pulmonary Disease NHLBI/WHO Workshop Report. www.goldcopd.com/workshop/index.html. 2001.

8. Anthonisen NR, Manfreda J, Warren CP, Hershfield ES, Harding GK, Nelson NA. Antibiotic therapy in exacerbations of chronic obstructive pulmonary disease. *Ann Intern Med* 1987;106:196–204

9. Rodriguez-Roisin R. Toward a consensus definition for COPD exacerbations. *Chest* 2000;117(Suppl 2):398-401S

10. Rohde G, Wiethege A, Borg I, Kauth M, Bauer TT, Gillissen A, *et al*. Respiratory viruses in exacerbations of chronic obstructive pulmonary disease requiring hospitalisation: a case–control study. *Thorax* 2003;58:37–42

11. White AJ, Gompertz S, Stockley RA. Chronic obstructive pulmonary disease. 6. The aetiology of exacerbations of chronic obstructive pulmonary disease. *Thorax* 2003;58:73–80

12. O'Driscoll BR, Taylor RJ, Horsley MG, Chambers DK, Bernstein A. Nebulised salbutamol with and without ipratropium bromide in acute airflow obstruction. *Lancet* 1989;1:1418–20

13. Backman R, Hellstrom PE. Fenoterol and ipratropium bromide for treatment of patients with chronic bronchitis. *Curr Ther Res* 1985;38:135–40

14. Karpel JP, Pesin J, Greenberg D. A comparison of the effects of ipratropium bromide and metaproterenol sulfate in acute exacerbations of COPD. *Chest* 1990;98:835–9

15. Zehner WJ, Jr, Scott JM, Iannolo PM, Ungaro A, Terndrup TE. Terbutaline vs albuterol for out-of-hospital respiratory distress: randomized, double-blind trial. *Acad Emerg Med* 1995;2:686–91

16. Emerman CL, Cydulka RK. Effect of different albuterol dosing regimens in the treatment of acute exacerbation of chronic obstructive pulmonary disease. *Ann Emerg Med* 1997;29:474–8

17. Cydulka RK, Emerman CL. Effects of combined treatment with glycopyrrolate and albuterol in acute exacerbation of asthma. *Ann Emerg Med* 1994;23:270–4

18. Shrestha M, O'Brien T, Haddox R, Gourlay HS, Reed G. Decreased duration of emergency department treatment of chronic obstructive pulmonary disease exacerbations with the addition of ipratropium bromide to beta-agonist therapy. *Ann Emerg Med* 1991;20:1206–9

19. Moayyedi P, Congleton J, Page RL, Pearson SB, Muers MF. Comparison of nebulised salbutamol and iprat-

ropium bromide with salbutamol alone in the treatment of chronic obstructive pulmonary disease. *Thorax* 1995;50:834–7

20. Patrick DM, Dales RE, Stark RM, Laliberte G, Dickinson G. Severe exacerbations of COPD and asthma. Incremental benefit of adding ipratropium to usual therapy. *Chest* 1990;98:295–7

21. Rebuck AS, Chapman KR, Abboud R, Pare PD, Kreisman H, Wolkove N, *et al.* Nebulised anticholinergic and sympathomimetic treatment of asthma and chronic obstructive airways disease in the emergency room. *Am J Med* 1987;82:59–64

22. Greene AB, Jr., Jackson CL. Terbutaline metered-dose inhalation vs metaproterenol by hand-held nebulization: a comparison in black inner-city COPD patients. *J Natl Med Assoc* 1988;80:393–6

23. Higgins RM, Cookson WO, Chadwick GA. Changes in blood gas levels after nebuhaler and nebulizer administration of terbutaline in severe chronic airway obstruction. *Bull Eur Physiopathol Respir* 1987;23:261–4

24. Barr RG, Rowe BH, Camargo CA, Jr. Methylxanthines for exacerbations of chronic obstructive pulmonary disease. *Cochrane Database Syst Rev* 2001:CD002168

25. Barr RG. Acute exacerbations of chronic obstructive pulmonary disease. *N Engl J Med* 2002;347:1533–4

26. Rice KL, Leatherman JW, Duane PG, Snyder LS, Harmon KR, Abel J, *et al.* Aminophylline for acute exacerbations of chronic obstructive pulmonary disease. A controlled trial. *Ann Intern Med* 1987;107:305–9

27. Seidenfeld JJ, Jones WN, Moss RE, Tremper J. Intravenous aminophylline in the treatment of acute bronchospastic exacerbations of chronic obstructive pulmonary disease. *Ann Emerg Med* 1984;13:248–52

28. McCrory DC, Brown CD. Inhaled short-acting beta2-agonists versus ipratropium for acute exacerbations of chronic obstructive pulmonary disease (Cochrane Review). *Cochrane Database Syst Rev* 2001;2:CD002984

29. Thompson WH, Nielson CP, Carvalho P, Charan NB, Crowley JJ. Controlled trial of oral prednisone in outpatients with acute COPD exacerbation. *Am J Respir Crit Care Med* 1996;154:407–12

30. Davies L, Angus RM, Calverley PM. Oral corticosteroids in patients admitted to hospital with exacerbations of chronic obstructive pulmonary disease: a prospective randomised controlled trial. *Lancet* 1999;354:456–60

31. Niewoehner DE, Erbland ML, Deupree RH, Collins D, Gross NJ, Light RW, *et al.* Effect of systemic glucocorticoids on exacerbations of chronic obstructive pulmonary disease. Department of Veterans

Affairs Cooperative Study Group. *N Engl J Med* 1999;340:1941–7

32. Emerman CL, Connors AF, Lukens TW, May ME, Effron D. A randomized controlled trial of methylprednisolone in the emergency treatment of acute exacerbations of COPD. *Chest* 1989;95:563–7

33. Albert RK, Martin TR, Lewis SW. Controlled clinical trial of methylprednisolone in patients with chronic bronchitis and acute respiratory insufficiency. *Ann Intern Med* 1980;92:753–8

34. Saetta M, Di Stefano A, Maestrelli P, Turato G, Ruggieri MP, Roggeri A, *et al.* Airway eosinophilia in chronic bronchitis during exacerbations. *Am J Respir Crit Care Med* 1994;150:1646–52

35. Paggiaro PL, Dahle R, Bakran I, Frith L, Hollingworth K, Efthimiou J. Multicentre randomised in placebo-controlled trial of inhaled fluticasone propionate in patients with chronic obstructive pulmonary disease. *Lancet* 1998;351: 773–80

36. Wood-Baker R, Walters EH, Gibson P. Oral corticosteroids for acute exacerbations of chronic obstructive pulmonary disease. *Cochrane Database Syst Rev* 2001(2):CD001288

37. Aaron SD, Vandemheen KL, Hebert P, *et al.* Outpatient oral prednisone after emergency treatment of chronic obstructive pulmonary disease. *N Engl J Med* 2003;348:2618–25

38. Saint S, Bent S, Vittinghoff E, Grady D. Antibiotics in chronic obstructive pulmonary disease exacerbations. A meta analysis. *J Am Med Assoc* 1995;273:957–60

39. Seemungal TA, Harper-Owen R, Bhowmik A, Jeffries DJ, Wedzicha JA. Detection of rhinovirus in induced sputum at exacerbation of chronic obstructive pulmonary disease. *Eur Respir J* 2000;16:677–83

40. Plant PK, Elliott MW. Chronic obstructive pulmonary disease. 9. Management of ventilatory failure in COPD. *Thorax* 2003;58:537–42

41. Bedon GA, Block AJ, Ball WC, Jr. The "28 percent" Venturi mask in obstructive airway disease. *Arch Intern Med* 1970;125:106–13

42. Bone RC, Pierce AK, Johnson RL, Jr. Controlled oxygen administration in acute respiratory failure in chronic obstructive pulmonary disease: a reappraisal. *Am J Med* 1978;65:896–902

43. Eldridge F, Gherman C. Studies of oxygen administration in respiratory failure. *Ann Intern Med* 1968;68:569–78

44. Warrell DA, Edwards RH, Godfrey S, Jones NL. Effect of controlled oxygen therapy on arterial blood gases in acute respiratory failure. *Br Med J* 1970;1:452–5

45. Barbe F, Togores B, Rubi M, Pons S, Maimo A, Agusti AG. Noninvasive ventilatory support does not facilitate recovery from acute respiratory failure in chronic obstructive pulmonary disease. *Eur Respir J* 1996;9:1240–5

46. Doherty MJ, Greenstone MA. Survey of non-invasive ventilation (NIPPV) in patients with acute exacerbations of chronic obstructive pulmonary disease (COPD) in the UK. *Thorax* 1998;53:863–6

47. Bott J, Carroll MP, Conway JH, Keilty SE, Ward EM, Brown AM, *et al*. Randomised controlled trial of nasal ventilation in acute ventilatory failure due to chronic obstructive airways disease. *Lancet* 1993;341:1555–7

48. Plant PK, Owen JL, Elliott MW. Early use of non-invasive ventilation for acute exacerbations of chronic obstructive pulmonary disease on general respiratory wards: a multicentre randomised controlled trial. *Lancet* 2000;355:1931–5

49. Brochard L, Mancebo J, Wysocki M, Lofaso F, Conti G, Rauss A, *et al*. Noninvasive ventilation for acute exacerbations of chronic obstructive pulmonary disease. *N Engl J Med* 1995;333:817–22

50. Kramer N, Meyer TJ, Meharg J, Cece RD, Hill NS. Randomized, prospective trial of noninvasive positive pressure ventilation in acute respiratory failure. *Am J Respir Crit Care Med* 1995;151:1799–806

51. Keenan SP, Kernerman PD, Cook DJ, Martin CM, McCormack D, Sibbald WJ. Effect of noninvasive positive pressure ventilation on mortality in patients admitted with acute respiratory failure: a meta-analysis. *Crit Care Med* 1997;25:1685–92

52. Bardi G, Pierotello R, Desideri M, Valdisserri L, Bottai M, Palla A. Nasal ventilation in COPD exacerbations: early and late results of a prospective, controlled study. *Eur Respir J* 2000;15:98–104

53. British Thoracic Society Standards of Care Committee. Non-invasive ventilation in acute respiratory failure. *Thorax* 2002;57:192–211

54. Dunn CJ, Goa KL. Zanamivir: a review of its use in influenza. *Drugs* 1999;58:761–84

55. Bardsley-Elliot A, Noble S. Oseltamivir. *Drugs* 1999;58:851–60

56. Poole PJ, Veale AG, Black PN. The effect of sustained-release morphine on breathlessness and quality of life in severe chronic obstructive pulmonary disease. *Am J Respir Crit Care Med* 1998;157:1877–80

7

Specialized treatment modalities: pulmonary rehabilitation, oxygen therapy and surgery

CONTENTS

Pulmonary rehabilitation
Cycle of consequences of COPD
Patient selection and benefits

Exercise
Exercise tests
Health-related quality of life
Exercise conditioning
Breathing control and posture
Inflammation

Nutrition
Immunology
Assessment of nutritional status
Prognosis
Dietary treatment

Sleep
Obstructive sleep apnea
Nocturnal hypoxia
Insomnia

Depression

Patient education

Pulmonary hypertension

Oxygen therapy and ventilatory support
Short-term oxygen therapy
Long-term oxygen therapy
Ambulatory oxygen
Oxygen during air travel
Oxygen supply
Oxygen delivery
Non-invasive positive pressure
    ventilation (NIPPV)
Invasive mechanical ventilation (IMV)

Surgery
Bullectomy
Lung volume reduction surgery
Lung transplantation

Palliative care

SUMMARY

Management of COPD requires integration of several clinical disciplines, using a variety of treatment approaches. This chapter considers a number of treatment modalities other than smoking cessation and pharmacotherapy.

Pulmonary rehabilitation is a multidisciplinary program of care that is employed to optimize physical and social performance in patients with COPD. Elements of pulmonary rehabilitation focus on exercise, nutrition, sleep, depression and patient education. A duration of at least 8 weeks for pulmonary rehabilitation programs is recommended in the GOLD (2003) guidelines.

Long-term oxygen therapy prolongs survival in patients with severe COPD, but should be given for at least 15 h/day. A variety of sources of oxygen and delivery systems are available and should be matched to individual patient's needs. Non-invasive positive pressure ventilation (NIPPV) has recently become established as effective therapy in acute hypercapnic exacerbations of COPD as well as in certain patients with hypercapnic chronic type II respiratory failure. NIPPV is increasingly performed as an effective alternative to invasive mechanical ventilation.

The major surgical procedures to consider for patients with COPD are bullectomy, lung volume reduction surgery and lung transplantation. Detailed evaluation is required to assess the risk of the surgical procedure in relation to potential benefits in terms of quality of life and survival of patients.

Patients with severe COPD have specialized needs for optimal standards of clinical and palliative care.

Figure 7.1   Pulmonary rehabilitation websites and useful videos

British Thoracic Society (BTS) guidelines on pulmonary rehabilitation — http://www.brit-thoracic.org.uk/guide/guidelines.html

Hartford Hospital pulmonary rehabilitation program (US) — http://www.harthosp.org/pulmonaryrehab/index.html

Cheshire Medical Center pulmonary rehabilitation program (US) — http://www.cheshire-med.com/programs/pulrehab/rehab.html

American Association for Respiratory Care (AARC) — http://www.aarc.org/patient education

American College of Chest Physicians — http://www.chestnet.org/education/patient

Milner Fenwick Patient Education Online (US) — http://www.milner-fenwick.com/pe/pulr.htm
Pulmonary Rehabilitation Video Series
- Breathing training and pulmonary illness
- Pulmonary medications and hygiene
- Stress and relaxation techniques for pulmonary patients
- Exercise for pulmonary patients
- Healthy choices for managing your pulmonary illness

PULMONARY REHABILITATION

An official statement from the American Thoracic Society in 1999 gave the following definition of pulmonary rehabilitation[1]:

'Pulmonary rehabilitation is a multidisciplinary program of care for patients with chronic respiratory impairment that is individually tailored and designed to optimize physical and social performance and autonomy.'

The principal goals of pulmonary rehabilitation[2] are to:

(1) Reduce symptoms, disability and handicap;

(2) Improve health-related quality of life;

(3) Improve functional independence, with maximal ability to perform a range of everyday activities;

(4) Increase physical, social and emotional well-being in everyday activities.

Several non-pharmacological approaches have been used in the management of COPD and may form part of a comprehensive pulmonary rehabilitation program[3,4]. Pulmonary rehabilitation programs are generally based on hospital outpatients, since there is the need for input from a team of health professionals. Important textbooks and special reports provide comprehensive coverage of pulmonary rehabilitation for patients with COPD[2,5–9]. Figure 7.1 lists websites and videos that contain useful material on pulmonary rehabilitation for patients and health professionals.

It is assumed that optimal medical management of the patient with COPD has been incorporated, including smoking cessation (Chapter 4), optimal use of bronchodilators and consideration for inhaled corticosteroids (Chapter 5). Rehabilitation involves a range of approaches, being a holistic approach to the well-being of the individual patient, and involving a multidisciplinary team:

(1) Exercise and physical training;

(2) Nutritional advice;

(3) Sleep studies for selected patients;

(4) Psychological assessment: depression;

(5) Disease education;

(6) Social and behavioral intervention.

Pulmonary rehabilitation includes physical exercise training to minimize deconditioning, disease education, physiotherapy and psychological and social support. Rehabilitation programs are successful in prospective randomized trials in terms of increased performance and quality of life[10–12]. The optimal length and frequency of rehabilitation programs are not known.

Cycle of consequences of COPD

Patients with COPD have a range of interlinked problems that are not just restricted to direct clinical consequences of pulmonary disease (Figure 7.2). These problems become a vicious circle of greater significance in patients with Stage II (moderate), Stage III (severe) and Stage IV (very severe) COPD and include:

(1) Pulmonary disease, primarily dyspnea, owing to obstructive airways disease, hyperinflation and respiratory failure;

(2) Systemic disease including weight loss[13] with muscle wasting and weakness[14,15]. Pulmonary hypertension, *cor pulmonale* and other smoking-related diseases (cardiovascular disease and malignancies) may also be prominent;

Figure 7.2   Clinical, physical, social and psychological features of COPD

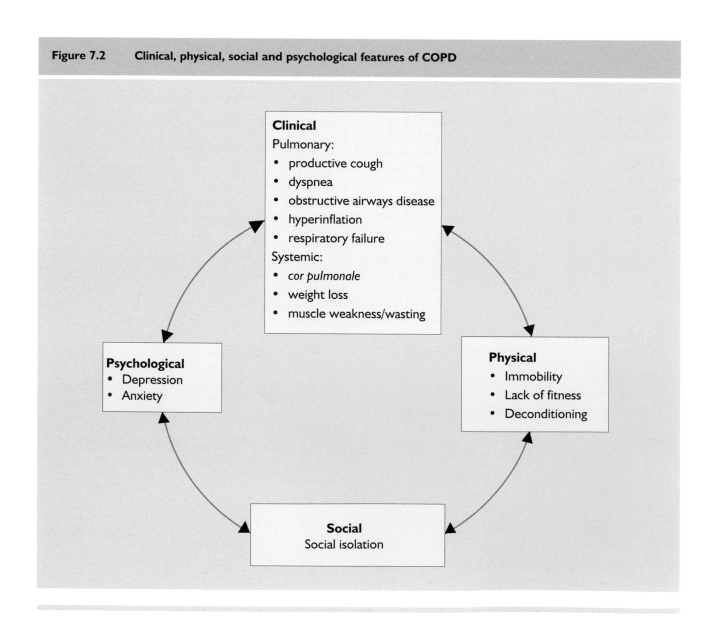

(3) Physical problems including immobility and exercise deconditioning;

(4) Social isolation;

(5) Depression[16].

Patient selection and benefits

Patients with moderate to very severe COPD are generally included in rehabilitation programs; however, more information on criteria for selecting patients is required[17]. Nevertheless, COPD patients of all GOLD stages from 0 (at risk) to stage IV (very severe) appear to benefit from participation in programs[18]. However, improvement in health status and exercise performance was best demonstrated in patients with moderate dyspnea[11]. A meta-analysis of randomized controlled trials of pulmonary rehabilitation has demonstrated improvement in dyspnea, with less obvious effects on exercise capacity[10]. Improvements in walking ability and quality of life have been demonstrated[12]. Maintenance by weekly telephone calls and monthly supervision sessions have only minor benefits[19].

GOLD (2003) recommends that pulmonary rehabilitation should be considered in patients with stages II, III and IV COPD (post-bronchoilator FEV_1 < 80%). The minimum length of an effective rehabilitation program is 7 weeks, with further benefits from longer programs[20]. Pulmonary rehabilitation has been shown to be effective when performed in hospitals, outpatient clinics and at home[21–24].

EXERCISE

Exercise tests

A variety of tests are available to assess exercise tolerance (Figure 7.3):

(1) The 6-min walk test is a self-paced timed walking test, that assesses the distance the patient can walk on a flat surface over 6 min, but requires at least one training session[25–28].

(2) The incremental shuttle walking test involves being supervised walking to-and-fro between two cones placed 10 m apart, the speed gradually being increased, generally to keep time with a pre-recorded audiotape[29–32].

(3) Bicycle ergometry and treadmill tests can also be performed in conjunction with cardiac monitoring, maximum oxygen consumption and maximum work performed[32,33].

Health-related quality of life

Health status has become a major feature of studies in COPD[17,34]. The St. George's Respiratory Questionnaire (SGRQ) is a standardized self-completed questionnaire for measuring health-related quality of life in airways disease[35–37]. The final version has 76 items divided into three sections: 'symptoms', 'activity' and 'impacts', and provides a total score. Scores range from 0 (perfect health) to 100 (worst possible state), with a four-point change in score considered a worthwhile treatment effect. The SGRQ and the Chronic Respiratory Disease Questionnaire (CRDQ) have been found to be equivalent in a comparative study[38]. Generic questionnaires have a place in COPD studies, but are relatively insensitive, and include the Sickness Impact Profile (SIP) and Short Form-36 Questionnaire (SF-36)[39,40].

Exercise conditioning

COPD patients of all degrees of severity appear to benefit from exercise training (Figure 7.3)[41–44].

(1) *Cardiorespiratory or exercise training* is generally helpful[45–48]. This may be performed on a weekly or daily basis, with a duration of 10 min to 1 h, with programs generally lasting 4–10 weeks. Patients are sometimes encouraged to achieve a predetermined target heart rate. When training to walk on flat surfaces, the patient may continue until symptom limitation, rest, and then continue until 20 min of walking is performed.

(2) *Upper limb exercises and strength training* can employ an upper limb ergometer or resistive training with weights[49]. This improves strength but does not improve health-related quality of life or exercise tolerance.

(3) *Ventilatory or respiratory muscle training* using resistive inspiratory loading may reduce breathlessness[50,51]. Maximal sustainable ventilation can be performed using a hand-held device for 15–30 min/day, providing targeted inspiratory muscle training. However, a meta-analysis of controlled studies of ventilatory muscle training alone has provided little evidence of overall benefit[45,52].

Figure 7.3   Exercise in pulmonary rehabilitation

Outcome measures

Testing methods
- 6-min walk test (6MWT)
- incremental shuttle walk test (ISWT)
- bicycle ergometry
- treadmill exercise

Health status questionnaire
- St. George's Respiratory Questionnaire (SGRQ)
- Chronic Respiratory Disease Questionnaire (CRDQ)
- Short Form-36 Questionnaire (SF-36) (general)

Dyspnea during exercise
- Visual analog and Borg rating scales
- Medical Research Council (MRC) scale
- Baseline and transitional dyspnea index (BDI and TDI)

Training

Breathing training (Figure 3.7)
- pursed lips on expiration: maintain pressure and patency of airways
- diaphragmatic breathing: expand abdomen on inspiration

Limb aerobic endurance and strength resistive training
- upper limb exercise: upper limb cycle ergometer

  resistance training with weights

  throwing ball against wall with raised arms
- lower limb exercise: walking 20 minutes daily for 4–10 weeks

  walk/rest/continue walking for 20 minutes

  cycling

  resistance training with weights

Ventilatory muscle training – controversial
- targeted inspiratory muscle training device
- maximal sustainable ventilation for 15 minutes
- add CO_2 to inspired air to maintain isocapnia during rapid ventilation

Breathing control and posture

Controlled breathing techniques, such as pursed-lip breathing and diaphragmatic breathing, have been claimed to result in reduced dyspnea in patients with COPD[53] (Figure 3.7). Pursed-lip breathing is a form of biofeedback that helps patients to reduce trans-airway pressure gradients and the tendency for small airways to collapse; it should be performed during the most strenuous part of a task such as lifting an object. Diaphragmatic breathing involves retraining the respiratory muscles for improved efficiency, so that the patient consciously relaxes to expand the abdominal wall during inspiration. However, attempts at diaphragmatic breathing can reduce the efficiency of breathing in chronic hyperinflation[54].

Forward-lean sitting can provide important postural relief in a patient with severe hyperinflation and a low flat diaphragm[55–57]. Passive fixation of the shoulder girdle by supporting the elbows and supported sitting may benefit individual patients.

Inflammation

Systemic inflammation is present in COPD[58] and this affects skeletal muscle morphology, metabolism and function[59,60].

NUTRITION

Patients with chronic bronchitis are more likely to be obese, while patients with emphysema are more likely to be underweight[61]. As part of a pulmonary rehabilitation program, it is important to perform assessment of nutritional state (Figure 3.28), to assess the patient's diet, to give dietary advice, and, in some cases, to institute dietary supplements (Figure 7.4)[62]. Inadequate diet may contribute to the development of COPD, owing to deficient supply of vitamins A, C and, possibly, E[63], and also due to insufficient fruit and vegetables[64–66]. In conditions of social isolation and decreased functional activities, it is important to establish that all patients with COPD have an adequate and balanced diet.

Immunology

Patients with COPD have an amplified inflammatory response in the lungs, and systemic inflammation with cachexia and skeletal muscle dysfunction may be present[13,67,68]. In patients with COPD and cachexia, there is enhanced whole body protein turnover[69] and increased nitrogen excretion with reduced fat-free mass[70]. In addition, there is a loss of circadian rhythm of circulating leptin[71–73] that may be independent of abnormalities in levels of serum tumor necrosis factor-α (TNF-α) and plasma soluble TNF receptor[74–76]. There is also weakness and atrophy of skeletal muscle[77], with abnormal skeletal muscle amino acid profiles[78] and increased skeletal muscle apoptosis[79–81].

Assessment of nutritional status: body mass index and fat-free mass

Body mass index (BMI, weight divided by (height)^2) can be used to classify patients as underweight, normal and overweight[62] (Figure 3.28). A BMI of < 21 kg/m^2 is generally regarded as underweight, being about 90% of ideal body weight. However, in elderly COPD patients, underweight may be < 25 kg/m^2.

Assessment of fat-free mass is a better indicator of nutritional depletion than body weight, BMI and percentage of ideal body weight[82]. Weight can be divided into fat mass and fat-free mass (water, protein and minerals). This water is distributed intra- and extracellularly. Depletion of fat-free mass in COPD is generally regarded as < 16 kg/m^2 in males and < 15 kg/m^2 in females.

Dual-energy X-ray absorptiometry (DEXA) scan allows assessment of whole body composition and the three compartments of lean body mass, fat body mass and bone mineral body mass[83]. Alternatively, bioelectrical impedance analysis is a simple and non-invasive means of measuring body composition and fat-free mass[84]. Mid-thigh muscle cross-sectional area is a predictor of mortality in COPD[85].

Prognosis

Nutritional depletion causes decreased exercise tolerance[86]. Reduced fat-free mass and low body mass index are associated with an increased mortality[87–91].

Dietary treatment

Points to consider for dietary treatment regimens include (Figure 7.4):

(1) *Obesity* Obese patients should lose weight, particularly if there are sleep disturbances such as obstructive sleep apnea.

(2) *Vitamins* Following dietary assessment, dietary advice and antioxidant vitamin supplements may be indicated.

(3) *Nutritional supplements* In selected patients with cachexia and COPD, low body weight can be reversed with a high calorie liquid supplement, sometimes with a short course of anabolic steroid[90,92,93]. However, food supplementation with high-calorie oral nutritional therapy has only modest benefits in the majority of patients[94], and a meta-analysis of nine trials has concluded that there is no effect on anthropometric measures, lung function or exercise capacity[95]. Non-response is associated with aging, relative anorexia and elevated systemic inflammation[96]. Nevertheless, slight but uniform benefits have been noted, and may be a prerequisite for exercise training[97].

(4) Megestrol acetate (a progestational agent)[98], anabolic steroids[99], growth hormone and therapy directed against TNF-α are potential therapies for cachexia in COPD that require clinical evaluation.

SLEEP

Sleep is a period of physiological disturbance in COPD, and patients with severe COPD generally

---

Figure 7.4   Nutrition in COPD

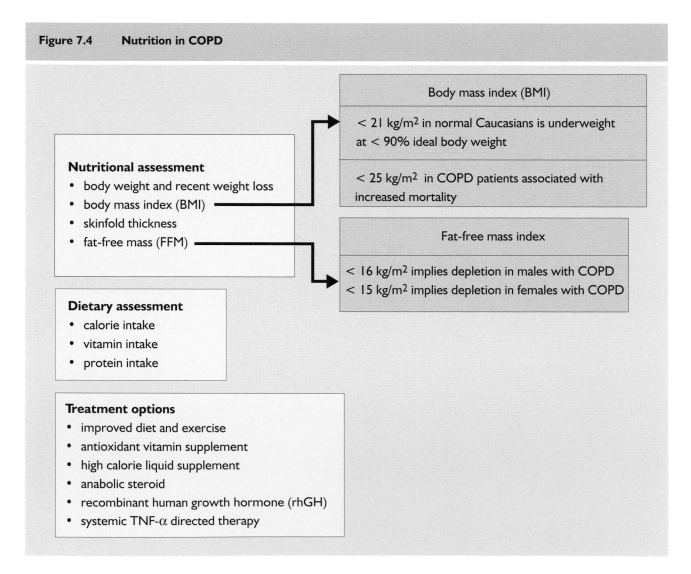

Based on Schols AMWT, Wouters EFM (Figure 14.1). In Hodgkin JE, Celli BR, Connors GL, eds. *Pulmonary Rehabilitation: Guidelines to Success.* Lippincott Williams & Wilkins, 3rd edition, 2000.

sleep badly and may have nocturnal hypoxemia[100–103](Figure 7.5).

Obstructive sleep apnea

In patients with suspected obstructive sleep apnea or sleep-related hypoxemia in the absence of obstructive sleep apnea, sleep studies with assessment of arterial blood gases should be performed[104]. A screening sleep study is performed by assessing nocturnal pulse oximetry in relation to heart rate[105]. A full overnight sleep test includes a polysomnogram and should be carried out at a specialized sleep center.

The Sleep Heart Study has recently shown that obstructive sleep apnea may coexist with COPD, but this is the result of chance alone, since both are common conditions[106]. Obstructive sleep apnea is present in up to 5% of men, who are typically but not always obese, loud snorers, with a short mandible, and in their fifties. Although not more common in COPD, obstructive sleep apnea may cause significant morbidity in COPD patients[103,107]. Obstructive sleep apnea is caused by multiple episodes of upper airway obstruction and arousal during sleep[108,109]. The obstruction is due to floppy pharyngeal walls collapsing after a series of ineffective but increasing inspiratory effects. After up to a minute of asphyxia, there is a bradycardia–tachycardia pattern, and arousal from sleep causes resumption of breathing and restoration of blood gases. The symptoms of obstructive sleep apnea may be described by the partner, while the patient with

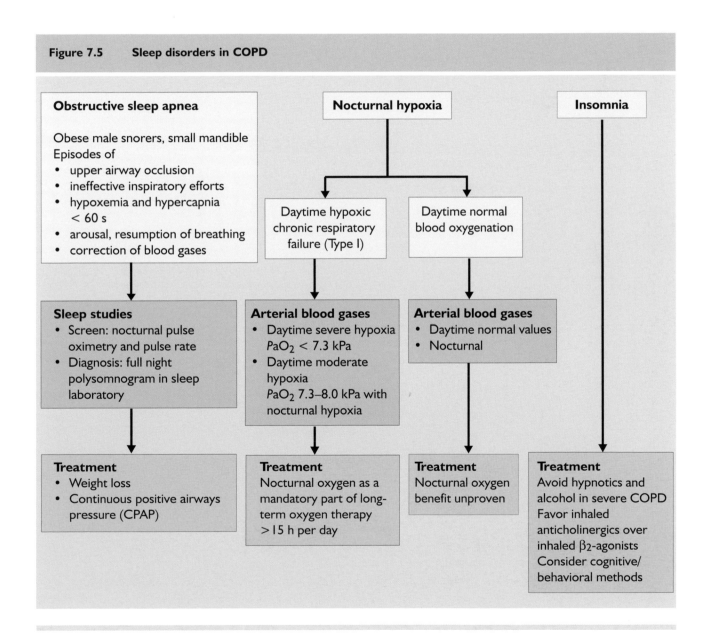

Figure 7.5   Sleep disorders in COPD

obstructive sleep apnea suffers sleep deprivation: excessive morning and daytime sleepiness, intellectual deterioration, memory loss and personality changes.

Continuous positive airways pressure (CPAP) has revolutionized the therapy of obstructive sleep apnea since being introduced in 1981[104], and criteria for therapy are being defined[110]. In patients with both COPD and obstructive sleep apnea, it is important adequately to treat both disorders, since CPAP with a full face mask is required for obstructive sleep apnea (Figure 7.6). CPAP involves giving compressed air to prevent collapse of small airways and alveoli.

Nocturnal hypoxia

COPD patients may have nocturnal oxygen desaturation that is not due to obstructive sleep apnea, and this can be detected by screening overnight pulse oximetry and sleep studies[105]. Treatment with nocturnal oxygen is given in those with both daytime and nocturnal hypoxemia, but nocturnal oxygen is not justified for those with isolated nocturnal hypoxemia[101,111]. Patients on long-term oxygen

therapy generally require supplemental oxygen at night to maintain therapy with oxygen > 15 h/day[112], and sleep is often the time with the worst gas exchange[103].

Insomnia

With increasingly severe COPD, more patients have difficulty going to sleep, more frequent awakenings and generalized insomnia. Anticholinergics are less likely to disturb sleep than β_2-agonists, and hypnotics and alcohol should be avoided in patients with severe COPD. Drug management of insomnia can be dangerous, especially in COPD patients with hypercarbia, and, in these patients, cognitive/behavioral methods are sometimes useful[113]. Sleep ventilation is common in hypercapnic COPD, and is related to baseline arterial carbon dioxide levels, body mass index and severity of airway obstruction[114].

DEPRESSION

Patients with severe COPD are at increased risk of developing depression, and this can occur in 25% of

---

Figure 7.6   Continuous positive airways pressure (CPAP)

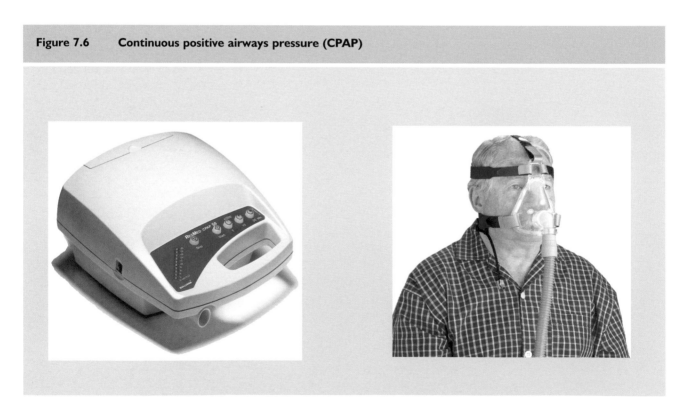

CPAP device (ResMed CPAP S6) and full face mask (Mirage series 2). Photographs by courtesy of ResMed Ltd, North Ryde, Australia

patients in general practice[115–117]. A systematic review of ten studies found only four to have a case–control design, and in these studies an association between COPD and depression was noted[16]. End-stage lung disease has considerable psychological impact[118], and this can interfere with health status[119–121]. However, patient acceptance of the antidepressant fluoxetine was poor, so this may not be an effective strategy[122], and pulmonary rehabilitation may significantly improve anxiety and depression[123].

PATIENT EDUCATION

Patient education alone does not improve exercise performance or lung function, but it does play a role in improving skills, ability to cope with illness and health status[124]. A systematic review was unable to make recommendations concerning self-management education for patients with COPD[125]. A range of topics for education should be considered at various stages in COPD:

(1) Smoking cessation and reducing risk factors: patient education regarding smoking cessation has the greatest capacity to influence the natural history of COPD (see Chapter 4);

(2) Learning about the causes and clinical outlook of COPD;

(3) Inhalers and medications: inhaler technique, the variety of inhaler devices, drugs and their actions and side-effects;

(4) Exacerbations: patient education may improve the patient's response;

(5) Strategies to minimize dyspnea;

(6) Complications: information on complications including *cor pulmonale* and cachexia;

(7) Oxygen treatment: education on the range of available options;

(8) End of life: discussions and education are important to alleviate issues for the patient and their family and carers.

There are a variety of educational materials, ranging from simple printed materials, to teaching sessions, and to management workshops. In general, passive use of printed materials is much less effective than interactive education in small workshops.

PULMONARY HYPERTENSION

Long-term oxygen therapy is the only treatment that slows down the progression of pulmonary hypertension in COPD[126]. Treatment with vasodilators such as calcium channel blockers is not recommended because they impair pulmonary gas exchange. Selective pulmonary vasodilators including 'pulsed' inhalation of nitric oxide with oxygen over a period of 3 months has recently been found to be safe and effective[127,128].

OXYGEN THERAPY AND VENTILATORY SUPPORT IN CHRONIC STABLE COPD

Short-term oxygen therapy

Poor oxygenation is a fundamental problem in more severe COPD and supplementary oxygen is an important part of therapy in patients with chronic stable COPD and hypoxemia[129,130] (Figures 7.7–7.9). See Chapter 6 for short-term oxygen therapy during steps 2–4 of an exacerbation of COPD requiring hospitalization.

Long-term oxygen therapy

Long-term home oxygen therapy (domiciliary oxygen) is indicated in selected patients with chronic stable COPD[131]. Two large multicenter trials have demonstrated that long-term oxygen administration (> 15 h daily) prolongs survival (by about 30%) in patients with very severe COPD[132,133]. Long-term oxygen therapy does not improve survival in patients with mild to moderate hypoxemia[10] or nocturnal oxygen desaturation alone.

Effects of long-term oxygen therapy

(1) Improvement in exercise capacity (increased endurance);

(2) Reduction in dyspnea;

(3) Reduction in pulmonary hypertension, by reducing hypoxic pulmonary vasoconstriction[134];

(4) Reduction in hematocrit by reducing erythropoietin levels;

(5) Improved quality of life[135] and neuropsychiatric function;

(6) Reduction in severe desaturation episodes during sleep.

Figure 7.7   Oxygen therapy and ventilatory support in chronic stable COPD

	Long-term oxygen therapy (LTOT)	Ambulatory and aircraft oxygen	Non-invasive positive pressure ventilation (NIPPV)
Indication	**Hypoxic chronic respiratory failure: Type I respiratory failure** **EITHER Severe hypoxia**[1] $PaO_2 < 7.3$ kPa (< 55 mmHg) corresponding to $SaO_2 < 88\%$ **OR Moderate hypoxia . . .** PaO_2 7.3–8.0 kPa (55–60 mmHg) corresponding to SaO_2 88–90% **with at least one of the following:** • Pulmonary hypertension • Peripheral edema • Polycythemia (hematocrit $> 55\%$) • Nocturnal hypoxemia If hypercapnia is present, consider NIPPV	**For temporary relief of hypoxia and dyspnea** • on exertion • on airline flights	**Hypercapnic respiratory failure: Type II respiratory failure** Hypoxia with hypercapnia $CO_2 > 6.0$ kPa (45 mmHg) Subject to contraindications (Figure 6.11) Treatment of choice for acute hypercapnic exacerbations of COPD (see Figure 6.11)
Delivery	• Nasal prongs/cannulae • Pulsed delivery system – delivery only on inspiration	• Venturi mask • Nasal prongs/cannulae	• Tight nasal mask (Figure 7.10) • Full facial mask
Oxygen source[2]	• Oxygen concentrator from room air • Compressed oxygen cylinders 24, 28, 35, 50% 2 l/min (cylinder lasts 2 h), 4 l/min • Liquid oxygen	• Compressed oxygen cylinders • Liquid oxygen • Aircraft oxygen	• Hospital gas supply • Oxygen concentrator • Compressed oxygen cylinders • Liquid oxygen In association with a NIPPV device to give positive pressure on inspiration (Figure 7.10)
Delivery regime	LTOT: at least 15 h/day for benefit	Prophylactically as required	Decreases work of breathing and decreases need for invasive mechanical ventilation (IMV)
Monitoring[2]	Arterial blood gases for levels of O_2, CO_2, pH, bicarbonate (HCO_3^-) Aim for arterial blood O_2 of $PaO_2 > 8.0$ kPa, > 60 mmHg $SaO_2 > 90\%$ while on oxygen therapy Pulse oximetry gives O_2 saturation (SaO_2) in pulsating blood vessels	Ambulatory assessment of oxygen desaturation on a standard walking test. Pre-flight assessment by: • prediction from arterial blood PaO_2 • hypoxic challenge test	Arterial blood gases for O_2, CO_2, pH, HCO_3^- Aim for arterial blood O_2 of $PaO_2 > 8.0$ kPa, > 60 mmHg $SaO_2 > 90\%$ while on NIPPV Aim for arterial blood CO_2 of < 6.0 kPa (45 mmHg)

[1] Normal PaO_2 11–13 kPa (80–100 mmHg), normal $PaCO_2$ 4.5–6.0 kPa (34–45 mmHg) (see Figure 6.6)

[2] Oxygen therapy must be controlled with monitoring of arterial blood gases, taking care to restore oxygenation but prevent the insidious onset of CO_2 retention: peripheral vasodilation, bounding pulse, retention flap and drowsiness

Figure 7.8   Supplementary oxygen products

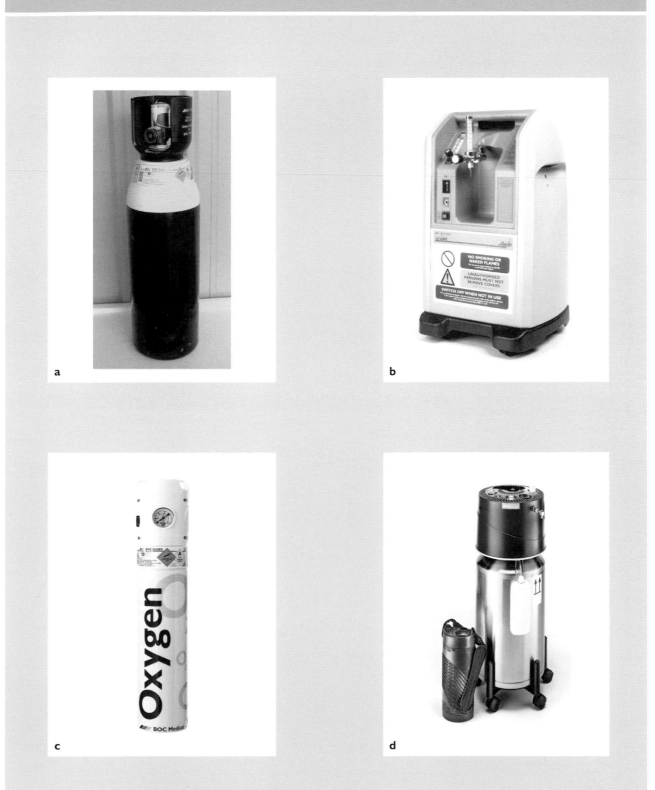

(a) Compressed oxygen cylinder containing medical oxygen (99.5%), given at medium flow rate (2 l/min) or high flow rate (4 l/min); (b) oxygen concentrator; (c) lightweight portable oxygen cylinder; (d) liquid oxygen in a base unit and a portable unit. Pictures by courtesy of BOC Medical (Vitalair, Manchester, UK).

Figure 7.9   Delivery of oxygen

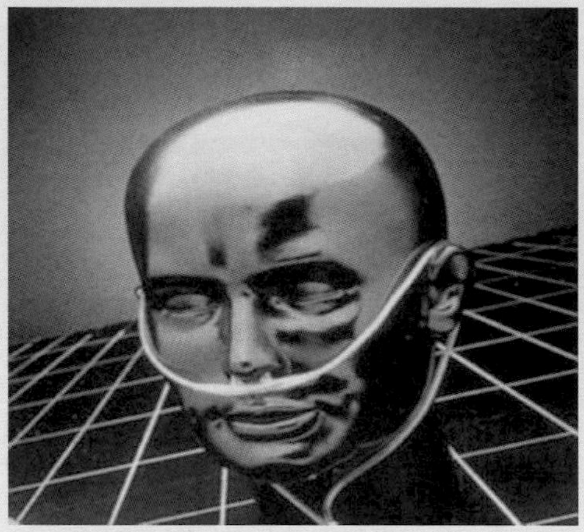

Nasal cannula

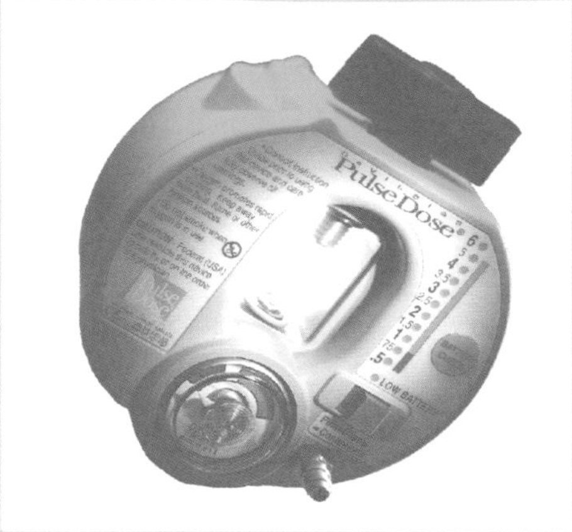

Pulsed delivery device

Picture of DeVilbiss Pulse Dose by courtesy of Sunrise Medical, Longmont, Colorado, USA.

Indications for long-term oxygen therapy (Figure 7.7)

As COPD becomes more severe, it is necessary for a respiratory specialist to consider long-term oxygen therapy in patients with chronic hypoxia. The UK Royal College of Physicians Clinical Guidelines give indications for patients to be given domiciliary oxygen[136,137]. Arterial blood gas measurements should be made when the patient is clinically stable and on optimal drug therapy for COPD on at least two occasions 3 weeks apart. Long-term oxygen therapy is hazardous for patients who continue to smoke, and special fire precautions are required.

(1) Long-term oxygen therapy should be prescribed for COPD patients with a PaO_2 of < 7.3 kPa (< 55 mmHg) when breathing air during a period of clinical stability. The level of $PaCO_2$ does not influence the need for long-term oxygen therapy, but is important in considering use of non-invasive ventilation (see below). Clinical stability is defined as absence of exacerbation of COPD and of peripheral edema for the previous 4 weeks.

(2) Long-term oxygen therapy should also be considered if PaO_2 is 7.3–8.0 kPa (55–60 mmHg) together with presence of at least one of the following: secondary polycythemia or nocturnal hypoxemia (defined as SaO_2 below 90% for at least 30% of the night), peripheral edema or pulmonary hypertension.

Provision of long-term oxygen therapy

Patients on long-term oxygen therapy should be reassessed regularly by measuring arterial blood gases. Blood gas measurements should be made when patients are on long-term oxygen therapy to ensure that PaO_2 is maintained at > 8.0 kPa (> 60 mmHg) without a rise in $PaCO_2$. The goal of oxygen therapy is to maintain $PaO_2 \geq 8.0$ kPa (≥ 60 mmHg) with SaO_2 (oxygen saturation) of $\geq 90\%$ with the patient resting at sea level. Increasing PaO_2 above 8.0 kPa (60 mmHg) has little further benefit and increases the risk of CO_2 retention[138]. Long-term oxygen therapy should be given for at least 15 h/day to achieve benefit; this generally involves nocturnal use (see Figure 7.5). Long-term oxygen therapy is most efficiently provided by an oxygen concentrator, set at a flow of 2–4 l/min, with delivery via nasal prongs.

Ambulatory oxygen

Portable systems need functional evaluation to see whether the patient can cope with a particular system.

Ambulatory oxygen may improve exercise tolerance and breathlessness in patients with severe COPD. Improvement is related to the degree of arterial oxygen desaturation on exercise[139]. Prescription of ambulatory oxygen should be based on documented desaturation on a standard walking test (> 4% fall in saturation below 90%). Portable oxygen is indicated in patients who desaturate during exercise and its efficacy needs to be assessed during a treadmill or 6-min walk test with patients wearing the portable oxygen cylinder. Portable oxygen may also be indicated in patients with severe exercise limitation irrespective of oxygen desaturation. Portable cylinders provide 2 h of oxygen at 2 l/min.

Oxygen during air travel

Supplementary oxygen may be needed for COPD patients during airline flights[140,141]. Screening to assess the fitness of patients to fly may be based on assessment of arterial blood oxygen levels (PaO_2), and then prediction of PaO_2 at altitude. Alternatively, the hypoxic challenge test involves simulation of the levels of oxygen in the aircraft cabin. If in doubt, always arrange for supplementary oxygen, by submitting a MEDIF form to the airline to give adequate advance warning, and by arranging oxygen for transit and at the destination.

Oxygen supply

There are several ways of providing supplementary oxygen (Figure 7.9):

(1) *Oxygen concentrators* are the most economic and convenient way of delivering long-term oxygen therapy at home[142].

(2) *Compressed gas cylinders* containing 99.5% oxygen are inconvenient as regular delivery is needed and the cylinders are large and heavy, but are still widely used. They are fitted with flow meters that are either medium (2 l/min) or high (4 l/min).

(3) *Liquid oxygen* is the most portable but most expensive form of supplementary oxygen. Lightweight devices weighing 3 kg can deliver oxygen for 14 h at 2 l/min.

Oxygen delivery

Oxygen may be delivered by a variety of delivery systems:

(1) *Face masks*: tight-fitting masks are the most efficient devices, but are uncomfortable and inconvenient for long-term use.

(2) *Nasal cannulae* are the most commonly used means of oxygen delivery and usually have no problems. A flow of 1.5–2.5 l/min is usually adequate to achieve a $PaO_2 > 8$ kPa (> 60 mmHg) (Figure 7.9).

(3) *Transtracheal catheter oxygen therapy* may be useful in some patients who cannot tolerate face masks or nasal cannulae, but catheters must be removed and cleaned frequently.

(4) *Pulsed delivery systems* use a thermistor or pressure valve to deliver oxygen only during the beginning of inspiration (Figure 7.9). These devices are expensive but reduce the amount of oxygen used by over one-third, so that the oxygen supply can be less heavy.

Non-invasive (or nasal intermittent) positive pressure ventilation

Non-invasive ventilation refers to ventilatory support using a mask and not a tracheal tube or tracheostomy. Non-invasive positive pressure ventilation (NIPPV) may incorporate PEEP (positive end expiratory pressure) to prevent small airway collapse on expiration (Figure 7.10). Remarkable progress has been made in establishing NIPPV for the treatment of both acute hypercapnic exacerbations of COPD[143–149] and chronic hypercapnic (type 2) respiratory failure[112,150–154]. Before starting NIPPV, it is important to consider indications and contraindications, equipment and monitoring[155]. Clinical indications for NIPPV use in COPD and a variety of lung disorders have been defined in a consensus conference report[156], while the British Thoracic Society has issued a guideline for use of non-invasive ventilation in acute respiratory failure[157].

Invasive positive pressure ventilation or invasive mechanical ventilation

Invasive positive pressure ventilation or invasive mechanical ventilation is employed in emergency cases, when invasive mechanical ventilation is

Figure 7.10   (a) Non-invasive positive pressure ventilator (NIPPV); (b) nasal mask

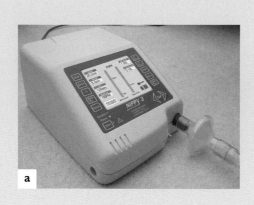
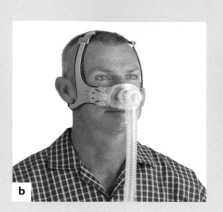

(a) The NIPPY 3 system has four modes of ventilation. Photograph by courtesy of B & D Electromedical, Stratford on Avon, UK. (b) Vista Mask. Photograph by courtesy of ResMed Ltd, North Ryde, Australia.

Figure 7.11   Surgery for COPD

	Bullectomy	Lung volume reduction surgery (LVRS)	Lung transplantation
Alternative procedures	Commonly by video-assisted thoracoscopic surgery (VATS)	1. Bilateral lung resection and stapling procedure through median sternotomy or by VATS 2. Unilateral bronchoscopic volume reduction with valve implant	1. Single lung transplantation (SLT) 2. Bilateral lung transplantation (BLT) 3. Heart–lung transplantation (HLT)
Indications	1. A localized large compressive bulla • >33% of a hemithorax • surrounded by normal/near normal lung parenchyma • tracheal displacement 2. Dyspnea and/or local symptoms: hemoptysis, infection or chest pain	1. Severe emphysema target zones in apices: heterogeneous not homogeneous distribution 2. Residual volume > 150%, signifying hyperinflation 3. FEV_1 20–40% of predicted	1. FEV_1 < 35% predicted 2. Hypoxia: oxygen-dependent (PaO_2 < 8 kPa, 60 mmHg) 3. Hypercapnia ($PaCO_2$ > 6.7 kPa, 50 mmHg) 4. Secondary pulmonary hypertension 5. Medical options exhausted and patient has prospect of better health-related quality of life and possibly survival with the operation
Age		Younger patients have a better prognosis	SLT < 65 years BLT < 60 years HLT < 55 years
Major cardiorespiratory contraindications	Generalized lung disease: 1. Hypoxia and hypercapnia 2. Decreased diffusion capacity (TLCO)	1. Hypoxia and hypercapnia 2. Pulmonary hypertension	Hypoxia, hypercapnia, and secondary pulmonary hypertension are indications and *not* contraindications.
Prognosis	Good symptomatic relief and improved health-related quality of life in carefully selected patients	Improved FEV_1 walking distance and health-related quality of life, but 5% perioperative mortality and overall survival not improved	Symptomatic and health-related quality of life improvement, but • 20% mortality at 1 year • 50% mortality at 5 years

required in a sedated patient (*see* Figures 6.12 and 6.13). Following invasive mechanical ventilation, there are frequently problems in weaning the patient[158].

SURGERY

There is a long history of surgery for COPD[159–161](Figure 7.11). Vagal nerve section and carotid body surgery are no longer performed, but, more recently, surgical techniques have been successfully applied to severe emphysema[162]. Detailed preoperative work-up may include complete lung function, arterial blood gases, radiology including computed tomographic (CT) scan, cardiology tests, incremental shuttle walk test, measurement of health-related quality of life, with assessment of social factors and level of motivation. Patients should have received pulmonary rehabilitation and optimization of pharmacological therapy. In addition, candidates for surgery should ideally be non-smokers for at least 6 months, and without alcohol or drug dependence.

Bullectomy

There is still controversy over the indications for bullectomy and good results depend on careful patient selection. The ideal patient is young with a large bulla, possibly with local complications such as hemoptysis and chest pain, and surrounding relatively normal lung. In patients with COPD, the problem is that surgical removal of one bulla may lead to growth of other bullae as the remaining emphysematous lung decompresses[163]. Favorable features for bullectomy are large bullae (> 1 l) with demonstration of surrounding lung compression, but a lack of generalized emphysema demonstrated by CT and a normal transfer coefficient (K_{CO})[164]. Another recommendation is that the bulla must occupy 50% or more of the hemithorax and produce definite displacement of the adjacent lung[165]. Bullectomy is commonly performed with video-assisted thoracoscopic surgery.

Lung volume reduction surgery

Recently, reduction of lung volume by excision has become popular for the treatment of heterogeneous emphysema with good target zones in the lung apices, accompanied by hyperinflation (residual volume > 150%)[166–169]. This involves resection of peripheral portions of both lungs using novel stapling techniques to prevent air leaks (Figure 7.12). The intention is to remove severely affected areas, thus allowing the remaining lung tissue to ventilate more effectively through restoration of chest wall dynamics[170–172]. CT scans help to characterize patients prior to surgery[173,174].

Major and relative contraindications to lung volume reduction surgery include:

(1) Acute illness or instability;

(2) Respiratory failure;

(3) Low forced expiratory volume in 1 s (FEV$_1$) (< 20%) and low CO diffusing capacity (T_{LCO}/D_{LCO}) (< 20%);

(4) Cardiac comorbidity, pulmonary hypertension, *cor pulmonale*;

(5) Pulmonary infection, hepatitis B and C, HIV;

(6) Active malignancy;

(7) Previous thoracic surgery;

(8) Major organ dysfunction, especially renal disease;

(9) Nutritional status: too fat or thin;

(10) Prednisolone > 10 mg orally per day;

(11) Symptomatic osteoporosis;

(12) Severe musculoskeletal disease.

Lung volume reduction surgery results in an increase in FEV$_1$ and a reduction in residual volume, with decreased dyspnea, improved exercise tolerance and improved quality of life[175–179]. However, the National Emphysema Treatment Trial (NETT) found that patients with a low FEV$_1$ (< 20% predicted) and either homogeneous emphysema or a very low carbon monoxide diffusing capacity (T_{LCO} or D_{LCO} < 20% predicted) are at high risk for death[180–182]. Lung volume reduction surgery has been shown to improve health-related quality of life[183] and exercise capacity but not survival when compared with medical therapy[184]. Hence, lung volume reduction surgery remains an unproven palliative surgical procedure. Lung volume reduction surgery may be cost-effective if benefits can be maintained over time[185]. Recently, lung volume reduction has been developed using unilateral bronchoscopically placed valve implants in patients with severe emphysema[186], and a preliminary report has shown a reduction in residual volume on CT scan in four of eight patients.

Figure 7.12   Lung volume reduction surgery

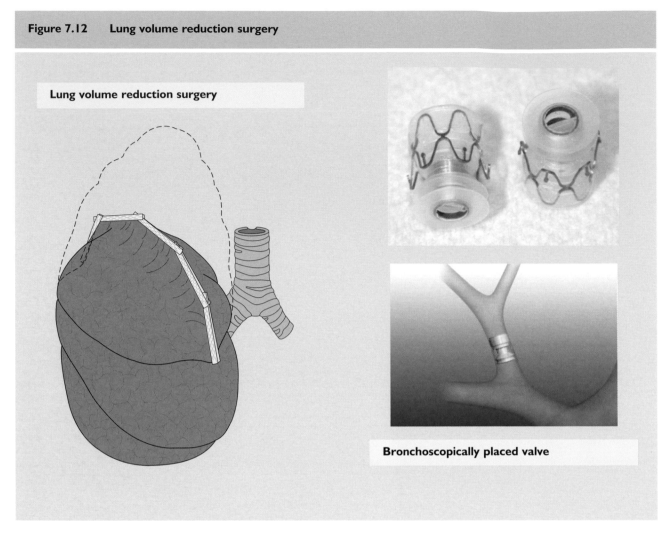

Lung volume reduction surgery

Bronchoscopically placed valve

Pictures by courtesy of Emphasys Medical, Inc. California, USA.

Lung transplantation

Heart–lung transplantation has been extensively performed in patients with end-stage emphysema[187,188]. More recently, single lung transplantation has become the favored technique, in view of the difficulty in obtaining donor organs and improvements in lung preservation and anesthetic management[189,190]. There is severely limited availability of donor lungs[191], and a long delay may occur prior to finding a suitable donor. Because of problems with residual infection in the remaining lung and of hyperinflation of the existing lung if there is extensive bullous disease, heart–lung transplantation or preferably bilateral sequential single lung transplantation is performed in patients with these complications.

Indications (Figure 7.11)

(1) $FEV_1 < 40\%$ predicted, $PaO_2 < 8.0$ kPa (< 60 mmHg), $PaCO_2 > 6.7$ kPa (50 mmHg) and secondary pulmonary hypertension[191,192]. Hence, patients generally have severe lung and heart disease;

(2) Deteriorating lung function, patients with a life expectancy of < 18 months, or onset of *cor pulmonale* with right ventricular failure;

(3) Patients should generally be under 60 years;

(4) Positive attitude and a supportive family are important.

Contraindications

(1) Recurrent or persistent sepsis;

(2) Active malignancy;

(3) Major organ dysfunction: poor renal and hepatic function;

(4) Bilateral extensive bullous disease is a contraindication to single lung transplantation;

(5) Previous thoracic surgery due to risk of hemorrhage;

(6) Oral prednisolone > 10 mg orally per day;

(7) Symptomatic osteoporosis.

Complications

(1) Early mortality owing to immediate postoperative complications, sepsis or diffuse alveolar damage;

(2) Acute lung rejection (confirmed by transbronchial biopsy);

(3) Lung infection (opportunistic infections due to immunosuppression);

(4) Chronic lung rejection (obliterative bronchiolitis).

Prognosis

(1) 1-year mortality of < 20%, 5-year mortality of 50%;

(2) Improvement in mortality has not been convincingly demonstrated, although marked improvement in quality of life and lung function can occur;

(3) 30% develop obliterative bronchiolitis within 5 years.

PALLIATIVE CARE

Patients dying from COPD have significantly impaired health-related quality of life that is not as well managed as in patients with lung cancer[193]. In particular, there are specialized needs for end-of-life care in the intensive care unit[194] as compared with at home. Ethical issues in patients with advanced lung disease include provision for intubation and mechanical ventilation[195]. It is also important to give patients with severe COPD advance care planning, special education and a framework for discussing actions with their families and health carers[196].

REFERENCES

1. Pulmonary rehabilitation-1999. American Thoracic Society. *Am J Respir Crit Care Med* 1999;159:1666–82

2. Pulmonary rehabilitation. *Thorax* 2001;56:827–34

3. Morgan MD, Britton JR. Chronic obstructive pulmonary disease. 8. Non-pharmacological management of COPD. *Thorax* 2003;58:453–7

4. MacNee W, Calverley PM. Chronic obstructive pulmonary disease. 7. Management of COPD. *Thorax* 2003;58:261–5

5. Hodgkin JE, Celli BR, Connors GL. *Pulmonary Rehabilitation: Guidelines to Success*. Philadelphia: Lippincott Williams & Wilkins, 2000

6. Morgan M, Singh S. *Practical Pulmonary Rehabilitation*. London, UK: Chapman & Hall, 1997

7. Simonds AK, Muir JF, Pierson DJ. *Pulmonary Rehabilitation*. London, UK: BMJ Publishing Group, 1996

8. Pulmonary rehabilitation. European Respiratory Society Journals, 2000

9. Pulmonary rehabilitation. ACCP/AACVPR Pulmonary Rehabilitation Guidelines Panel. American College of Chest Physicians. American Association of Cardiovascular and Pulmonary Rehabilitation. *Chest* 1997;112:1363–96

10. Lacasse Y, Wong E, Guyatt GH, King D, Cook DJ, Goldstein RS. Meta-analysis of respiratory rehabilitation in chronic obstructive pulmonary disease. *Lancet* 1996;348:1115–19

11. Wedzicha JA, Bestall JC, Garrod R, Garnham R, Paul EA, Jones PW. Randomized controlled trial of pulmonary rehabilitation in severe chronic obstructive pulmonary disease patients, stratified with the MRC dyspnoea scale. *Eur Respir J* 1998;12:363–9

12. Griffiths TL, Burr ML, Campbell IA, *et al.* Results at 1 year of outpatient multidisciplinary pulmonary rehabilitation: a randomised controlled trial. *Lancet* 2000;355:362–8

13. Wouters EF. Chronic obstructive pulmonary disease: systemic effects of COPD. *Thorax* 2002;57:1067–70

14. Gosselink R, Troosters T, Decramer M. Peripheral muscle weakness contributes to exercise limitation in COPD. *Am J Respir Crit Care Med* 1996;153:976–80

15. Debigare R, Cote CH, Maltais F. Peripheral muscle wasting in chronic obstructive pulmonary disease. Clinical relevance and mechanisms. *Am J Respir Crit Care Med* 2001;164:1712–17

16. van Ede L, Yzermans CJ, Brouwer HJ. Prevalence of depression in patients with chronic obstructive pulmonary disease: a systemic review. *Thorax* 1999;54:688–92

17. Buist AS, Sullivan SD, Weiss K, eds. Measurement and evaluation of outcomes in COPD. *Eur Respir J* 2003;21(Suppl):1–53s

18. Berry MJ, Rejeski WJ, Adair NE, Zaccaro D. Exercise rehabilitation and chronic obstructive pulmonary disease stage. *Am J Respir Crit Care Med* 1999;160:1248–53

19. Ries AL, Kaplan RM, Myers R, Prewitt LM. Maintenance after pulmonary rehabilitation in chronic lung disease: a randomized trial. *Am J Respir Crit Care Med* 2003;167:880–8

20. Green RH, Singh SJ, Williams J, Morgan MD. A randomised controlled trial of four weeks versus seven weeks of pulmonary rehabilitation in chronic obstructive pulmonary disease. *Thorax* 2001;56:143–5

21. Goldstein RS, Gort EH, Stubbing D, Avendano MA, Guyatt GH. Randomised controlled trial of respiratory rehabilitation. *Lancet* 1994;344:1394–7

22. Behnke M, Taube C, Kirsten D, Lehnigk B, Jorres RA, Magnussen H. Home-based exercise is capable of preserving hospital-based improvements in severe chronic obstructive pulmonary disease. *Respir Med* 2000;94:1184–91

23. Finnerty JP, Keeping I, Bullough I, Jones J. The effectiveness of outpatient pulmonary rehabilitation in chronic lung disease: a randomized controlled trial. *Chest* 2001;119:1705–10

24. Wijkstra PJ, Van Altena R, Kraan J, Otten V, Postma DS, Koeter GH. Quality of life in patients with chronic obstructive pulmonary disease improves after rehabilitation at home. *Eur Respir J* 1994;7:269–73

25. ATS. ATS statement: guidelines for the six-minute walk test. *Am J Respir Crit Care Med* 2002;166:111–7

26. Marin JM, Carrizo SJ, Gascon M, Sanchez A, Gallego B, Celli BR. Inspiratory capacity, dynamic hyperinflation, breathlessness, and exercise performance during the 6-minute-walk test in chronic obstructive pulmonary disease. *Am J Respir Crit Care Med* 2001;163:1395–9

27. Troosters T, Vilaro J, Rabinovich R, *et al.* Physiological responses to the 6-min walk test in patients with chronic obstructive pulmonary disease. *Eur Respir J* 2002;20:564–9

28. Enright PL, Sherrill DL. Reference equations for the six-minute walk in healthy adults. *Am J Respir Crit Care Med* 1998;158:1384–7

29. Singh SJ, Morgan MD, Scott S, Walters D, Hardman AE. Development of a shuttle walking test of disability in patients with chronic airways obstruction. *Thorax* 1992;47:1019–24

30. Booth S, Adams L. The shuttle walking test: a reproducible method for evaluating the impact of shortness of breath on functional capacity in patients with advanced cancer. *Thorax* 2001;56:146–50

31. Dyer CA, Singh SJ, Stockley RA, Sinclair AJ, Hill SL. The incremental shuttle walking test in elderly people with chronic airflow limitation. *Thorax* 2002;57:34–8

32. O'Donnell DE, Lam M, Webb KA. Measurement of symptoms, lung hyperinflation, and endurance during exercise in chronic obstructive pulmonary disease. *Am J Respir Crit Care Med* 1998;158:1557–65

33. Hughes PD, Hart N, Hamnegard CH, *et al.* Inspiratory muscle relaxation rate slows during exhaustive treadmill walking in patients with chronic heart failure. *Am J Respir Crit Care Med* 2001;163:1400–3

34. Jones PW, Mahler DA. Key outcomes in COPD: health-related quality of life. Proceedings of an expert round table held July 20–22, 2001 in Boston, Massachusetts, USA. *Eur Respir Rev* 2002;12

35. Jones PW, Quirk FH, Baveystock CM. The St George's Respiratory Questionnaire. *Respir Med* 1991;85(Suppl B):25–31

36. Jones PW, Quirk FH, Baveystock CM, Littlejohns P. A self-complete measure of health status for chronic airflow limitation. The St. George's Respiratory Questionnaire. *Am Rev Respir Dis* 1992;145:1321–7

37. Jones PW. Health status measurement in chronic obstructive pulmonary disease. *Thorax* 2001;56:880–7

38. Rutten-van Molken MP, Roos B, van Noord JA. An empirical comparison of the St George's respiratory questionnaire (SGRQ) and the chronic respiratory disease questionnaire (CRQ) in a clinical trial setting. Thorax 1999;54:995–1003

39. Mahler DA, Mackowiak JI. Evaluation of the short-form 36-item questionnaire to measure health-related quality of life in patients with COPD. *Chest* 1995;107:1585–9

40. Engstrom CP, Persson LO, Larsson S, Sullivan M. Health-related quality of life in COPD: why both

disease-specific and generic measures should be used. *Eur Respir J* 2001;18:69–76

41. Celli BR. Exercise in the rehabilitation of patients with respiratory disease. In Hodgkin JE, Celli BR, Connors GL, eds. *Pulmonary Rehabilitation: Guidelines to Success*. Lippincott Williams & Wilkins, 2000:147–63

42. Morgan MDL. Preventing hospital admissions for COPD: role of physical activity. *Thorax* 2003;58:95–6

43. Garcia-Aymerich J, Farrero E, Felez MA, Izquierdo J, Marrades RM, Anto JM. Risk factors of readmission to hospital for a COPD exacerbation: a prospective study. *Thorax* 2003;58:100–5

44. Oga T, Nishimura K, Tsukino M, Sato S, Hajiro T. Analysis of the factors related to mortality in chronic obstructive pulmonary disease: role of exercise capacity and health status. *Am J Respir Crit Care Med* 2003;167:544–9

45. Smith K, Cook D, Guyatt GH, Madhavan J, Oxman AD. Respiratory muscle training in chronic airflow limitation: a meta-analysis. *Am Rev Respir Dis* 1992;145:533–9

46. Clark CJ, Cochrane LM, Mackay E, Paton B. Skeletal muscle strength and endurance in patients with mild COPD and the effects of weight training. *Eur Respir J* 2000;15:92–7

47. Ortega F, Toral J, Cejudo P, *et al.* Comparison of effects of strength and endurance training in patients with chronic obstructive pulmonary disease. *Am J Respir Crit Care Med* 2002;166:669–74

48. Cooper CB. Exercise in chronic pulmonary disease: limitations and rehabilitation. *Med Sci Sports Exerc* 2001;33(Suppl 7):S643–6

49. Clark CJ, Cochrane LM, Mackay E, Paton B. Skeletal muscle strength and endurance in patients with mild COPD and the effects of weight training. *Eur Respir J* 2000;15:92–7

50. Mahler DA. Ventilatory muscle training. In Hodgkin JE, Celli BR, Connors GL, eds. *Pulmonary Rehabilitation: Guidelines to Success*. Baltimore, MD: Lippincott Williams & Wilkins, 2000:165–72

51. Ramirez-Sarmiento A, Orozco-Levi M, Guell R, *et al.* Inspiratory muscle training in patients with chronic obstructive pulmonary disease: structural adaptation and physiologic outcomes. *Am J Respir Crit Care Med* 2002;166:1491–7

52. Smith K, Cook D, Guyatt GH, Madhavan J, Oxman AD. Respiratory muscle training in chronic airflow limitation: a meta-analysis. *Am Rev Respir Dis* 1992;145:533–9

53. Miller WF. Historical perspective of pulmonary rehabilitation. In Hodgkin JE, Celli BR, Connors GL, eds. *Pulmonary Rehabilitation: Guidelines to Success*. Baltimore, MD: Lippincott Williams & Wilkins, 2000:1–20

54. Gosselink RA, Wagenaar RC, Rijswijk H, Sargeant AJ, Decramer ML. Diaphragmatic breathing reduces efficiency of breathing in patients with chronic obstructive pulmonary disease. *Am J Respir Crit Care Med* 1995;151:1136–42

55. Sharp JT, Drutz WS, Moisan T, Foster J, Machnach W. Postural relief of dyspnea in severe chronic obstructive pulmonary disease. *Am Rev Respir Dis* 1980;122:201–11

56. O'Neill S, McCarthy DS. Postural relief of dyspnoea in severe chronic airflow limitation: relationship to respiratory muscle strength. *Thorax* 1983;38:595–600

57. Bott J, Agent P, Callaghan S. Physiotherapy and nursing during non-invasive positive pressure. In Simonds AK, ed. *Non-invasive Respiratory Support: a Practical Handbook*. New York: Arnold, 2001:230–54

58. Agusti AGN, Noguera A, Sauleda J, Busquets X. Systemic inflammation in chronic respiratory disease. In Wouters EFM, Schols AM, eds. *Nutrition and Metabolism in Chronic Respiratory Disease*. European Respiratory Society Journals, 2003:46–55

59. Langen RC. Effects of inflammation on skeletal muscle. In Wouters EFM, Schols AM, eds. *Nutrition and Metabolism in Chronic Respiratory Disease*. European Respiratory Society Journals, 2003:68–85

60. Gorselink M, Drost MR, van der Vusse GJ. Muscle morphology, metabolism and muscle function: general principles. In Wouters EFM, Schols AM, eds. *Nutrition and Metabolism in Chronic Respiratory Disease. European Respiratory Society Journals*, 2003:86–98

61. Guerra S, Sherrill DL, Bobadilla A, Martinez FD, Barbee RA. The relation of body mass index to asthma, chronic bronchitis, and emphysema. *Chest* 2002;122(4):1256-63.

62. Schols AM, Wouters EFM. Nutritional assessment and support. In Hodgkin JE, Celli BR, Connors GL, eds. *Pulmonary Rehabilitation: Guidelines to Success*. Baltimore, MD: Lippincott Williams & Wilkins, 2000:247–59

63. Romieu I, Trenga C. Diet and obstructive lung diseases. *Epidemiol Rev* 2001;23:268–87

64. Britton JR, Pavord ID, Richards KA, *et al.* Dietary antioxidant vitamin intake and lung function in the

general population. *Am J Respir Crit Care Med* 1995;151:1383–7

65. Tabak C, Arts IC, Smit HA, Heederik D, Kromhout D. Chronic obstructive pulmonary disease and intake of catechins, flavonols, and flavones: the MORGEN Study. *Am J Respir Crit Care Med* 2001;164:61–4

66. Watson L, Margetts B, Howarth P, Dorward M, Thompson R, Little P. The association between diet and chronic obstructive pulmonary disease in subjects selected from general practice. *Eur Respir J* 2002;20:313–18

67. Wouters EF, Creutzberg EC, Schols AM. Systemic effects in COPD. *Chest* 2002;121(Suppl 5):127S–30S

68. Agusti AGN, Noguera A, Sauleda J, Sala E, Pons J, Busquets X. Systemic effects of chronic obstructive pulmonary disease. *Eur Respir J* 2003;21:347–60

69. Engelen MP, Deutz NE, Wouters EF, Schols AM. Enhanced levels of whole-body protein turnover in patients with chronic obstructive pulmonary disease. *Am J Respir Crit Care Med* 2000;162:1488–92

70. Eid AA, Ionescu AA, Nixon LS, *et al.* Inflammatory response and body composition in chronic obstructive pulmonary disease. *Am J Respir Crit Care Med* 2001;164:1414–8

71. Takabatake N, Nakamura H, Minamihaba O, *et al.* A novel pathophysiologic phenomenon in cachexic patients with chronic obstructive pulmonary disease: the relationship between the circadian rhythm of circulating leptin and the very low-frequency component of heart rate variability. *Am J Respir Crit Care Med* 2001;163:1314–19

72. Creutzberg EC, Wouters EF, Vanderhoven-Augustin IM, Dentener MA, Schols AM. Disturbances in leptin metabolism are related to energy imbalance during acute exacerbations of chronic obstructive pulmonary disease. *Am J Respir Crit Care Med* 2000;162:1239–45

73. Creutzberg EC. Leptin in relation to systematic inflammation and regulation of the energy balance. In Wouters EFM, Schols AM, eds. *Nutrition and Metabolism in Chronic Respiratory Disease. European Respiratory Society Journals*, 2003:56–67

74. Di Francia M, Barbier D, Mege JL, Orehek J. Tumor necrosis factor-alpha levels and weight loss in chronic obstructive pulmonary disease. *Am J Respir Crit Care Med* 1994;150:1453–5

75. de G, I, Donahoe M, Calhoun WJ, Mancino J, Rogers RM. Elevated TNF-alpha production by peripheral blood monocytes of weight-losing COPD patients. *Am J Respir Crit Care Med* 1996;153:633–7

76. Vernooy JH, Kucukaycan M, Jacobs JA, *et al.* Local and systemic inflammation in patients with chronic obstructive pulmonary disease: soluble tumor necrosis factor receptors are increased in sputum. *Am J Respir Crit Care Med* 2002;166:1218–24

77. Bernard S, LeBlanc P, Whittom F, *et al.* Peripheral muscle weakness in patients with chronic obstructive pulmonary disease. *Am J Respir Crit Care Med* 1998;158:629–34

78. Engelen MP, Wouters EF, Deutz NE, Menheere PP, Schols AM. Factors contributing to alterations in skeletal muscle and plasma amino acid profiles in patients with chronic obstructive pulmonary disease. *Am J Clin Nutr* 2000;72:1480–7

79. Agusti AG, Sauleda J, Miralles C, *et al.* Skeletal muscle apoptosis and weight loss in chronic obstructive pulmonary disease. *Am J Respir Crit Care Med* 2002;166:485–9

80. Lewis MI. Apoptosis as a potential mechanism of muscle cachexia in chronic obstructive pulmonary disease. *Am J Respir Crit Care Med* 2002;166:434–6

81. Reid MB. COPD as a muscle disease. *Am J Respir Crit Care Med* 2001;164:1101-2

82. Schols AM, Soeters PB, Dingemans AM, Mostert R, Frantzen PJ, Wouters EF. Prevalence and characteristics of nutritional depletion in patients with stable COPD eligible for pulmonary rehabilitation. *Am Rev Respir Dis* 1993;147:1151–6

83. Slosman DO, Casez JP, Pichard C, *et al.* Assessment of whole-body composition with dual-energy x-ray absorptiometry. *Radiology* 1992;185:593–8

84. Kyle UG, Pichard C, Rochat T, Slosman DO, Fitting JW, Thiebaud D. New bioelectrical impedance formula for patients with respiratory insufficiency: comparison to dual-energy X-ray absorptiometry. *Eur Respir J* 1998;12:960–6

85. Marquis K, Debigare R, Lacasse Y, *et al.* Midthigh muscle cross-sectional area is a better predictor of mortality than body mass index in patients with chronic obstructive pulmonary disease. *Am J Respir Crit Care Med* 2002;166:809–13

86. Palange P. Effects of nutritional depletion on exercise tolerance. In Wouters EFM, Schols AM, eds. *Nutrition and Metabolism in Chronic Respiratory Disease. European Respiratory Society Journal*, 2003:123–31

87. Gray-Donald K, Gibbons L, Shapiro SH, Macklem PT, Martin JG. Nutritional status and mortality in chronic obstructive pulmonary disease. *Am J Respir Crit Care Med* 1996;153:961–6

88. Landbo C, Prescott E, Lange P, Vestbo J, Almdal TP. Prognostic value of nutritional status in chronic

obstructive pulmonary disease. *Am J Respir Crit Care Med* 1999;160:1856

89. Prescott E, Almdal T, Mikkelsen KL, Tofteng CL, Vestbo J, Lange P. Prognostic value of weight change in chronic obstructive pulmonary disease: results from the Copenhagen City Heart Study. *Eur Respir J* 2002;20:539–44

90. Schols AM, Slangen J, Volovics L, Wouters EF. Weight loss is a reversible factor in the prognosis of chronic obstructive pulmonary disease. *Am J Respir Crit Care Med* 1998;157:1791–7

91. Landbo C, Prescott E, Lange P, Vestbo J, Almdal TP. Prognostic value of nutritional status in chronic obstructive pulmonary disease. *Am J Respir Crit Care Med* 1999;160:1856–61

92. Schols AM, Soeters PB, Mostert R, Pluymers RJ, Wouters EF. Physiologic effects of nutritional support and anabolic steroids in patients with chronic obstructive pulmonary disease. A placebo-controlled randomized trial. *Am J Respir Crit Care Med* 1995;152:1268–74

93. Schols AM, Brug J. Efficacy of nutritional intervention in chronic obstructive pulmonary disease. In Wouters EFM, Schols AM, eds. *Nutrition and Metabolism in Chronic Respiratory Disease. European Respiratory Society Journals*, 2003:142–52

94. Rogers RM, Donahoe M, Costantino J. Physiologic effects of oral supplemental feeding in malnourished patients with chronic obstructive pulmonary disease. A randomized control study. *Am Rev Respir Dis* 1992;146:1511–17

95. Ferreira IM, Brooks D, Lacasse Y, Goldstein RS. Nutritional support for individuals with COPD: a meta-analysis. *Chest* 2000;117:672–8

96. Creutzberg EC, Schols AM, Weling-Scheepers CA, Buurman WA, Wouters EF. Characterization of nonresponse to high caloric oral nutritional therapy in depleted patients with chronic obstructive pulmonary disease. *Am J Respir Crit Care Med* 2000;161:745–52

97. Slinde F, Gronberg AM, Engstrom CR, Rossander-Hulthen L, Larsson S. Individual dietary intervention in patients with COPD during multidisciplinary rehabilitation. *Respir Med* 2002;96:330–6

98. Weisberg J, Wanger J, Olson J, *et al*. Megestrol acetate stimulates weight gain and ventilation in underweight COPD patients. *Chest* 2002;121:1070–8

99. Creutzberg EC. Anabolic steroids in acute and chronic disease. In Wouters EFM, Schols AM, eds. *Nutrition and Metabolism in Chronic Respiratory*

Disease. European Respiratory Society Journals, 2003:163–80

100. Fleetham JA. Is chronic obstructive pulmonary disease related to sleep apnea-hypopnea syndrome? *Am J Respir Crit Care Med* 2003;167:3–4

101. Weitzenblum E, Chaouat A, Charpentier C, *et al*. Sleep-related hypoxaemia in chronic obstructive pulmonary disease: causes, consequences and treatment. *Respiration* 1997;64:187–93

102. Brown LK. Sleep-related disorders and chronic obsructive pulmonary disease. *Respir Care Clin N Am* 1998;4:493–512

103. Rodenstein DO. Sleep disorders in pulmonary patients. In Hodgkin JE, Celli BR, Connors GL, eds. *Pulmonary Rehabilitation: Guidelines to Success* 3rd edn. Balitimore, USA: Lippincott Williams & Wilkins, 2000:479–93

104. Simonds AK. Continuous positive airway pressure (CPAP) therapy. In Simonds AK, ed. *Non-invasive Respiratory Support: a Practical Handbook*. New York: Arnold, 2001:203–29

105. De Angelis G, Sposato B, Mazzei L, *et al*. Predictive indexes of nocturnal desaturation in COPD patients not treated with long term oxygen therapy. *Eur Rev Med Pharmacol Sci* 2001;5:173–9

106. Sanders MH, Newman AB, Haggerty CL, *et al*. Sleep and sleep-disordered breathing in adults with predominantly mild obstructive airway disease. *Am J Respir Crit Care Med* 2003;167:7–14

107. Young T, Peppard PE, Gottlieb DJ. Epidemiology of obstructive sleep apnea: a population health perspective. *Am J Respir Crit Care Med* 2002;165:1217–39

108. Krieger J. Clinical presentations of sleep apnoea. *Eur Respir Mon* 1998;10:75–105

109. Hedner J, Grote L. Cardiovascular consequences of obstructive sleep apnoea. *Eur Respir Mon* 1998;10:227–65

110. Engleman H. When does 'mild' obstructive sleep apnea/hypopnea syndrome merit continuous positive airway pressure treatment? [Editorial]. *Am J Respir Crit Care Med* 2002;165:743–4

111. Connaughton JJ, Catterall JR, Elton RA, Stradling JR, Douglas NJ. Do sleep studies contribute to the management of patients with severe chronic obstructive pulmonary disease? *Am Rev Respir Dis* 1988;138:341–4

112. Simonds AK. *Non-Invasive Respiratory Support: a Practical Handbook*. New York: Arnold, 2001

113. George CF, Bayliff CD. Management of insomnia in patients with chronic obstructive pulmonary disease. *Drugs* 2003;63:379–87

114. O'Donoghue FJ, Catcheside PG, Ellis EE, Grunstein RR, Pierce RJ, Rowland LS, *et al.* Sleep hypoventilation in hypercapnic chronic obstrucitve pulmonary disease: prevalence and associated factors. *Eur Respir J* 2003;21:977–84

115. van Manen JG, Bindels PJ, Dekker FW, IJzermans CJ, van der Zee JS, Schade E. Risk of depression in patients with chronic obstructive pulmonary disease and its determinants. *Thorax* 2002;57:412–16

116. Clary GL, Palmer SM, Doraiswamy PM. Mood disorders and chronic obstructive pulmonary disease: current research and future needs. *Curr Psychiatry Rep* 2002;4:213–21

117. Yohannes AM, Baldwin RC, Connolly MJ. Depression and anxiety in elderly outpatients with chronic obstructive pulmonary disease: prevalence, and validation of the BASDEC screening questionnaire. *Int J Geriatr.Psychiatry* 2000;15:1090–6

118. Singer HK, Ruchinskas RA, Riley KC, Broshek DK, Barth JT. The psychological impact of end-stage lung disease. *Chest* 2001;120:1246–52

119. Gift AG, McCrone SH. Depression in patients with COPD. *Heart Lung* 1993;22:289–97

120. Lacasse Y, Rousseau L, Maltais F. Prevalence of depressive symptoms and depression in patients with severe oxygen-dependent chronic obstructive pulmonary disease. *J Cardiopulm Rehabil* 2001;21:80–6

121. Crockett AJ, Cranston JM, Moss JR, Alpers JH. The impact of anxiety, depression and living alone in chronic obstructive pulmonary disease. *Qual Life Res* 2002;11:309–16

122. Yohannes AM, Connolly MJ, Baldwin RC. A feasibility study of antidepressant drug therapy in depressed elderly patients with chronic obstructive pulmonary disease. *Int J Geriatr Psychiatry* 2001;16:451–4

123. Withers NJ, Rudkin ST, White RJ. Anxiety and depression in severe chronic obstructive pulmonary disease: the effects of pulmonary rehabilitation. *J Cardiopulm Rehabil* 1999;19:362–5

124. Lareau SC, Insel KC. Patient and family education. In Hodgkin JE, Celli BR, Connors GL, eds. *Pulmonary Rehabilitation: Guidelines to Success*. Lippincott Williams & Wilkins, 2000:91–101

125. Monninkhof E, van d, V, van der PJ, van Herwaarden C, Partridge MR, Zielhuis G. Self-management education for patients with chronic obstructive

126. Barbera JA, Peinado VI, Santos S. Pulmonary hypertension in chronic obstructive pulmonary disease. *Eur Respir J* 2003;21:892–905

127. Vonbank K, Ziesche R, Higenbottam TW, Stiebellehner L, Petkov V, Schenk P, *et al.* Controlled prospective randomised trial on the effects on pulmonary haemodynamics of the ambulatory long term use of nitric oxide and oxygen in patients with severe COPD. *Thorax* 2003;58:289–93

128. Pepke-Zaba J, Morrell NW. Pulmonary hypertension in patients with COPD: NO treatment? *Thorax* 2003;58:283–4

129. Tarpy SP, Celli B. Long-term oxygen therapy. *N Engl J Med* 1995;333:710–4

130. O'Donohue WJ Jr. Oxygen therapy in pulmonary rehabilitation. In Hodgkin JE, Celli BR, Connors GL, eds. *Pulmonary Rehabilitation: Guidelines to Success*. Lippincott Williams & Wilkins; 2000:135–46

131. Restrick LJ, Paul EA, Braid GM, Cullinan P, Moore-Gillon J, Wedzicha JA. Assessment and follow up of patients prescribed long term oxygen treatment. *Thorax* 1993;48:708–13

132. Nocturnal Oxygen Therapy Group. Continuous or nocturnal oxygen therapy in hypoxemic chronic obstructive lung disease: a clinical trial. *Ann Int Med* 1980;93:391–8

133. Report of the Medical Research Council Working Party. Long-term domiciliary oxygen therapy in chronic hypoxic cor pulmonale complicating chronic bronchitis and emphysema. *Lancet* 1981;1:681–6

134. Weitzenblum E, Sautegeau A, Ehrhart M, Mammosser M, Pelletier A. Long-term oxygen therapy can reverse the progression of pulmonary hypertension in patients with chronic obstructive pulmonary disease. *Am Rev Respir Dis* 1985;131:493–8

135. Wedzicha JA. Effects of long-term oxygen therapy on neuropsychiatric function and quality of life. *Respir Care* 2000;45:119–24

136. Rudolf M, Wedzicha JA, Calverley PMA, *et al.* *Domiciliary Oxygen Therapy Services: cinical Guidelines and Advice for Prescribers. A report of the Royal College of Physicians*. London, Royal College of Physicians,

137. Wedzicha JA. Domiciliary oxygen therapy services: clinical guidelines and advice for prescribers. Summary of a report of the Royal College of Physicians. *J R Coll Physicians Lond* 1999;33:445–7

138. Georgopoulos D, Anthonisen NR. Continuous oxygen therapy for the chronically hypoxemic patient. *Annu Rev Med* 1990;41:223–30

139. Lock SH, Paul EA, Rudd RM, Wedzicha JA. Portable oxygen therapy: assessment and usage. *Respir Med* 1991;85:407–12

140. British Thoracic Society Standards of Care Committee. Managing passengers with respiratory disease planning air travel: British Thoracic Society recommendations. *Thorax* 2002;57:289–304

141. Johnson AOC. Chronic obstructive pulmonary disease. 11. Fitness to fly with COPD. *Thorax* 2003;58:729–32

142. Walshaw MJ, Lim R, Evans CC, Hind CR. Prescription of oxygen concentrators for long term oxygen treatment: reassessment in one district. *Br Med J* 1988;297:1030–2

143. Elliott MW. Non-invasive ventilation in acute exacerbations of COPD. In Simonds AK, ed. *Non-invasive Respiratory Support: a Practical Handbook*. New York: Arnold, 2001:30–46

144. Brochard L, Mancebo J, Wysocki M, *et al.* Noninvasive ventilation for acute exacerbations of chronic obstructive pulmonary disease [Comments]. *N Engl J Med* 1995;333:817–22

145. Bott J, Carroll MP, Conway JH, *et al.* Randomised controlled trial of nasal ventilation in acute ventilatory failure due to chronic obstructive airways disease. *Lancet* 1993;341:1555–7

146. Bardi G, Pierotello R, Desideri M, Valdisserri L, Bottai M, Palla A. Nasal ventilation in COPD exacerbations: early and late results of a prospective, controlled study. *Eur Respir J* 2000;15:98–104

147. Plant PK, Owen JL, Elliott MW. Early use of non-invasive ventilation for acute exacerbations of chronic obstructive pulmonary disease on general respiratory wards: a multicentre randomised controlled trial. *Lancet* 2000;355:1931–5

148. Doherty MJ, Greenstone MA. Survey of non-invasive ventilation (NIPPV) in patients with acute exacerbations of chronic obstructive pulmonary disease (COPD) in the UK. *Thorax* 1998;53:863–6

149. Davidson AC. The pulmonary physician in critical care. 11: critical care management of respiratory failure resulting from COPD. *Thorax* 2002;57:1079–84

150. Simonds AK. Selection of patients for home ventilation. In Simonds AK, editor. *Non-invasive Respiratory Support: a Practical Handbook*. New York: Arnold, 2001:119–32

151. Elliott MW. Domiciliary non-invasive ventilation in COPD. In Simonds AK, ed. *Non-invasive Respiratory Support: a Practical Handbook*. New York: Arnold, 2001:146–59

152. Elliott MW. Noninvasive ventilation in chronic ventilatory failure due to chronic obstructive pulmonary disease. *Eur Respir J* 2002;20:511–14

153. Wedzicha JA, Muir JF. Noninvasive ventilation in chronic obstructive pulmonary disease, bronchiectasis and cystic fibrosis. *Eur Respir J* 2002;20:777–84

154. Jones SE, Packham S, Hebden M, Smith AP. Domiciliary nocturnal intermittent positive pressure ventilation in patients with respiratory failure due to severe COPD: long-term follow up and effect on survival. *Thorax* 1998;53:495–8

155. Simonds AK. Starting NIPPV: practical aspects. In Simonds AK, ed. *Non-invasive Respiratory Support: a Practical Handbook*. New York: Arnold, 2001:58–75

156. Clinical indications for noninvasive positive pressure ventilation in chronic respiratory failure due to restrictive lung disease, COPD, and nocturnal hypoventilation – a consensus conference report. *Chest* 1999;116:521–34

157. British Thoracic Society Standards of Care Committee. Non-invasive ventilation in acute respiratory failure. *Thorax* 2002;57:192–211

158. Vitacca M, Vianello A, Colombo D, *et al.* Comparison of two methods for weaning patients with chronic obstructive pulmonary disease requiring mechanical ventilation for more than 15 days. *Am J Respir Crit Care Med* 2001;164:225–30

159. Cooper JD. The history of surgical procedures for emphysema. *Ann Thorac Surg* 1997;63:312–19

160. Martinez FJ. Surgical Therapy for COPD. In Hodgkin JE, Celli BR, Connors GL, eds. *Pulmonary Rehabilitation: Guidelines to Success*. Lippincott Williams & Wilkins, 2000:415–51

161. Meyers BF, Patterson GA. Chronic obstructive pulmonary disease. 10. Bullectomy, lung volume reduction surgery, and transplantation for patients with chronic obstructive pulmonary disease. *Thorax* 2003;58:634–8

162. Edelman JD, Kotloff RM. Surgical approaches to advanced emphysema. *Respir Care Clin N Am* 1998;4:513–39

163. Mehran RJ, Deslauriers J. Indications for surgery and patient work-up for bullectomy. *Chest Surg Clin N Am* 1995;5:717–34

164. Hughes JA, MacArthur AM, Hutchison DC, Hugh-Jones P. Long term changes in lung function after

surgical treatment of bullous emphysema in smokers and ex-smokers. *Thorax* 1984;39:140–2

165. Laros CD, Gelissen HJ, Bergstein PG, *et al.* Bullectomy for giant bullae in emphysema. *J Thorac Cardiovasc Surg* 1986;91:63–70

166. Dark JH. Lung volume reduction surgery and lung transplantation for COPD. In: Wedzicha JA, ed. *The Effective Management of COPD*. 2001:81–95

167. Cooper JD, Trulock EP, Triantafillou AN, *et al.* Bilateral pneumonectomy (volume reduction) for chronic obstructive pulmonary disease. *J Thorac Cardiovasc Surg* 2002;109:106–16

168. Cooper JD, Patterson GA, Sundaresan RS, *et al.* Results of 150 consecutive bilateral lung volume reduction procedures in patients with severe emphysema. *J Thorac Cardiovasc Surg* 1996;112:1319–29

169. Russi EW, Stammberger U, Weder W. Lung volume reduction surgery for emphysema. *Eur Respir J* 1997;10:208–18

170. Martinez FJ, de Oca MM, Whyte RI, Stetz J, Gay SE, Celli BR. Lung-volume reduction improves dyspnea, dynamic hyperinflation, and respiratory muscle function. *Am J Respir Crit Care Med* 1997;155:1984–90

171. Criner G, Cordova FC, Leyenson V, *et al.* Effect of lung volume reduction surgery on diaphragm strength. *Am J Respir Crit Care Med* 1998;157:1578–85

172. Fessler HE, Permutt S. Lung volume reduction surgery and airflow limitation. *Am J Respir Crit Care Med* 1998;157:715–22

173. Russi EW, Bloch KE, Weder W. Functional and morphological heterogeneity of emphysema and its implication for selection of patients for lung volume reduction surgery. *Eur Respir J* 1999;14:230–6

174. Gevenois PA, Estenne M. Can computed tomography predict functional benefit from lung volume reduction surgery for emphysema? *Am J Respir Crit Care Med* 2001;164:2137–8

175. Gelb AF, McKenna RJ Jr, Brenner M, Epstein JD, Zamel N. Lung function 5 yr after lung volume reduction surgery for emphysema. *Am J Respir Crit Care Med* 2001;163:1562–6

176. Brenner M, McKenna RJ Jr, Gelb AF, Fischel RJ, Wilson AF. Rate of FEV1 change following lung volume reduction surgery. *Chest* 1998;113:652–9

177. Doyle RL, Mark JB. Lung volume reduction surgery for the treatment of chronic obstructive pulmonary disease. *Adv Intern Med* 1998;43:233–52

178. Geddes D, Davies M, Koyama H, *et al.* Effect of lung-volume-reduction surgery in patients with severe emphysema. *N Engl J Med* 2000;343:239–45

179. Meyers BF, Yusen RD, Lefrak SS, Cooper JD. Improved long-term survival seen after lung volume reduction surgery compared to continued medical therapy for emphysema. *Ann Thorac Surg* 2001;71:2081

180. Rationale and design of The National Emphysema Treatment Trial: a prospective randomized trial of lung volume reduction surgery. The National Emphysema Treatment Trial Research Group. *Chest* 1999;116:1750–61

181. National Emphysema Treatment Trial Research Group. Patients at high risk of death after lung-volume-reduction surgery. *N Engl J Med* 2001;345:1075–83

182. Drazen JM. Surgery for emphysema – not for everyone. *N Engl J Med* 2001;345:1126–7

183. Goldstein RS, Todd TR, Guyatt G, Keshavjee S, Dolmage TE, van Rooy S, *et al.* Influence of lung volume reduction surgery (LVRS) on health related quality of life in patients with chronic obstructive pulmonary disease. *Thorax* 2003;58:405–10

184. Fishman A, Martinez F, Naunheim K, Piantadosi S, Wise R, Ries A, *et al.* National Emphysema Treatment Trial Research Group. A randomized trial comparing lung-volume-reduction surgery with medical therapy for severe emphysema. *N Engl J Med* 2003;348:2059–73

185. Ramsey SD, Berry K, Etzioni R, Kaplan RM, Sullivan SD, Wood DE. National Emphysema Treatment Trial Research Group. Cost effectiveness of lung-volume-reduction surgery for patients with severe emphysema. *N Engl J Med* 2003;348:2092–102

186. Toma TP, Hopkinson NS, Hillier J, *et al.* Bronchoscopic volume reduction with valve implants in patients with severe emphysema. *Lancet* 2003;361:931–3

187. Trulock EP. Lung transplantation. *Am J Respir Crit Care Med* 1997;155:789–818

188. Theodore J, Lewiston N. Lung transplantation comes of age. *N Engl J Med* 1990;322:772–4

189. Cassivi SD, Meyers BF, Battafarano RJ, *et al.* Thirteen-year experience in lung transplantation for emphysema. *Ann Thorac Surg* 2002;74:1663–9

190. Trulock EP III. Lung transplantation for COPD. *Chest* 1998;113(Suppl 4):269S–76S

191. Maurer JR, Frost AE, Estenne M, Higenbottam T, Glanville AR. International guidelines for the selec-

178. Geddes D, Davies M, Koyama H, *et al*. Effect of lung-volume-reduction surgery in patients with severe emphysema. *N Engl J Med* 2000;343:239–45

179. Meyers BF, Yusen RD, Lefrak SS, Cooper JD. Improved long-term survival seen after lung volume reduction surgery compared to continued medical therapy for emphysema. *Ann Thorac Surg* 2001;71:2081

180. Rationale and design of The National Emphysema Treatment Trial: a prospective randomized trial of lung volume reduction surgery. The National Emphysema Treatment Trial Research Group. *Chest* 1999;116:1750–61

181. National Emphysema Treatment Trial Research Group. Patients at high risk of death after lung-volume-reduction surgery. *N Engl J Med* 2001;345:1075–83

182. Drazen JM. Surgery for emphysema – not for everyone. *N Engl J Med* 2001;345:1126–7

183. Goldstein RS, Todd TR, Guyatt G, Keshavjee S, Dolmage TE, van Rooy S, *et al*. Influence of lung volume reduction surgery (LVRS) on health related quality of life in patients with chronic obstructive pulmonary disease. *Thorax* 2003;58:405–10

8

New drugs for COPD

SUMMARY

There is a major need to develop new drugs for patients with COPD, and a large number of targets have been defined for therapy[1–3] (Figure 8.1). It is fundamental to stop patients smoking and to provide safer cigarettes, and new aids to smoking cessation are being developed. Bronchodilators are the basis of current drug therapy for COPD, although there is only minor reversibility of FEV_1 in COPD, and tiotropium and long-acting β_2-agonists have been considerable therapeutic advances.

Clinical research is ongoing to define the role of inhaled steroids, as well as combined inhaled steroids with long-acting β_2-agonists, for certain patients with COPD. However, the efficacy of inhaled corticosteroids in stable COPD is limited. Since there is amplified inflammation in the airways and lung parenchyma of patients with COPD, a range of therapies are being assessed that address the particular inflammatory cells that are prominent in COPD: neutrophils, macrophages and CD8+ T cells.

Promising clinical trial data are available for two PDE4 inhibitors in COPD, cilomilast and roflumilast, and PDE4B holds promise of being an important target for anti-inflammatory effects. Leukotriene B_4 inhibitors, chemokine receptor inhibitors (CXCR2 and CCR2), and a range of therapy directed against TNF-α also has considerable potential. Among various programs to inhibit protease activity, those to selectively develop inhibitors of MMP-9 look most attractive. A variety of approaches can regulate the production of mucus, including tachykinin antagonists and agents to inhibit tachykinin release, but the role of mucus in the pathophysiology of COPD is still not defined. A more ambitious approach is to accelerate alveolar repair and regeneration using agents such as retinoic acid derivatives and hepatic growth factor.

Apart from identification of novel targets and drugs, it is also necessary to improve drug delivery, establish designs for clinical trials in limited numbers of patients with COPD, develop biomarkers and non-invasive monitoring techniques, and better understand the pathophysiology of COPD.

Figure 8.1   Targets for future COPD therapy

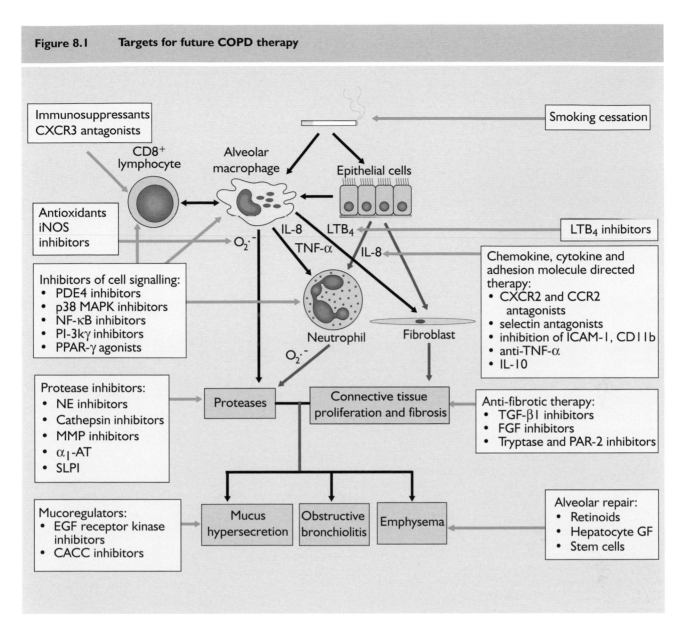

The various targets for novel drugs to treat COPD are rationally based on understanding of the oxidant, inflammatory, fibrotic, proteolytic and regenerative processes that occur in the airways and lung parenchyma. Pathogenic pathways are shown in pink, while potential therapies are in green. Oxidants within cigarette smoke, as well as other irritants, activate epithelial cells and macrophages in the respiratory tract which release neutrophil chemotactic factors, including interleukin-8 (IL-8) and leukotriene B₄ (LTB₄). The IL-8 family causes chemotaxis of neutrophils via the cysteine-X-cysteine receptor 2 (CXCR2), while monocyte chemotactic peptide-1 (MCP-1) binds to cysteine-cysteine receptor 2 (CCR2). Cytotoxic CD8+ T cells may also be involved in the inflammatory cascade. Neutrophils and tissue macrophages are a potent source of oxidants (O_2^-) and proteases, the latter being normally inhibited by a panel of endogenous protease inhibitors. Proteases include neutrophil elastase (NE), cathepsins and various matrix metalloproteinases (MMPs). Protease inhibitors include α_1-antitrypsin (α_1-AT), secretory leukoprotease inhibitor (SLPI) and tissue inhibitor of matrix metalloproteinases (TIMP). Fibroblasts are a prominent feature in the pathology of bronchiolitis and emphysema, and regenerative healing processes, as well as tissue remodelling, occur in COPD. Vascular endothelial cells, pneumocytes and mast cells may also contribute to the pathogenesis of COPD. CACC, calcium activated chloride channel; EGF, epidermal growth factor; FGF, fibroblast growth factors; GF, hepatocyte growth factor; iNOS, inducible nitric oxide synthase; ICAM-1, intercellular adhesion molecule-1; IL-10, interleukin-10; MAPKs, mitogen-activated protein kinases; NF-κB, nuclear factor kappa B; PPAR-γ, peroxisome proliferator-activated receptor-γ; PDE4, phosphodiesterase type 4; PI-3Kγ, phosphoinositide-3 kinase γ; PAR, protease activated receptor; TGF-β, transforming growth factor-β; TNF-α, tumor necrosis factor-α.

INTRODUCTION

COPD is characterized by a particular type of inflammation, with increased numbers of macrophages, neutrophils and cytotoxic CD8+ T cells in the airways. These changes may persist for a long time in ex-smokers. Corticosteroids have limited efficacy in the treatment of COPD, prompting the search for new anti-inflammatory drugs. Several inflammatory cells and mediators are involved in the pathophysiology of COPD and antagonists to individual elements are in development (Figure 8.1). Because there is a different profile of cells and mediators in COPD compared with asthma, it is probable that different drugs are likely to be effective for the treatment of COPD. Leukotriene B_4 (LTB_4), interleukin-8 (IL-8), tumor necrosis factor-α (TNF-α) , oxidants and nitric oxide (NO) are mediator targets among a variety of other anti-inflammatory approaches, summarized in Figure 8.2.

SMOKING CESSATION

Smoking cessation is the only therapeutic intervention that has been clearly demonstrated to reduce disease progression in COPD. A major issue with smoking cessation is that the patient has become addicted to nicotine. Despite the use of behavioral approaches, counselling and nicotine replacement therapy, the overall rates of smoking cessation are only 5–15%. The most effective treatment to aid smoking cessation is the antidepressant bupropion slow-release (SR) (Zyban®, GlaxoSmithKline)[4], which, when given as a short course of 7 weeks, caused a point prevalence quit rate of 23% at 12 months[5]. The point cessation rate at 12 months can be increased to 35% when used with nicotine patches[6]. However, in this 1999 study, the continued smoking cessation rate in the bupropion SR group at 12-month follow-up was 18.4%[6,7]. In smokers with COPD, bupropion SR caused a 16% continuous abstinence rate from weeks 4 to 26[8]. Bupropion SR should be used with caution since it may cause headache, sleeplessness and agitation, and epilepsy has been reported in approximately 0.1% of patients, mainly in patients with a previous history of epilepsy. To minimize the risk of adverse effects, a modified dose titration scheme has been introduced, involving 150 mg once daily for 6 days, increasing to 150 mg twice daily on day 7. Better understanding of the neuropharmacology of nicotine addiction is likely to lead to novel drugs to aid smoking cessation. Efforts have also been made to provide 'safer cigarettes' that provide the flavor and nicotine of cigarettes without the oxidants and tar.

NEW BRONCHODILATORS

Bronchodilators are the mainstay of current management of COPD and the major recent advances have been in the development of long-acting bronchodilators. Tiotropium bromide (Spiriva®) is a newly licensed once-daily anticholinergic bronchodilator that has recently been recommended in the GOLD guidelines as a first-line bronchodilator alongside long-acting β_2-agonists for COPD of Stages II–IV[9]. The long-acting inhaled β_2-agonists, salmeterol and formoterol, are given twice daily in patients with COPD, and are now established in the management of chronic stable COPD[10–17]. Viozan® (AR-C68397AA) is a dual agonist of β_2-adrenergic and dopamine D_2 receptors, the rationale being that D_2-agonists may activate receptors on airway sensory nerves to inhibit cough and reflex mucus secretion, but, due to tolerance on repeat dosing, this drug has now been discontinued[18,19].

The mechanism of action of β_2-agonists on the smooth muscle cell is well established at a molecular level[20,21] (Figure 8.3). Following triggering of the β_2-adrenoceptor, there is Gαs stimulation of adenylyl cyclase (AC), production of cyclic adenosine monophosphate (cAMP), and protein kinase A (PKA), before inhibition of calcium levels and myosin light chain kinase (MLCK) to cause bronchodilation. In contrast, acetylcholine stimulates the M3 muscarinic receptor to activate Gαq, which activates phospholipase Cβ (PLCβ) to act on the phosphoinositol pathway and stimulate protein kinase C. This causes bronchoconstriction due to calcium release and myosin ATPase stimulation[21].

INHALED CORTICOSTEROIDS

Inhaled corticosteroids have been studied in 3-year long-term studies in COPD. They have been shown to have no significant effect on the natural history of loss of FEV_1, but to have effects on health status and prevention of exacerbations[22–25]. Furthermore, regular use of inhaled fluticasone alone or in combination with salmeterol was associated with increased survival in patients with COPD[26]. The TRISTAN

Figure 8.2 **Potential new drugs for COPD**

Target	Candidate therapies
Smoking cessation	
Phosphodiesterase type 4 (PDE-4)	PDE-4 inhibitors Cilomilast (SB 207499, Ariflo, GSK) Roflumilast (BY 217, Altana)
Leukotrienes	LTB$_4$ antagonists (LY 29311, SC-53228, CP-105696, SB 201146, BIL284) 5'-lipoxygenase inhibitors (zileuton, Bay x1005)
Chemokines	Interleukin-8 receptor antagonists (CXCR2 antagonists, e.g. SB 225002) MCP receptor antagonists (CCR2 antagonists) CXCR3 receptor antagonists
Adhesion molecules	Anti CD11/CD18, anti-ICAM-1, E-selectin inhibitors
Cytokines	TNF-inhibitors (monoclonal antibodies (infliximab, Remicade), soluble receptors (etanercept, Enbrel), TNF-α converting enzyme (TACE) inhibitors) Interleukin-10 and analogues
Kinases and transcription factors	p38 MAP kinase inhibitors (SB 203580, SB 220025) PI-3 kinase-γ inhibitors NF-κB inhibitors (proteasome inhibitors, IκB kinase inhibitors, IκB-α gene transfer) PPAR activators
Oxidants	Antioxidants (e.g. stable glutathione analogues) Resveratrol Inducible nitric oxide synthase (iNOS) inhibitors (e.g. SC-51, prodrug for L-NIL)
Proteases	Endogenous antiproteases: α1-AT, SLPI, TIMPs, elafin Neutrophil elastase inhibitors Cysteine protease inhibitors Matrix metalloprotease (MMP) inhibitors: inhaled marimastat
Mucoregulation	EGF receptor kinase inhibitors: Gefitinib Calcium activated chloride channel (CACC) inhibitors: niflumic acid and MSI 1956
Fibrosis	TGF-β_1 inhibitors (TGF-β_1 receptor kinase inhibitors) Fibroblast growth factor inhibitors Tryptase and protease-activated receptor (PAR)-2 inhibition
Lung regeneration	Retinoic acid (all trans retinoic acid) and γ-retinoids Hepatocyte growth factor Stem cells

L-NIL, 1-N6-(1-iminoethyl) lysine; LTB$_4$, leukotriene B$_4$; MCP, monocyte chemotactic protein; TNF, tumor necrosis factor; TGF, transforming growth factor; EGF, epithelium-derived growth factor; COX, cyclo-oxygenase; iNOS, inducible nitric oxide synthase; NF-κB, nuclear factor-κB; IκB, inhibitor of NF-κB; MAP, mitogen-activated protein; PI, phosphoinositide; PPAR, peroxisome proliferation activated receptor.

study group has found that inhaled combined corticosteroid (fluticasone) with long-acting β_2-agonist (salmeterol) has promising efficacy in COPD[27,28].

Inhaled corticosteroids do not seem to affect markers of inflammation in sputum[29,30], nor inhibit neutrophilic inflammation induced by ozone[31]. There may be an active resistance to corticosteroids due to an inhibitory effect of cigarette smoke on histone deacetylase, which is required for steroids to switch off inflammatory genes[32]. Therapeutic strategies that unlock the molecular mechanism of resistance might be possible, for example drugs that increase histone deacetylase activity may resensitize cells to the effects of steroids.

PHOSPHODIESTERASE-4 INHIBITORS

Phosphodiesterases (PDEs) break down cyclic nucleotides (cyclic AMP and cyclic GMP) which regulate cellular activity (Figure 8.4). Inhibition of these enzymes results in inhibition of inflammatory cells and relaxation of smooth muscle[33–37]. Eleven families of PDEs are now recognized, but the family most relevant to COPD inflammation is PDE4, since PDE4 is the predominant PDE expressed in neutrophils, macrophages and CD8+ T cells[38,39]. Recently, genetic analysis has demonstrated that there are four isoenzymes of PDE4 itself; these are

---

Figure 8.3   Molecular actions of bronchodilators

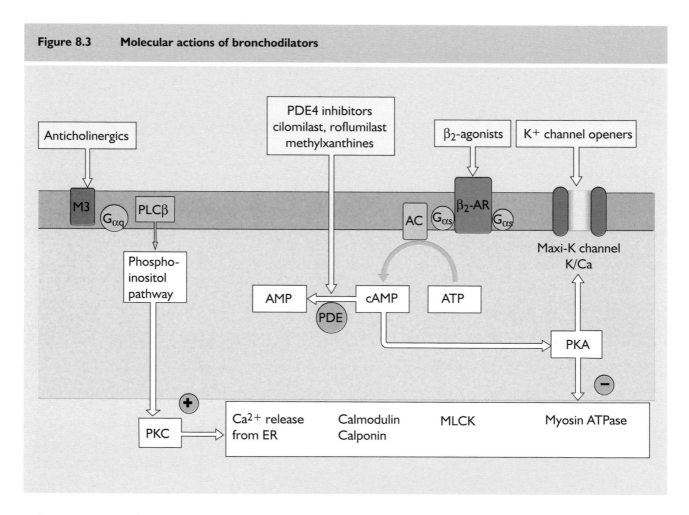

β_2-agonists act on the β_2-adrenoceptor (β_2-AR) that is coupled to $G_{\alpha s}$. Stimulation of the receptor causes GTP-bound $G_{\alpha s}$ to stimulate adenylyl cyclase (AC), resulting in the conversion of ATP to cAMP. Increased cytosolic cAMP activates protein kinase A (PKA), which in turn phosphorylates myosin light chain kinase (MLCK) and causes relaxation of smooth muscle. Anticholinergics act on the M_3-muscarinic receptor, which links to $G_{\alpha q}$. The agonists acetylcholine and methacholine cause GTP-bound $G_{\alpha q}$ to stimulate phospholipase Cβ (PLCβ) which has activity on the phospho-inositol pathway and protein kinase C (PKC). There is then release of Ca^{2+} from endoplasmic reticulum (ER) into the cytosol, liberating Ca^{2+} binding to calmodulin and activating MLCK, with bronchoconstriction. For further details see Johnson EN, Druey KM, *J Allergy Clin Immunol* 2002;109:592–602.

termed PDE A–D, and there is further complexity due to alternative splicing in some cells.

Cilomilast (Ariflo®, GlaxoSmithKline) was developed based on the selectivity for the conformation of PDE4 that binds to the low-affinity rather than the high-affinity rolipram binding site[40]. This was in an effort to minimize the amount of nausea caused in general by PDE4 inhibitors, but cilomilast may be selective for PDE4D, which may contribute to nausea. Cilomilast has been demonstrated to be effective in animal models of inflammation[41]. Preliminary studies have also demonstrated beneficial clinical effects of cilomilast in a 12-week study in COPD patients[40] (Figure 8.5) and larger studies are currently underway.

Roflumilast is under clinical development from Altana, and may have the advantage over cilomilast of being non-selective for PDE4 isoenzymes A–D. The efficacy of roflumilast has been demonstrated in animal models[42] as well as in studies with human blood cells[43]. Roflumilast has effects on exercise–induced asthma[44] and allergic rhinitis[45], and inhibits early and late asthmatic reactions following inhaled allergen challenge[46]. Abstracts have recently been presented that demonstrate effects of roflumilast on FEV_1 in a 6-month study in COPD[47,48].

The effects of PDE4 inhibitors may still currently be limited by side-effects, particularly nausea and other gastrointestinal effects, but it might be possible

---

Figure 8.4   Phosphodiesterase (PDE) 4 inhibitors

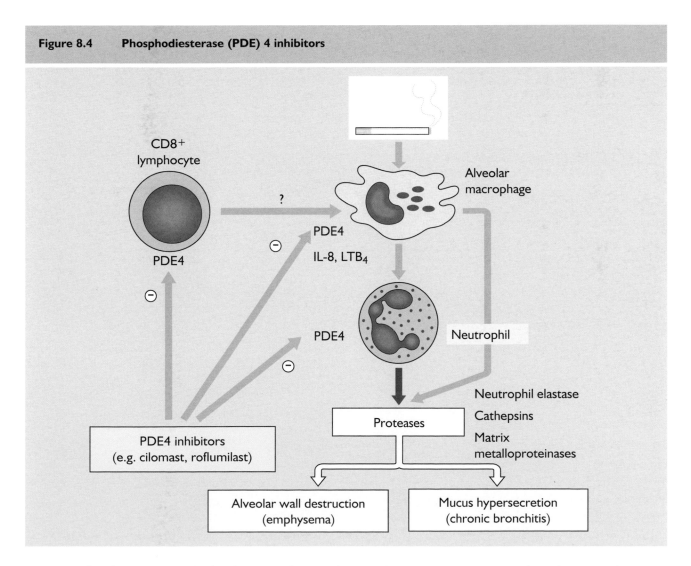

PDE4 is found in CD8+ T-cells, alveolar macrophages and neutrophils. PDE4 is a promising target for COPD therapy. PDE4B is believed to be selectively expressed in these inflammatory cells. Leukotriene B4 (LTB_4) and interleukin-8 (IL-8) are generated by macrophages.

Figure 8.5   Effect of a PDE4 inhibitor, cilomilast, in COPD

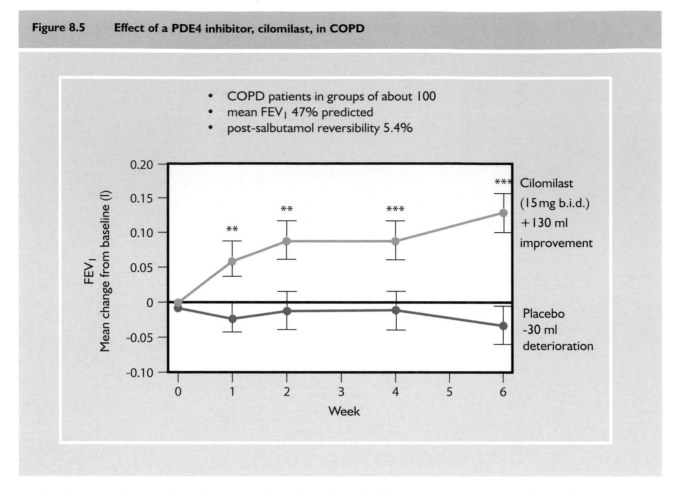

- COPD patients in groups of about 100
- mean FEV_1 47% predicted
- post-salbutamol reversibility 5.4%

Cilomilast caused a significantly improved trough prebronchodilator FEV_1 compared with placebo at week 6 (p < 0.0001). Adapted from Compton CH et al. Lancet 2001;358:265–70.

to develop in the future isoenzyme subtype or splice variant selective inhibitors which are not dose-limited by adverse effects.

LEUKOTRIENE B₄ INHIBITORS

Leukotriene B_4 (LTB_4) is a potent chemoattractant of neutrophils and is increased in the sputum of patients with COPD[49]. It is probably derived from alveolar macrophages, as well as neutrophils, and may be synergistic with IL-8. Two subtypes of receptor for LTB_4 have been described: BLT_1 receptors are mainly expressed on granulocytes and monocytes, whereas BLT_2 receptors are expressed on T cells[50] (Figure 8.6).

- Selective LTB_4 receptor (BLT receptor) antagonists have now been developed. A potent LTB_4 antagonist (LY293111) is ineffective against

allergen challenge in asthmatic patients, although it inhibits the neutrophil recruitment into the airways during the late response, indicating the capacity to inhibit neutrophil chemotaxis in the airways[51,52]. In addition, LY293111 inhibits the neutrophil chemotactic activity of sputum from COPD patients[53]. Several potent LTB_4 antagonists are now in development (including SC-53228, CP-105696, SB 201146, BIIL284).

- LTB_4 is synthesized by 5'-lipoxygenase (5-LO), of which there are now several potent inhibitors. 5-LO inhibitors, such as zileuton, are now available in some countries for the treatment of asthma, since they also inhibit the synthesis of cysteinyl-leukotrienes. However, there have been problems with hepatotoxicity, and it is not known whether they are effective in COPD.

Figure 8.6   Inhibition of leukotriene B₄ (LTB₄)

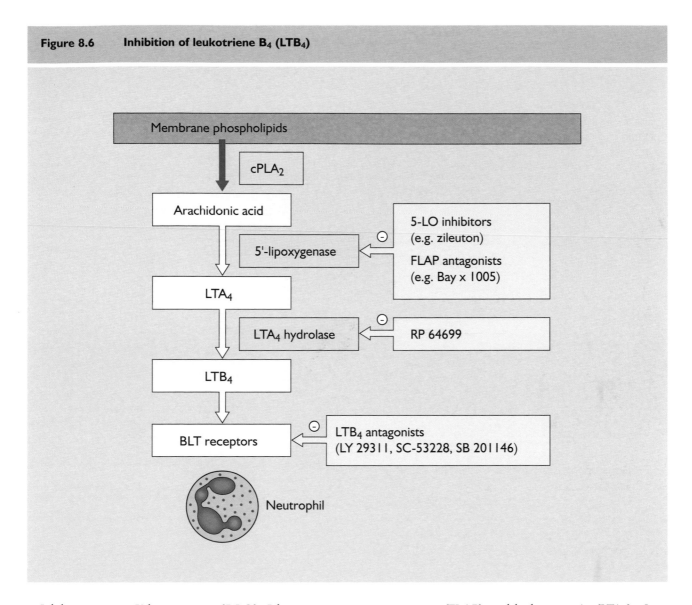

Inhibitors act on 5'-lipoxygenase (5-LO), 5-lipoxygenase activating protein (FLAP), and leukotriene A₄ (LTA₄). In addition, there are agents to antagonize LTB₄ receptors (BLT).

- LTA$_4$ hydrolase inhibitors that selectively inhibit the synthesis of LTB$_4$ have also been developed.

- Members of the 15-lipoxygenase enzyme family are proinflammatory and present in elevated amounts in inflamed epithelial cells[54].

CHEMOKINE INHIBITORS

Several chemotactic cytokines (chemokines) are involved in neutrophil, monocyte and T lymphocyte chemotaxis[55–57] (Figure 8.7). These belong to the CXC family of chemokines, the most prominent member of which is IL-8, which is markedly elevated in the sputum of patients with COPD[58–61]. Fully human monoclonal antibodies against IL-8 block neutrophil CD11b upregulation and chemotaxis in experimental animals[62]. In addition, a monoclonal antibody against IL-8 blocks the chemotactic response of neutrophils within sputum from patients with chronic bronchitis[63].

IL-8 activates neutrophils via a specific low-affinity G protein-coupled specific receptor (CXCR1). A high-affinity receptor (CXCR2) is activated by IL-8 and other members of the CXC chemokine family[56] (Figure 8.8). A potent non-peptide inhibitor of IL-8 has been developed[64,65].

Figure 8.7   Therapy directed against adhesion molecules, chemokines and cytokines

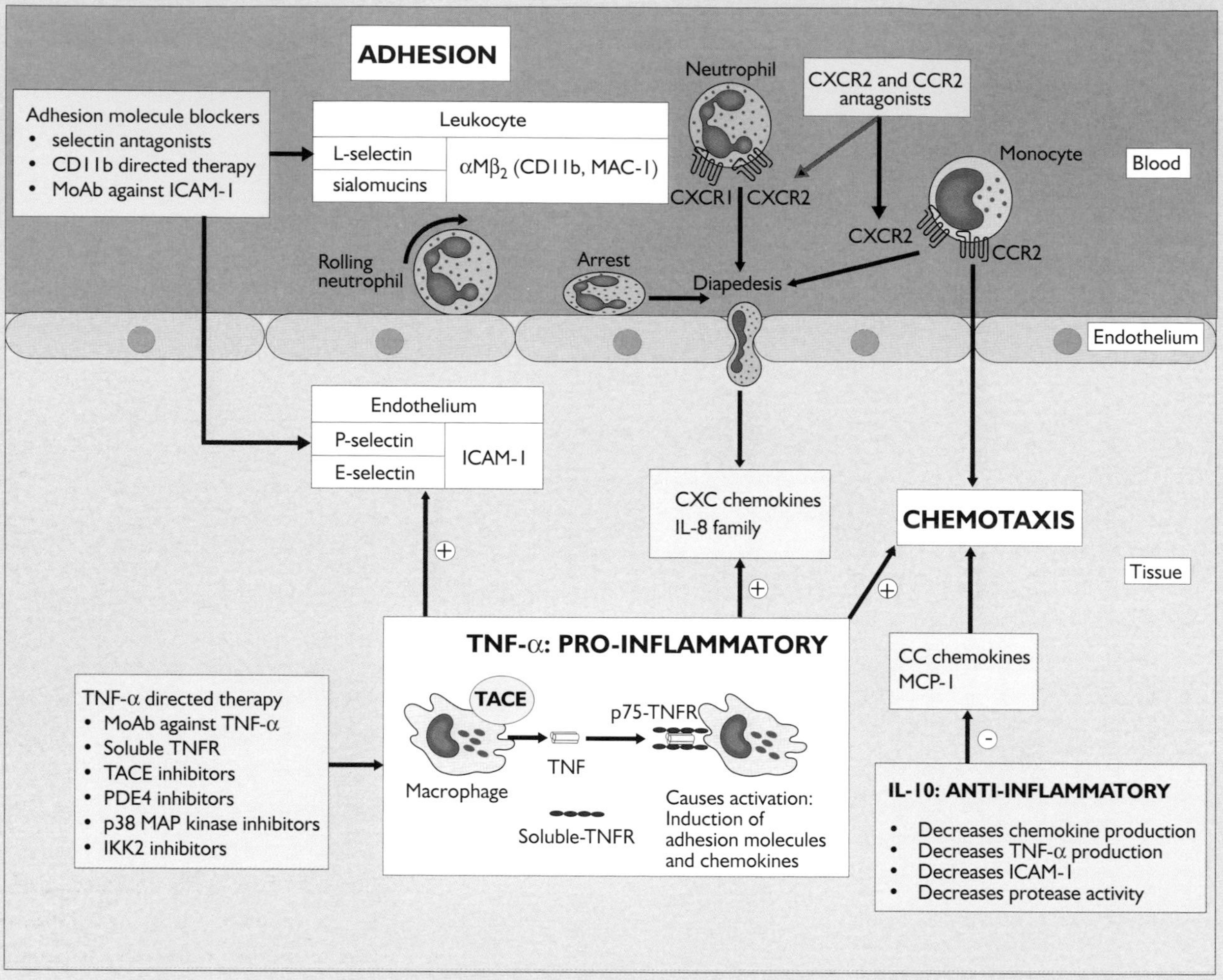

This figure represents the passage of neutrophils and monocytes from blood to lung tissue, with potential therapeutics show in green. Endothelial cell adhesion molecules are induced in response to inflammatory stimuli, and include P- and E-selectin, intercellular adhesion molecule-1 and -2 (ICAM-1 and -2). Neutrophils and monocytes express a variety of adhesion molecules including L-selectin, sialomucins and $\alpha M\beta 2$ (CD11b, Mac-1), which bind to endothelial cells through adhesion molecule interactions. Interleukin-8 (IL-8) is a member of the CXC family of chemokines, and binds to CXCR1 as well as CXCR2 on neutrophils. Monocyte chemotactic peptide-1 (MCP-1) is a CC chemokine that binds to CCR2 on monocytes. Tumor necrosis factor-α (TNF-α) is a pro-inflammatory cytokine whose production is influenced by phosphodiesterase type 4 (PDE4) activity, and whose release from cells is governed by TNF-α converting enzyme (TACE). TNF-α is present as a homotrimer that binds to membrane-bound TNF receptors (TNFR) on a variety of different cells. Interleukin-10 (IL-10) is an endogenous anti-inflammatory cytokine that decreases the expression of chemokines such as interleukin-8 (IL-8) and monocyte chemotactic protein (MCP). In addition, subcutaneous IL-10 decreases levels of TNF-α and matrix metalloproteinases (MMPs), while increasing levels of tissue inhibitors of MMPs (TIMPs).

Figure 8.8   Neutrophil inhibition

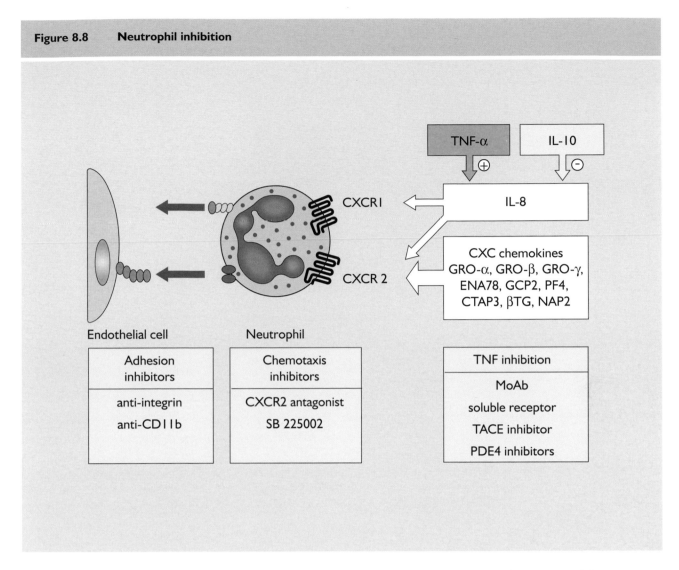

Interleukin-8 (IL-8) activates both the low-affinity chemokine receptor CXCR1, which mediates neutrophil activation, and high-affinity receptor CXCR2, which mediates chemotaxis. CXCR2 is also activated by other CXC-chemokines that might also be involved in COPD. CTAP3, connective tissue-activating peptide III; ENA, epithelial neutrophil-activating protein; GCP2, granulocyte chemotatic protein 2; GRO, growth-related oncoprotein; NAP2, neutrophil-activating peptide 2; PF4, platelet factor 4; βTG, β-thromboglobulin.

Other CXC chemokines, such as GRO-α, are also elevated in COPD[66], and therefore a CXCR2 antagonist is likely to be more useful than a CXCR1 antagonist, particularly as CXCR2 is also expressed on monocytes. Small molecule inhibitors of CXCR2, such as SB225002, have now been developed[64,65]. There is also involvement of C-C chemokines in COPD, since there is increased expression of monocyte chemotactic protein-1 and its receptor CCR2 by macrophages and epithelial cells in COPD. Small molecule inhibitors of CCR2 are now in development.

ADHESION MOLECULE BLOCKERS

Recruitment of neutrophils, monocytes and cytotoxic T cells into the lungs and respiratory tract is dependent on adhesion molecules expressed on these cells and on endothelial cells in the pulmonary and bronchial circulations (Figure 8.9). Several adhesion molecules can now be inhibited pharmacologically. For example, E-selectin on endothelial cells interacts with sialyl-Lewis[x] on neutrophils. A mimic of sialyl-Lewis[x], TBC 1269, blocks selectins and inhibits granulocyte adhesion, with preferential

Figure 8.9   Adhesion molecule blockers in COPD

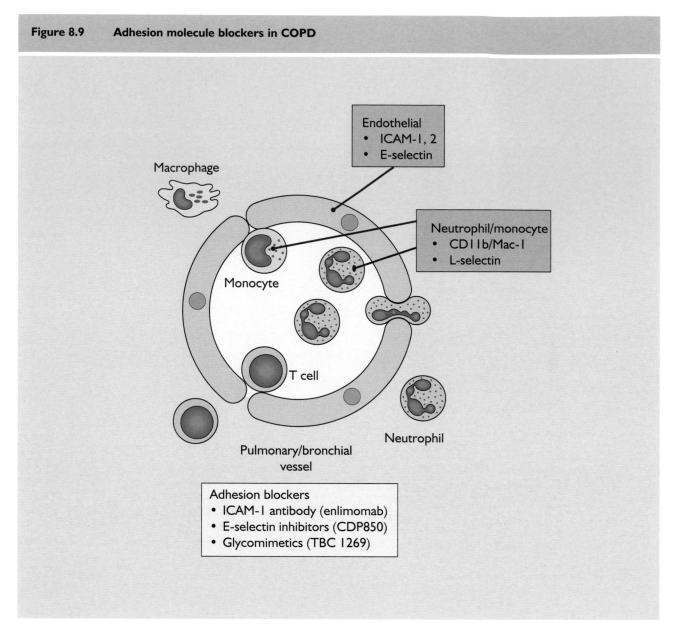

Endothelial cell adhesion molecules are induced in response to inflammatory stimuli, and include intercellular adhesion molecule-1 and -2 (ICAM-1 and -2). Neutrophils and monocytes express a variety of adhesion molecules, including CD11b (Mac-1) and L-selectin, and bind to endothelial cells through adhesion molecule interactions.

effects on neutrophils[67]. However, there are concerns about this therapeutic approach for a chronic disease, as an impaired neutrophilic response may increase the susceptibility to infection. Chemotaxis, as well as the expression of Mac-1 (CD11b/CD18), is increased on neutrophils of patients with COPD[68,69], suggesting that targeting this adhesion molecule, which is also expressed on monocytes and macrophages, might be beneficial.

TUMOR NECROSIS FACTOR-α INHIBITORS

Tumor necrosis factor-α (TNF-α) levels are raised in the sputum of COPD patients[58], and increased TNF-α may cause skeletal muscle apoptosis and the severe wasting in some patients with advanced COPD[70]. Humanized monoclonal TNF antibodies (Remicade, Infliximab, Centocor) and soluble TNF receptors (Etanercept, Amgen), which are effective

Figure 8.10   Tumor necrosis factor-α (TNF-α) as a target in COPD

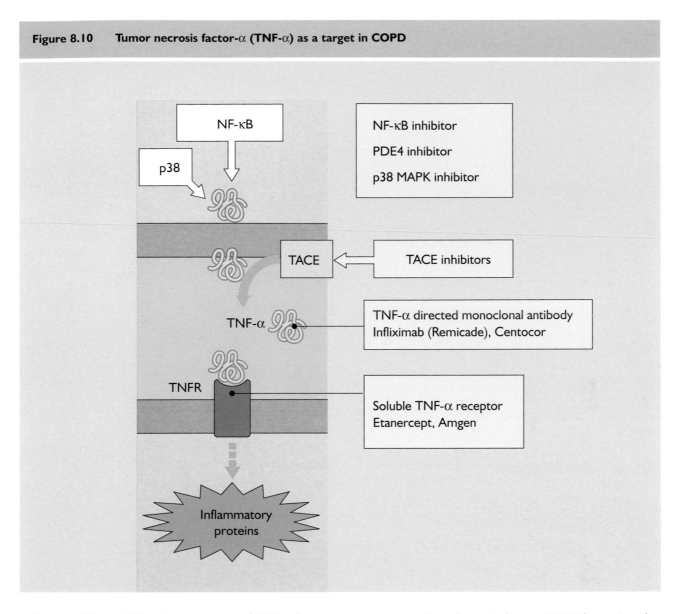

It is possible to inhibit the generation of TNF-α by acting on mitogen-activated protein kinases (MAP kinases) and nuclear factor-κB (NF-κB). In addition, phosphodiesterase 4 (PDE4) inhibitors affect TNF-α synthesis. TNF-α release is governed by tumor necrosis factor-α converting enzyme (TACE), while tumor necrosis factor receptor (TNFR) mediates the action of TNF-α on cells.

in other chronic inflammatory diseases, such as rheumatoid arthritis and Crohn's disease, should also be effective in COPD[71,72] (Figure 8.10). Caution is required in the treatment of COPD due to the potential for reactivation of tuberculosis and aggravation of heart failure. TNF-α converting enzyme (TACE), which is required for the release of soluble TNF-α, may be a more attractive target, as it is possible to discover small molecule TACE inhibitors, some of which are also matrix metalloproteinase inhibitors[73,74]. General anti-inflammatory drugs such as phosphodiesterase 4 (PDE4) inhibitors and p38 inhibitors also potently inhibit TNF-α expression.

INTERLEUKIN-10

Interleukin-10 (IL-10) is a cytokine with a wide spectrum of anti-inflammatory actions (Figure 8.11). It inhibits the secretion of TNF-α and IL-8 from

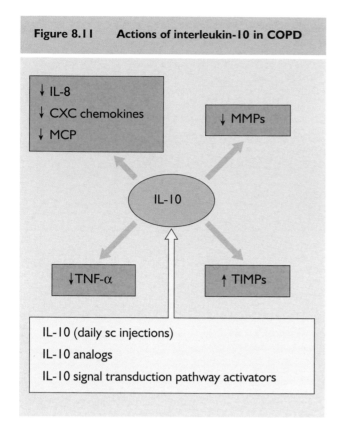

Figure 8.11   Actions of interleukin-10 in COPD

Interleukin-10 (IL-10) is an endogenous anti-inflammatory cytokine that decreases the expression of chemokines such as interleukin-8 (IL-8) and monocyte chemotactic protein (MCP). In addition, IL-10 decreases levels of tumor necrosis factor-α (TNF-α) and matrix metalloproteinases (MMPs), while increasing levels of tissue inhibitors of MMPs (TIMPs). IL-10 is administered subcutaneously (sc).

macrophages, but tips the balance in favor of antiproteases, by decreasing the expression of matrix metalloproteinases, while increasing the expression of endogenous tissue inhibitors of matrix metalloproteinases (TIMP). IL-10 concentrations are reduced in induced sputum from patients with COPD, so that this may be a mechanism for increasing lung inflammation[75]. IL-10 is currently in clinical trials for other chronic inflammatory diseases (inflammatory bowel disease, rheumatoid arthritis and psoriasis), including patients with steroid resistance, but IL-10 may cause hematological side-effects[76]. Treatment with daily injections of IL-10 over several weeks has been well tolerated. IL-10 may have therapeutic potential in COPD, especially if a selective activator of IL-10 receptors or signal transduction pathways can be developed.

DRUGS ACTING ON TRANSCRIPTION FACTORS

NF-κB inhibitors

The transcription factor NF-κB regulates the expression of IL-8 and other chemokines, in addition to TNF-α and some matrix metalloproteinases (MMPs). One approach to inhibition of NF-κB involves gene transfer of the inhibitor of NF-κB (IκB); alternatively, there are inhibitors of IκB kinases (IKK), and drugs that inhibit the degradation of IκB[77] (Figure 8.12). In addition, NF-κB-inducing kinase (NIK) and IκB ubiquitin ligase regulate the activity of NF-κB. The most promising approach may be the inhibition of IKKβ by small molecule inhibitors. A putative selective IKK inhibitor, hypoestoxide, is a component of an African folk remedy for inflammatory disorders. One concern about long-term inhibition of NF-κB is that effective inhibitors may result in immune suppression and impair host defences, since knock-out mice which lack NF-κB proteins succumb to septicemia. However, there are alternative pathways of NF-κB activation that might be more important in inflammatory disease[78].

p38 MAP kinase inhibitors

Mitogen-activated protein (MAP) kinases play a key role in chronic inflammation and several complex enzyme cascades have now been defined (Figure 8.13). One of these, the p38 MAP kinase pathway, is involved in the expression of inflammatory cytokines, including IL-8, TNF-α and MMPs[79,80]. Non-peptide inhibitors of p38 MAP kinase, such as SB 203580, SB 239063 and RWJ 67657, have now been developed and these drugs have a broad range of anti-inflammatory effects[81]. SB 239063 reduces neutrophil infiltration after inhaled endotoxin and the concentrations of IL-6 and MMP-9 in bronchoalveolar lavage fluid of rats, indicating its potential as an anti-inflammatory agent in COPD[82]. It is likely that such a broad-spectrum anti-inflammatory drug will have some toxicity, but inhalation may be a feasible therapeutic approach.

Phosphoinositide 3-kinase inhibitors

Phosphoinositide 3-kinase inhibitors (PI-3Ks) are a family of enzymes that lead to the generation of lipid second messengers which regulate a number of cellu-

Figure 8.12   Inhibitors of cell signalling

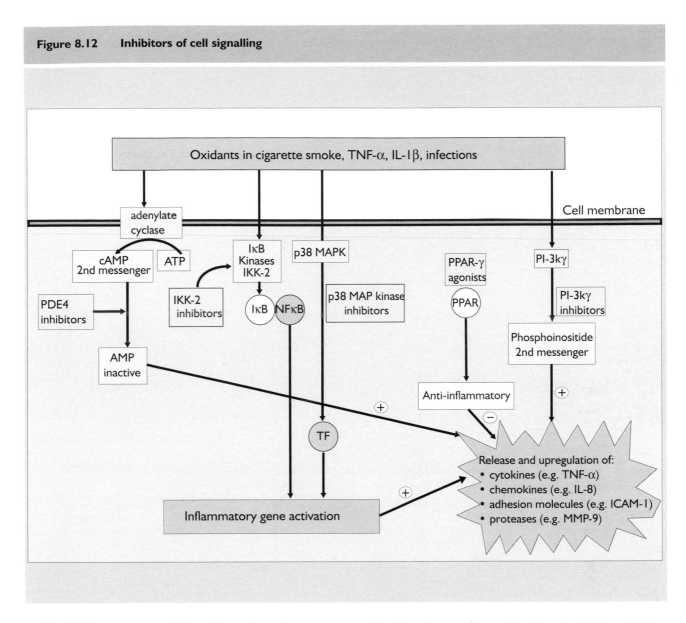

Phosphodiesterase type 4 (PDE4) catalyzes the inactivation of cyclic adenosine monophosphate (cAMP) to AMP, cAMP being an active second messenger within the cell. Multiple pathways mediate kinase then transcription factor (TF) activity in relation to inflammatory gene expression, including a system acting on nuclear factor kappa B (NF-kB). Inhibitor of NF-κB (IκB) kinases (IKK-2) and p38 mitogen-activated protein kinases (MAPKs) are involved. Inflammatory gene activation causes synthesis of cytokines, chemokines, adhesion molecules and proteases (for abbreviations see footnote to Figure 8.1). Peroxisome proliferator-activated receptors (PPARs) are a family of hormone receptors that belong to the steroid superfamily, and PPAR-γ has anti-inflammatory activity. Phosphoinositide-3 (PI-3) kinase causes activation of cells through generation of phosphoinositide second messengers.

lar events. A particular isoform, PI-3Kγ, is involved in neutrophil recruitment and activation. Knock-out of the PI-3Kγ gene results in inhibition of neutrophil migration and activation, as well as impaired T lymphocyte and macrophage function[83]. This suggests that selective PI-3Kγ inhibitors may have relevant anti-inflammatory activity in COPD.

ANTIOXIDANTS

Oxidative stress is especially important during exacerbations of COPD[84–86], and antioxidants may be of use in the therapy of COPD (Figure 8.14). *N*-acetyl cysteine (NAC) provides cysteine for enhanced production of glutathione (GSH) and has antioxidant

Figure 8.13   Mitogen-activated protein kinase (MAPK) inhibitors in COPD

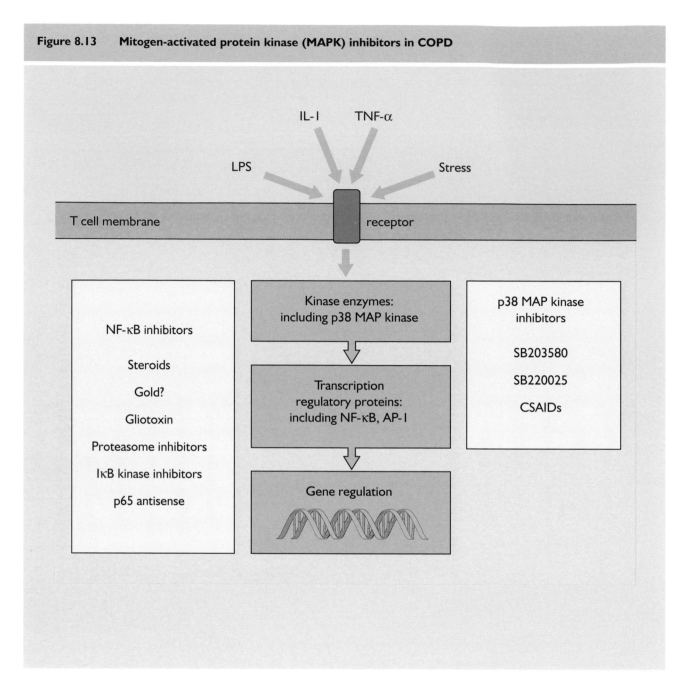

Lipopolysaccharide (LPS), interleukin-1 (IL-1), tumor necrosis factor-α (TNF-α) and stress activate receptors which in turn activate kinase enzymes, including p38 MAP kinase. There is then activation of nuclear factor-κB (NF-κB) and activator protein-1 (AP-1).

effects *in vitro* and *in vivo*. Recent systematic reviews of studies with oral NAC in COPD suggest small but significant reductions in exacerbations[87,88]. More effective antioxidants, including stable glutathione compounds, analogs of superoxide dismutase (SOD) and selenium-based drugs, are now in development for clinical use[89].

INDUCIBLE NITRIC OXIDE INHIBITORS

Oxidative stress and increased nitric oxide release from expression of inducible nitric oxide synthase (iNOS) may result in the formation of peroxynitrite, which is a potent radical and may nitrate proteins, resulting in altered function[90]. Hence, the presence

Figure 8.14   Oxidative stress in COPD

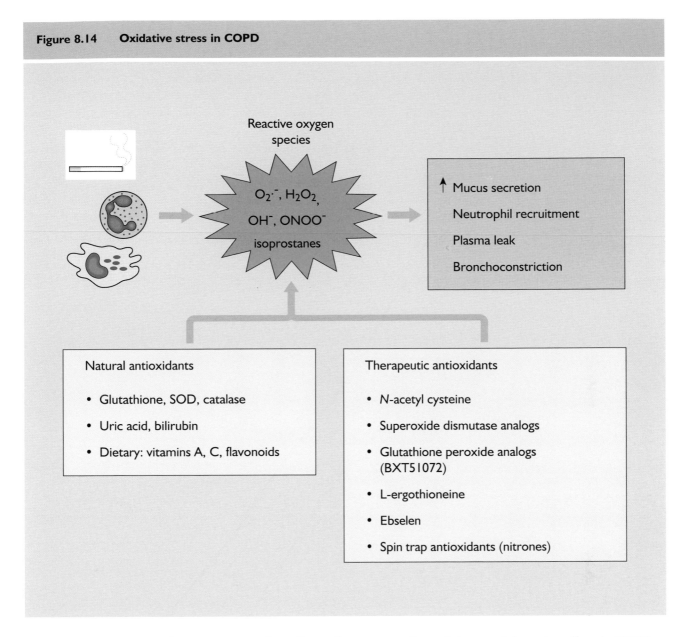

Reactive oxygen species from cigarette smoke or from inflammatory cells result in several damaging effects in COPD, including decreased antiprotease defences, activation of nuclear factor-κB (NF-κB), resulting in increased secretion of isoprostanes and direct effects on airway functions. $O_2{}^{\cdot-}$, superoxide anion; H_2O_2, hydrogen peroxide; $ONOO^-$, peroxynitrite; SLPI, secretory leukoprotease inhibitor; α_1-AT, α_1-antitrypsin.

of 3-nitrotyrosine (3NT) may indicate local peroxynitrite formation, and 3NT is markedly increased in sputum macrophages of patients with COPD[91]. Selective inhibitors of iNOS are now in development[92]. Single doses of a selective iNOS inhibitor (SD 3651) were well tolerated in healthy volunteers and patients with mild asthma, and 200 mg caused pronounced inhibition of exhaled breath nitric oxide for 72 h after administration[93,94].

PROTEASE INHIBITORS

There is compelling evidence in COPD for an imbalance between proteases that digest elastin (and other structural proteins) and antiproteases that protect against this. This suggests that either inhibiting these proteolytic enzymes or increasing the number of antiproteases may be beneficial and theoretically should prevent the progression of airflow obstruction in COPD. Considerable progress has been made in identifying the enzymes involved in elastolytic activity in emphysema and in characterizing the endogenous antiproteases that counteract this activity[95,96]. One approach is to give endogenous antiproteases including α_1-antitrypsin (α_1-AT), tissue inhibitor of metalloproteinases (TIMP-1), elafin, or secretory leukoprotease inhibitor (SLPI) (Figure 8.15).

Neutrophil elastase inhibitors

As neutrophil elastase (NE) is a major constituent of lung elastolytic activity and also potently stimulates mucus secretion, it is a potential target for inhibition. Several potent NE inhibitors have been developed, including small molecule inhibitors, such as ONO 5046 and FR90127[97,98]. These drugs inhibit NE-induced lung injury in experimental animals,

---

Figure 8.15   Protease inhibition in COPD

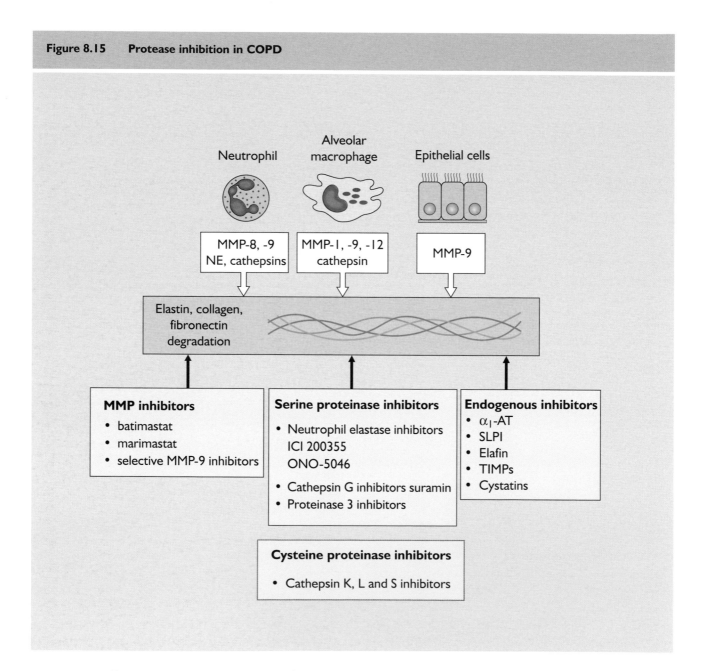

Matrix metalloproteases (MMP), neutrophil elastase (NE) and cathepsin catalyze the degradation of extracellular matrix proteins such as elastin, collagen and fibronectin. Endogenous protease inhibitors include α_1-antitrypsin (α_1-AT), secretory leukoprotease inhibitor (SLPI) and tissue inhibitor of matrix metalloproteinases (TIMP).

whether given by inhalation or systemically, and also inhibit the other serine proteases released from neutrophils (cathepsin G and proteinase-3). Small molecule inhibitors of NE are now entering clinical trials, but there is concern that NE may not play a critical role in emphysema, and that other proteases are more important in elastolysis. There are few clinical studies in COPD; the NE inhibitor MR889 administered for 4 weeks showed no overall effect on plasma elastin-derived peptides or urinary desmosine (markers of elastolytic activity)[99]. It may be difficult to inhibit enzyme activity, since neutrophils adhere to connective tissue, so that access of the enzyme inhibitor may be a problem. Intracellular inhibitors may be more effective. Although NE is likely to be the major mechanism mediating elastolysis in patients with α_1-AT deficiency, NE may not play a critical role in emphysema. Inhibitors of elastolytic cysteine proteases, such as cathepsins K, S and L which are released from macrophages, are also in development[100,101].

Matrix metalloproteinase inhibitors

MMPs derived from macrophages, neutrophils and epithelial cells may also play a role in connective tissue destruction, suggesting that MMP inhibitors may be beneficial. There are several approaches to inhibiting MMPs[102]:

(1) One approach is to enhance the secretion of the tissue inhibitors of MMPs, TIMPs;

(2) Another is to develop enzyme inhibitors, such as batimastat (BB-94) and the orally active marimastat (BB-2516). These are non-selective inhibitors and have considerable side-effects;

(3) Selective inhibitors of individual MMPs, such as MMP-9 and MMP-12 (metalloelastase) could have less toxicity, and are now in development. MMP-9 is markedly overexpressed by alveolar macrophages from patients with COPD[103], suggesting a selective MMP-9 inhibitor could be useful in emphysema.

α_1-Antitrypsin

The association of α_1-AT deficiency with early-onset emphysema suggested that this endogenous inhibitor of neutrophil elastase may be of therapeutic benefit in COPD.

(1) Extraction of α_1-AT from human plasma is very expensive and extracted α_1-AT is only available in a few countries. This treatment has to be given intravenously and has a half-life of only 5 days. Human α_1-AT has now been available for over 10 years, but, even in patients with severe α_1-AT deficiency and emphysema, there is only a marginal effect on the rate of decline in FEV_1[104].

(2) Recombinant α_1-AT from yeast lacks the three carbohydrate side-chains and has an additional amino-terminal methionine. When given intravenously, it has a much shorter plasma half-life than natural α_1-AT. Inhaled α_1-AT may be more effective than intravenously administered α_1-AT[105,106], and Arriva in conjunction with Baxter are co-developing inhaled yeast recombinant α_1-AT. Inhaled α_1-AT may be effective in COPD because, in mice exposed to cigarette smoke, α_1-AT inhibits connective tissue breakdown mediated by neutrophils[107]. Furthermore, inhaled α_1-AT may replace α_1-AT stocks inactivated by cigarette smoking[108], has potential anti-inflammatory actions[109], and may reduce airway hyperreactivity[110].

Serpins

Other serum protease inhibitors (serpins), such as elafin, may also be important in counteracting elastolytic activity in the lung. Elafin, an elastase-specific inhibitor, is found in bronchoalveolar lavage and is synthesized by epithelial cells in response to inflammatory stimuli[111]. Serpins may not be able to inhibit neutrophil elastase at the sites of elastin destruction, due to tight adherence of the inflammatory cell to connective tissue. Furthermore, these proteins may become inactivated by the inflammatory process and the action of oxidants, so that they may not be able to adequately counteract elastolytic activity in the lung unless used in conjunction with other therapies.

Secretory leukoprotease inhibitor

Secretory leukoprotease inhibitor (SLPI) is a 12-kDa serpin that appears to be a major inhibitor of elastase activity in the airways. It is secreted by epithelial cells[111]. *In vitro* recombinant human SLPI is more effective at inhibiting neutrophil-mediated proteolysis than α_1-AT[112]. Recombinant human SLPI given by aerosolization increases anti-neutrophil elastase activity in epithelial lining fluid for over 12 h, indicating a potential therapeutic use[113].

MUCOREGULATORS

Increased secretion of mucus is found in all patients who smoke heavily, irrespective of airflow obstruction. However, while mucus hypersecretion (GOLD stage 0) has been found to be associated with a more rapid decline in FEV_1[114], a study over 15 years found that GOLD stage 0 does not identify subsequent airway obstruction, possibly because GOLD stage 0 is not a stable feature[115]. This questions the rationale

of developing drugs that inhibit the hypersecretion of mucus. It is also important not to suppress normal levels of mucus secretion or impair mucociliary clearance. There are several types of mucoregulatory drugs in development (see Figure 8.16).

Tachykinin antagonists

Tachykinins are sensory neuropeptides that potently stimulate mucus secretion from submucosal glands

Figure 8.16   Potential therapy directed against mucus hypersecretion in COPD

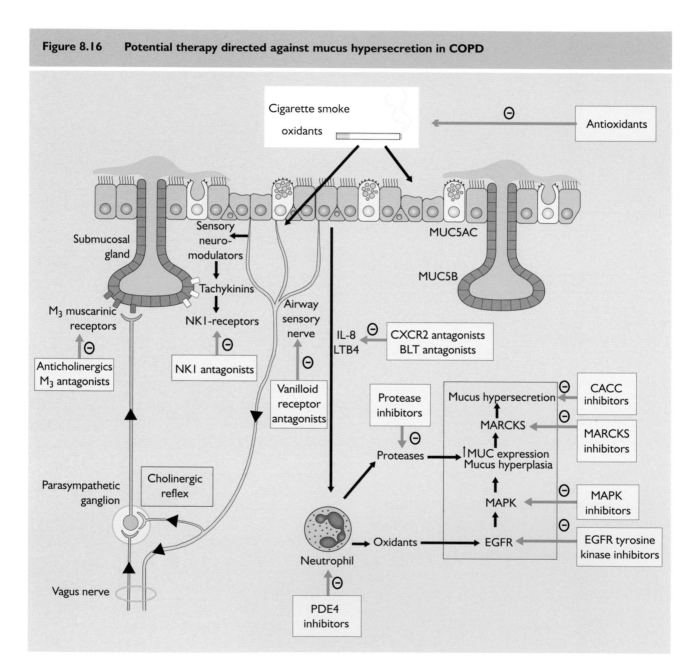

CACC, calcium-activated chloride channel; EGFR, epidermal growth factor receptor; IL-8, interleukin-8; LTB4, leukotriene B4; MAPK, mitogen-activated protein kinase; MARCKS, myristoylated alanine-rich C kinase substrate; NK1, neurokinin 1; PDE4, phosphodiesterase 4

and goblet cells in human and animal airways and act via NK$_1$-receptors. In animal studies, cigarette smoke induces airway mucus secretion via release of tachykinins from sensory nerves through a local axon reflex mechanism[116]. NK$_1$-antagonists markedly inhibit neurogenic mucus secretion and may therefore have potential as mucoregulators in cigarette smoke-induced chronic bronchitis. Several potent non-peptide NK$_1$-receptor antagonists, such as CP-99,994 and SR 140333, are now in clinical development, and might have a role as regulators of mucus hypersecretion in COPD.

Opioids and potassium channel openers

Another approach to blocking tachykinin-mediated effects is to inhibit the release of tachykinins from sensory nerve endings, via activation of pre-junctional receptors[117]. Of these receptors, μ-opioid receptors are most effective and the μ-opioid agonist morphine potently inhibits cigarette smoke-induced mucus secretion in animal airways. In human airways, *in vitro* morphine inhibits mucus secretion activated via stimulation of sensory nerves[118]. While morphine itself may not be useful as a therapeutic agent because of addiction, peripherally acting opioid agonists that do not cross the blood–brain barrier, such as BW443, might be of use. Many pre-junctional receptors appear to operate via the opening of a common potassium (K$^+$) channel, suggesting that K$^+$ channel openers may be useful in blocking mucus secretion. Openers of ATP-dependent K channels, such as levcromakalim, have an inhibitory effect on cigarette smoke-induced mucus secretion in animals[119].

Mediator and enzyme inhibitors

Many mediators stimulate mucus secretion from submucosal glands and/or goblet cells and may therefore contribute to increased mucus secretion in COPD[120]. It is unlikely, however, that any mediator antagonists (e.g. anti-leukotrienes) would have a major effect on mucus secretion. Neutrophil elastase, proteinase-3 and other proteases are potent stimulants of submucosal gland and goblet cell secretion, suggesting that protease inhibitors may have inhibitory effects on mucus secretion, as well as inhibiting lung destruction. Inhalation of the cyclooxygenase inhibitor, indomethacin, is reported to reduce mucus hypersecretion in patients with COPD[121], but long-term trials of cyclooxygenase inhibitors have not yet been undertaken.

MUC gene suppressors

Nine MUC genes that code for mucin synthesis have already been cloned and many are expressed in human airways[122]. MUC5AC (particularly in goblet cells), MUC5B (particularly in submucosal glands), MUC4 and MUC8 appear to be important in airway mucus. MUC5AC may be up-regulated by inflammatory cytokines and inhibited by glucocorticoids[123]. It is possible that drugs may be developed that inhibit the abnormally increased expression of MUC genes in COPD, while preserving baseline secretion of MUC2. Such drugs, other than corticosteroids, have not yet been developed.

Macrolide antibiotics

Erythromycin inhibits mucin secretion from human airways *in vitro* and appears to be interactive with corticosteroids[124]. This property does not appear to be related to their antibiotic activity and is consistent with other studies demonstrating an inhibitory action of erythromycin on cell secretion. The molecular mechanisms involved in these effects need to be defined, and controlled studies in COPD may be indicated.

Epidermal growth factor antagonists

Epidermal growth factor (EGF) appears to play an important role in mucus secretion and increased expression of MUC genes[125,126], suggesting that inhibition of EGF receptors or signalling pathways may be effective treatments for mucus hypersecretion.

LUNG REGENERATION: REMODELLING

A major mechanism of airway obstruction in COPD is loss of elastic recoil due to proteolytic destruction of lung parenchyma and alveolar attachments. An ambitious target for drugs is to cause lung repair and regeneration of parenchymal tissue (Figure 8.17). However, it might be possible to reduce the rate of progression by preventing the inflammatory and enzymatic disease process.

(1) Retinoic acid increases the number of alveoli in rats and, remarkably, reverses the histological and physiological changes induced by elastase treatment[127,128]. It is not certain whether such alveolar proliferation is possible in adult human lungs, however. Inhalation of retinoic acid or

Figure 8.17   Regeneration of lung parenchyma

Retinoic acid prevents elastase-induced emphysema in rats

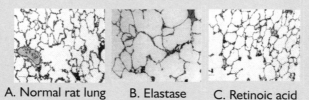

A. Normal rat lung   B. Elastase   C. Retinoic acid

Elastase instilled into rat lungs causes features of human emphysema, which can be reversed by therapy with retinoic acid. Massaro G, Massaro D, *Nature Med* 1997;3:675–7

Agents with capacity to regenerate lung parenchyma:

- Retinoic acid
  Retinoids: selective RARγ agonists
- Hepatocyte growth factor (scatter factor)
- Stem cells

derivates may be preferred, as side-effects are likely to be problem with repeated administrations[129]. Retinoic acid activates intracellular retinoic acid receptors, which act as transcription factors to regulate the expression of many genes. A particular subtype of retinoic acid receptor appears to mediate this effect, so that selective agonists, which would be safer than *all-trans* retinoic acid, are in development[128]. The molecular mechanisms involved and whether this can be extrapolated to humans are not yet known, but retinoic acid inhibits elastase-induced injury in human lung epithelial cell lines[130,131]. Several retinoic acid receptor subtype agonists have now been developed that may have a greater selectivity for this effect. A short-term trial of *all-trans* retinoic acid in patients with emphysema failed to show improvement in clinical parameters[132].

(2) Hepatocyte growth factor (scatter factor) appears to be a major growth factor responsible for alveolar development[133]. If responsiveness could be restored in adult lung parenchyma, this might be a strategy for repairing damaged lung.

OTHER ADVANCES

Drug delivery

Bronchodilators are currently given using inhalers, metered dose inhalers or dry powder inhalers that have been optimized to deliver drugs to the respiratory tract in asthma. But, in emphysema, the inflammatory and destructive process takes place in the lung parenchyma, while, in chronic obstructive bronchiolitis, the predominant irreversible changes take place in the small airways. This implies that, if a drug is to be delivered by inhalation, it should have a lower mass median diameter, so that there is preferential deposition in the lung periphery. It may be more appropriate to give therapy parenterally, as it will need to reach the lung parenchyma via the pulmonary circulation, but parenteral administration may increase the risk of systemic side-effects. In the future, targeted delivery may be more effective with a reduced risk of side-effects. For example, drugs may be delivered that are selectively phagocytosed by macrophages or released from inactive prodrugs by elastases. This would reduce the risk of side-effects that may be quite high for drugs such as

NF-κB, protease inhibitors and p38 MAP kinase inhibitors.

Animal models of COPD

Animal models for chronic bronchitis and COPD have proved difficult to develop[134-136]. Emphysema may be induced by challenge with exogenous agents such as irritants and cigarette smoke, as well as with proteinases. More recently, there has been extensive research on genetic mutant mouse strains and genetically engineered mice with enlarged air spaces[137].

New technologies

Artificial ventilation devices have improved enormously. Non-invasive ventilation using *non-invasive intermittent positive pressure ventilation* (NIPPV) has been an important advance in the management of acute exacerbations of COPD in hospital and, more recently, in the control of hypercapnic respiratory failure at home, thus reducing the need for hospitalization[138]. NIPPV corrects the hypercapnia and respiratory acidosis, while resting the respiratory muscles. Excellent results in management of acute exacerbations have been reported, with significant reduction in mortality and time spent in hospital.

Genetic risk factors

It is likely that several genetic polymorphisms will be discovered that will confer risk on smokers for the development of COPD and emphysema[139-142], so that it will eventually be possible to identify at-risk patients and focus more effective therapies on these patients before their lung function becomes too impaired[143]. The development of gene chip technologies that allow the detection of multiple polymorphisms may provide a simple way to detect the risk in individual patients, as well as to identify new target genes. It may also predict the risk of developing pulmonary hypertension and *cor pulmonale*.

Early detection

One of the most important developments in the future will be the detection of COPD at an earlier stage, before symptoms appear. This will depend on screening of cigarette smokers in the community and instituting preventive measures (smoking cessation plans and possible drug therapy). More rigorous attempts to prevent smoking, particularly in teenagers, are needed, with a complete ban on cigarette advertising and increased taxation of tobacco. In the future, it may be possible to detect the genetic polymorphisms that predetermine whether a patient will develop COPD with cigarette smoking. The development of small lungs in neonates, due to malnutrition and smoking in pregnancy, may increase the risk of COPD in cigarette smoking and emphasizes the importance of trying to prevent cigarette smoking in pregnant women.

Surrogate markers in sputum and breath

Several drugs are now in development that may be useful for patients with COPD. However, it will be difficult to demonstrate the efficacy of such treatments, as determination of the effect of any drug on the rate of decline in lung function will require large studies over at least 2 years. There is an urgent need to develop surrogate markers, based on non-invasive sampling techniques. Analysis of sputum parameters (cells, mediators, enzymes) may predict the clinical usefulness of such drugs in smaller studies[144,145]. Analyses of exhaled breath nitric oxide (NO) with volatile gases measured in breath condensate are promising techniques[84,146-148] (Figure 8.18).

Lung function, health status, body mass and imaging techniques

Sophisticated lung function techniques, in conjunction with exercise responses, can be used to assess dynamic hyperinflation, and have proved useful in the assessment of bronchodilators. Assessment of health status, or health-related quality of life, is an important feature of modern clinical trials in COPD[149]. In addition, testing responses to exercise as a 6-minute walk test or incremental shuttle walk test are validated models to test exercise capacity[150,151]. For patients with COPD and cachexia, it is important to assess fat-free mass and to perform tests of metabolism and muscle function[152,153]. CT scanning is proving useful in discrimination of large and small airways, as well as parenchymal disease, and is likely to become increasingly important in the assessment of individual patients[154].

CONCLUSIONS

There is an urgent need for new drugs for the treatment of COPD. While preventing and quitting

Figure 8.18   Exhaled breath analysis

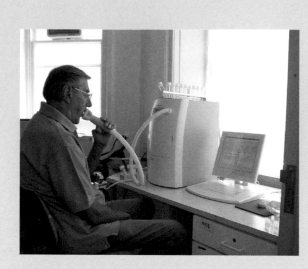

Exhaled breath nitric oxide analysis
NIOX Analyser from Aerocrine, Soha, Sweden

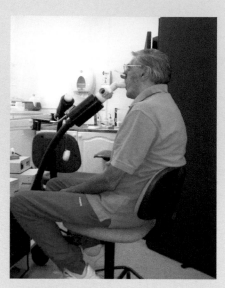

Breath condenser
ECoScreen from Jaeger, Erlangen,
Germany

smoking is the obvious preferred approach, this has proved to be very difficult for the majority of patients. More research on the basic physiological, pathological, cellular and molecular mechanisms of COPD and emphysema is required. These efforts are likely to result in the successful introduction of new therapeutics for patients with COPD in the near future.

REFERENCES

1.   Barnes PJ. New treatments for COPD. *Nat Rev Drug Discov* 2002;1:437–46

2.   Barnes PJ. Therapy of chronic obstructive pulmonary disease. *Pharmacol Ther* 2003;97:87–94

3.   Hansel TT, Barnes PJ, eds. *New Drugs for Asthma, Allergy and COPD*. Basel: Karger, 2001

4.   Holm KJ, Spencer CM. Bupropion: a review of its use in the management of smoking cessation. *Drugs* 2000;59:1007–24

5.   Hurt RD, Sachs DP, Glover ED, Offord KP, Johnston JA, Dale LC, *et al*. A comparison of sustained-release bupropion and placebo for smoking cessation. *N Engl J Med* 1997;337:1195–202

6.   Jorenby DE, Leischow SJ, Nides MA, Rennard SI, Johnston JA, Hughes AR, *et al*. A controlled trial of sustained-release bupropion, a nicotine patch, or both for smoking cessation. *N Engl J Med* 1999;340:685–91

7.   Huibers MJ, Chavannes NH, Wagena EJ, van Schayck CP. Antidepressants for smoking cessation: a promising new approach? *Eur Respir J* 2000;16:379–80

8.   Tashkin D, Kanner R, Bailey W, Buist S, Anderson P, Nides M, *et al*. Smoking cessation in patients with chronic obstructive pulmonary disease: a double-blind, placebo-controlled, randomised trial. *Lancet* 2001;357:1571–5

9.   Hansel TT, Barnes PJ. Tiotropium bromide: a novel once-daily anticholinergic bronchodilator for the treatment of COPD. *Drugs Today* 2002;38:585–600

10.   Cazzola M, Donner CF. Long-acting beta2 agonists in the management of stable chronic obstructive pulmonary disease. *Drugs* 2000;60:307–20

11.   Mahler DA, Donohue JF, Barbee RA, Goldman MD, Gross NJ, Wisniewski ME, *et al*. Efficacy of salmeterol xinafoate in the treatment of COPD. *Chest* 1999;115:957–65

12. Rennard SI, Anderson W, ZuWallack R, Broughton J, Bailey W, Friedman M, et al. Use of a long-acting inhaled beta2-adrenergic agonist, salmeterol xinafoate, in patients with chronic obstructive pulmonary disease. Am J Respir Crit Care Med 2001;163:1087–92

13. Boyd G, Morice AH, Pounsford JC, Siebert M, Peslis N, Crawford C. An evaluation of salmeterol in the treatment of chronic obstructive pulmonary disease (COPD). Eur Respir J 1997;10:815–21

14. Jarvis B, Markham A. Inhaled salmeterol: a review of its efficacy in chronic obstructive pulmonary disease. Drugs Aging 2001;18:441–72

15. Albers R, Ayres J, Backer V, Decramer M, Lier PA, Magyar P, et al. Formoterol in patients with chronic obstructive pulmonary disease: a randomized, controlled, 3-month trial. Eur Respir J 2002;19: 936–43

16. Dahl R, Greefhorst LA, Nowak D, Nonikov V, Byrne AM, Thomson MH, et al. Inhaled formoterol dry powder versus ipratropium bromide in chronic obstructive pulmonary disease. Am J Respir Crit Care Med 2001;164:778–84

17. Rossi A, Kristufek P, Levine BE, Thomson MH, Till D, Kottakis J, et al. Comparison of the efficacy, tolerability, and safety of formoterol dry powder and oral, slow-release theophylline in the treatment of COPD. Chest 2002;121:1058–69

18. Newbold P, Jackson DM, Young A. Dual D2 dopamine receptor and beta2-adrenoceptor agonists for the modulation of sensory nerves in COPD. In Hansel TT, Barnes PJ, eds. New Drugs for Asthma and COPD. Basel: Karger, 2001:68–71

19. Bonnert RV, Brown RC, Chapman D, Cheshire DR, Dixon J, Ince F, et al. Dual D2-receptor and beta2-adrenoceptor agonists for the treatment of airway diseases. 1. Discovery and biological evaluation of some 7-(2-aminoethyl)-4-hydroxybenzothiazol-2 (3H)-one analogues. J Med Chem 1998;41:4915–17

20. Johnson M. Beta2-adrenoceptors: mechanisms of action of beta2-agonists. Paediatr Respir Rev 2001;2:57–62

21. Johnson EN, Druey KM. Heterotrimeric G protein signaling: role in asthma and allergic inflammation. J Allergy Clin Immunol 2002;109:592–602

22. Vestbo J, Sorensen T, Lange P, Brix A, Torre P, Viskum K. Long-term effect of inhaled budesonide in mild and moderate chronic obstructive pulmonary disease: a randomised controlled trial. Lancet 1999;353:1819–23

23. Pauwels RA, Lofdahl CG, Laitinen LA, Schouten JP, Postma DS, Pride NB, et al. Long-term treatment with inhaled budesonide in persons with mild chronic obstructive pulmonary disease who continue smoking. European Respiratory Society Study on Chronic Obstructive Pulmonary Disease. N Engl J Med 1999;340:1948–53

24. Burge PS, Calverley PM, Jones PW, Spencer S, Anderson JA, Maslen TK. Randomised, double blind, placebo controlled study of fluticasone propionate in patients with moderate to severe chronic obstructive pulmonary disease: the ISOLDE trial. Br Med J 2000;320:1297–303

25. Lung Health Study Research Group. Effect of inhaled triamcinolone on the decline in pulmonary function in chronic obstructive pulmonary disease. N Engl J Med 2000;343:1902–9

26. Soriano JB, Vestbo J, Pride NB, Kiri V, Maden C, Maier WC. Survival in COPD patients after regular use of fluticasone propionate and salmeterol in general practice. Eur Respir J 2002;20:819–25

27. Mahler DA, Wire P, Horstman D, Chang CN, Yates J, Fischer T, et al. Effectiveness of fluticasone propionate and salmeterol combination delivered via the diskus device in the treatment of chronic obstructive pulmonary disease. Am J Respir Crit Care Med 2002;166:1084–91

28. Calverley P, Pauwels R, Vestbo J, Jones P, Pride N, Gulsvik A, Anderson J, Maden C, for the TRISTAN Study Group. Combined salmeteral and fluticasone in the treatment of chronic obstructive pulmonary disease: a randomized controlled trial. Lancet 2003;361:449–56

29. Keatings VM, Jatakanon A, Worsdell YM, Barnes PJ. Effects of inhaled and oral glucocorticoids on inflammatory indices in asthma and COPD. Am J Respir Crit Care Med 1997;155:542–8

30. Culpitt SV, Maziak W, Loukidis S, Nightingale JA, Matthews JL, Barnes PJ. Effect of high dose inhaled steroid on cells, cytokines, and proteases in induced sputum in chronic obstructive pulmonary disease. Am J Respir Crit Care Med 1999;160:1635–9

31. Nightingale JA, Rogers DF, Fan CK, Barnes PJ. No effect of inhaled budesonide on the response to inhaled ozone in normal subjects. Am J Respir Crit Care Med 2000;161:479–86

32. Ito K, Lim S, Caramori G, Chung KF, Barnes PJ, Adcock IM. Cigarette smoking reduces histone deacetylase 2 expression, enhances cytokine expression and inhibits glucocorticoid actions in alveolar macrophages. FASEB J 2001;15:1100–2

33. Huang Z, Ducharme Y, MacDonald D, Robichaud A. The next generation of PDE4 inhibitors. *Curr Opin Chem Biol* 2001;5:432–8

34. Giembycz MA. Development status of second generation PDE4 inhibitors for asthma and COPD: the story so far. *Monaldi Arch Chest Dis* 2002;57: 48–64

35. Essayan DM. Cyclic nucleotide phosphodiesterases. *J Allergy Clin Immunol* 2001;108:671–80

36. Dyke HJ, Montana JG. The therapeutic potential of PDE4 inhibitors. *Exp Opin Invest Drugs* 1999;8: 1301–25

37. Giembycz MA. Phosphodiesterase 4 inhibitors and the treatment of asthma: where are we now and where do we go from here? *Drugs* 2000;59:193–212

38. Torphy TJ. Phosphodiesterase isozymes: molecular targets for novel antiasthma agents. *Am J Respir Crit Care Med* 1998;157:351–70

39. Souness JE, Aldous D, Sargent C. Immuno-suppressive and anti-inflammatory effects of cyclic AMP phosphodiesterase (PDE) type 4 inhibitors. *Immunopharmacology* 2000;47:127–62

40. Compton CH, Gubb J, Nieman R, Edelson J, Amit O, Bakst A, *et al.* Cilomilast, a selective phosphodi-esterase-4 inhibitor for treatment of patients with chronic obstructive pulmonary disease: a randomised, dose-ranging study. *Lancet* 2001;358: 265–70

41. Spond J, Chapman R, Fine J, Jones H, Kreutner W, Kung TT, *et al.* Comparison of PDE 4 inhibitors, rolipram and SB 207499 (Ariflo), in a rat model of pulmonary neutrophilia. *Pulm Pharmacol Ther* 2001; 14:157–64

42. Bundschuh DS, Eltze M, Barsig J, Wollin L, Hatzelmann A, Beume R. *In vivo* efficacy in airway disease models of roflumilast, a novel orally active PDE4 inhibitor. *J Pharmacol Exp Ther* 2001;297: 280–90

43. Hatzelmann A, Schudt C. Anti-inflammatory and immunomodulatory potential of the novel PDE4 inhibitor roflumilast *in vitro*. *J Pharmacol Exp Ther* 2001;297:267–79

44. Timmer W, Leclerc V, Birraux G, Neuhauser M, Hatzelmann A, Bethke T, *et al.* The new phosphodi-esterase 4 inhibitor roflumilast is efficacious in exer-cise-induced asthma and leads to suppression of LPS-stimulated TNF-alpha *ex vivo*. *J Clin Pharmacol* 2002;42:297–303

45. Schmidt BM, Kusma M, Feuring M, Timmer WE, Neuhauser M, Bethke T, *et al.* The phosphodiesterase

4 inhibitor roflumilast is effective in the treatment of allergic rhinitis. *J Allergy Clin Immunol* 2001;108: 530–6

46. van Schalkwyk EM, van Heerden K, Bredenbroker D, Leichtl S, Wurst W, Venter L, *et al.* Dose-dependent inhibitory effect of roflumilast, a new, orally active, selective phosphodieterase 4 inhibitor, on allergen-induced early and late asthmatic reaction. *Eur Resp J* 2002;20:110S

47. Bredenbroker D, Syed J, Leichtl S, Rathgeb F, Wurst W. Roflumilast, a new orally active, selective phos-phodiesterase 4 inhibitor, is effective in the treat-ment of chronic obstructive pulmonary disease. *Eur Resp J* 2002;20:374S

48. Leichtl S, Syed J, Bredenbroker D, Rathgeb F, Wurst W. Roflumilast, a new orally active, selective phos-phodiesterase 4 inhibitor, is safe and well tolerated in patients with chronic obstructive pulmonary disease. *Eur Resp J* 2002;20:303S

49. Hill AT, Campbell EJ, Hill SL, Bayley DL, Stockley RA. Association between airway bacterial load and markers of airway inflammation in patients with stable chronic bronchitis. *Am J Med* 2000;109: 288–95

50. Yokomizo T, Kato K, Terawaki K, Izumi T, Shimizu T. A second leukotriene B(4) receptor, BLT2. A new therapeutic target in inflammation and immunologi-cal disorders. *J Exp Med* 2000;192:421–32

51. Evans DJ, Barnes PJ, Spaethe SM, van Alstyne EL, Mitchell MI, O'Connor BJ. Effect of a leukotriene B4 receptor antagonist, LY293111, on allergen induced responses in asthma. *Thorax* 1996;51:1178–84

52. Silbaugh SA, Stengel PW, Cockerham SL, Froelich LL, Bendele AM, Spaethe SM, *et al.* Pharmacologic actions of the second generation leukotriene B4 receptor antagonist LY29311: *in vivo* pulmonary studies. *Naunyn Schmiedebergs Arch Pharmacol* 2000;361:397–404

53. Crooks SW, Bayley DL, Hill SL, Stockley RA. Bronchial inflammation in acute bacterial exacerba-tions of chronic bronchitis: the role of leukotriene B4. *Eur Respir J* 2000;15:274–80

54. Chanez P, Bonnans C, Chavis C, Vachier I. 15-lipoxy-genase: a Janus enzyme? *Am J Respir Cell Mol Biol* 2002;27:655–8

55. Luster AD. Chemokines – chemotactic cytokines that mediate inflammation. *N Engl J Med* 1998;338: 436–45

56. Rossi D, Zlotnik A. The biology of chemokines and their receptors. *Ann Rev Immunol* 2000;18:217–42

57. Hay DWP, Sarau HM. Interleukin-8 receptor antagonists in pulmonary diseases. *Curr Opin Pharm* 2001;1:242–7

58. Keatings VM, Collins PD, Scott DM, Barnes PJ. Differences in interleukin-8 and tumor necrosis factor-alpha in induced sputum from patients with chronic obstructive pulmonary disease or asthma. *Am J Respir Crit Care Med* 1996;153:530–4

59. Hill AT, Bayley DL, Campbell EJ, Hill SL, Stockley RA. Airways inflammation in chronic bronchitis: the effects of smoking and alpha1-antitrypsin deficiency. *Eur Respir J* 2000;15:886–90

60. Hill AT, Bayley DL, Stockley RA. The interrelationship of sputum inflammatory markers in patients with chronic bronchitis. *Am J Respir Crit Care Med* 1999;160:893–8

61. Yamamoto C, Yoneda T, Yoshikawa M, Fu A, Tokuyama T, Tsukaguchi K, et al. Airway inflammation in COPD assessed by sputum levels of interleukin-8. *Chest* 1997;112:505–10

62. Yang XD, Corvalan JR, Wang P, Roy CM, Davis CG. Fully human anti-interleukin-8 monoclonal antibodies: potential therapeutics for the treatment of inflammatory disease states. *J Leukoc Biol* 1999;66:401–10

63. Richman-Eisenstat JB, Jorens PG, Hebert CA, Ueki I, Nadel JA. Interleukin-8: an important chemoattractant in sputum of patients with chronic inflammatory airway diseases. *Am J Physiol* 1993;264:L413–18

64. White JR, Lee JM, Young PR, Hertzberg RP, Jurewicz AJ, Chaikin MA, et al. Identification of a potent, selective non-peptide CXCR2 antagonist that inhibits interleukin-8-induced neutrophil migration. *J Biol Chem* 1998;273:10095–8

65. Hay DW, Sarau HM. Interleukin-8 receptor antagonists in pulmonary diseases. *Curr Opin Pharmacol* 2001;1:242–7

66. Traves SL, Culpitt SV, Russell RE, Barnes PJ, Donnelly LE. Increased levels of the chemokines GROalpha and MCP-1 in sputum samples from patients with COPD. *Thorax* 2002;57:590–5

67. Davenpeck KL, Berens KL, Dixon RA, Dupre B, Bochner BS. Inhibition of adhesion of human neutrophils and eosinophils to P-selectin by the sialyl Lewis antagonist TBC1269: preferential activity against neutrophil adhesion *in vitro*. *J Allergy Clin Immunol* 2000;105:769–75

68. Burnett D, Chamba A, Hill SL, Stockley RA. Neutrophils from subjects with chronic obstructive lung disease show enhanced chemotaxis and extracellular proteolysis. *Lancet* 1987;2:1043–6

69. Noguera A, Busquets X, Sauleda J, Villaverde JM, MacNee W, Agusti AG. Expression of adhesion molecules and G proteins in circulating neutrophils in chronic obstructive pulmonary disease. *Am J Respir Crit Care Med* 1998;158:1664–8

70. de Godoy I, Donahoe M, Calhoun WJ, Mancino J, Rogers RM. Elevated TNF-alpha production by peripheral blood monocytes of weight-losing COPD patients. *Am J Respir Crit Care Med* 1996;153:633–7

71. Markham A, Lamb HM. Infliximab: a review of its use in the management of rheumatoid arthritis. *Drugs* 2000;59:1341–59

72. Jarvis B, Faulds D. Etanercept: a review of its use in rheumatoid arthritis. *Drugs* 1999;57:945–66

73. Barlaam B, Bird TG, Lambert-Van Der Brempt C, Campbell D, Foster SJ, Maciewicz R. New alpha-substituted succinate-based hydroxamic acids as TNFalpha convertase inhibitors. *J Med Chem* 1999;42:4890–908

74. Rabinowitz MH, Andrews RC, Becherer JD, Bickett DM, Bubacz DG, Conway JG, et al. Design of selective and soluble inhibitors of tumor necrosis factor-alpha converting enzyme (TACE). *J Med Chem* 2001;44:4252–67

75. Takanashi S, Hasegawa Y, Kanehira Y, Yamamoto K, Fujimoto K, Satoh K, et al. Interleukin-10 level in sputum is reduced in bronchial asthma, COPD and in smokers. *Eur Respir J* 1999;14:309–14

76. Fedorak RN, Gangl A, Elson CO, Rutgeerts P, Schreiber S, Wild G, et al. Recombinant human interleukin 10 in the treatment of patients with mild to moderately active Crohn's disease. The Interleukin 10 Inflammatory Bowel Disease Cooperative Study Group. *Gastroenterology* 2000;119:1473–82

77. Delhase M, Li N, Karin M. Kinase regulation in inflammatory response. *Nature* 2000;406:367–8

78. Nasuhara Y, Adcock IM, Catley M, Barnes PJ, Newton R. Differential IkappaB kinase activation and IkappaBalpha degradation by interleukin-1beta and tumor necrosis factor-alpha in human U937 monocytic cells. Evidence for additional regulatory steps in kappaB-dependent transcription. *J Biol Chem* 1999;274:19965–72

79. Carter AB, Monick MM, Hunninghake GW. Both Erk and p38 kinases are necessary for cytokine gene transcription. *Am J Respir Cell Mol Biol* 1999;20:751–8

80. Meja KK, Seldon PM, Nasuhara Y, Ito K, Barnes PJ, Lindsay MA, *et al.* p38 MAP kinase and MKK-1 co-operate in the generation of GM-CSF from LPS-stimulated human monocytes by an NF-kappa B-independent mechanism. *Br J Pharmacol* 2000;131: 1143–53

81. Lee JC, Kumar S, Griswold DE, Underwood DC, Votta BJ, Adams JL. Inhibition of p38 MAP kinase as a therapeutic strategy. *Immunopharmacology* 2000; 47:185–201

82. Underwood DC, Osborn RR, Bochnowicz S, Webb EF, Rieman DJ, Lee JC, *et al.* SB 239063, a p38 MAPK inhibitor, reduces neutrophilia, inflammatory cytokines, MMP-9, and fibrosis in lung. *Am J Physiol Lung Cell Mol Physiol* 2000;279:L895–L902

83. Sasaki T, Irie-Sasaki J, Jones RG, Oliveira-dos-Santos AJ, Stanford WL, Bolon B, *et al.* Function of PI3Kgamma in thymocyte development, T cell activation, and neutrophil migration. *Science* 2000;287: 1040–6

84. Montuschi P, Collins JV, Ciabattoni G, Lazzeri N, Corradi M, Kharitonov SA, *et al.* Exhaled 8-isoprostane as an *in vivo* biomarker of lung oxidative stress in patients with COPD and healthy smokers. *Am J Respir Crit Care Med* 2000;162:1175–7

85. Paredi P, Kharitonov SA, Leak D, Ward S, Cramer D, Barnes PJ. Exhaled ethane, a marker of lipid peroxidation, is elevated in chronic obstructive pulmonary disease. *Am J Respir Crit Care Med* 2000;162: 369–73

86. MacNee W. Oxidants/antioxidants and COPD. *Chest* 2000;117:303–17S

87. Grandjean EM, Berthet P, Ruffmann R, Leuenberger P. Efficacy of oral long-term N-acetylcysteine in chronic bronchopulmonary disease: a meta-analysis of published double-blind, placebo-controlled clinical trials. *Clin Ther* 2000;22:209–21

88. Poole PJ, Black PN. Oral mucolytic drugs for exacerbations of chronic obstructive pulmonary disease: systematic review. *Br Med J* 2001;322:1271–4

89. Cuzzocrea S, Riley DP, Caputi AP, Salvemini D. Antioxidant therapy: a new pharmacological approach in shock, inflammation, and ischemia/reperfusion injury. *Pharmacol Rev* 2001;53:135–59

90. Ricciardolo FLM. Multiple roles of nitric oxide in the airways. *Thorax* 2003;58:175–82

91. Ichinose M, Sugiura H, Yamagata S, Koarai A, Shirato K. Increase in reactive nitrogen species production in chronic obstructive pulmonary disease airways. *Am J Respir Crit Care Med* 2000;162:701–6

92. Hobbs AJ, Higgs A, Moncada S. Inhibition of nitric oxide synthase as a potential therapeutic target. *Ann Rev Pharmacol Toxicol* 1999;39:191–220

93. Hansel TT, Kharitonov SA, Donnelly LE, Erin EM, Currie MG, Moore WM, *et al.* A selective inhibitor of inducible nitric oxide synthase (iNOS) inhibits exhaled breath nitric oxide (NO) in asthma. *FASEB J* 2003;17:1298–300

94. Maestrelli P, Paska C, Saetta M, Turato G, Nowicki Y, Monti S, *et al.* Decreased haem oxygenase-1 and increased inducible nitric oxide synthase in the lung of severe COPD patients. *Eur Respir J* 2003;21: 971–6

95. Stockley RA. Neutrophils and protease/antiprotease imbalance. *Am J Respir Crit Care Med* 1999;160: S49–S52

96. Shapiro SD, Senior RM. Matrix metalloproteinases. Matrix degradation and more. *Am J Respir Cell Mol Biol* 1999;20:1100–2

97. Kawabata K, Suzuki M, Sugitani M, Imaki K, Toda M, Miyamoto T. ONO-5046, a novel inhibitor of human neutrophil elastase. *Biochem Biophys Res Commun* 1991;177:814–20

98. Fujie K, Shinguh Y, Yamazaki A, Hatanaka H, Okamoto M, Okuhara M. Inhibition of elastase-induced acute inflammation and pulmonary emphysema in hamsters by a novel neutrophil elastase inhibitor FR901277. *Inflamm Res* 1999;48:160–7

99. Luisetti M, Sturani C, Sella D, Madonini E, Galavotti V, Bruno G, *et al.* MR889, a neutrophil elastase inhibitor, in patients with chronic obstructive pulmonary disease: a double-blind, randomized, placebo-controlled clinical trial. *Eur Respir J* 1996;9: 1482–6

100. Punturieri A, Filippov S, Allen E, Caras I, Murray R, Reddy V, *et al.* Regulation of elastinolytic cysteine proteinase activity in normal and cathepsin K-deficient human macrophages. *J Exp Med* 2000;192: 789–99

101. Leung-Toung R, Li W, Tam TF, Karimian K. Thiol-dependent enzymes and their inhibitors: a review. *Curr Med Chem* 2002;9:979–1002

102. Cawston TE. Metalloproteinase inhibitors and the prevention of connective tissue breakdown. *Pharmacol Ther* 1996;70:163–82

103. Russell RE, Culpitt SV, DeMatos C, Donnelly L, Smith M, Wiggins J, *et al.* Release and activity of matrix metalloproteinase-9 and tissue inhibitor of metalloproteinase-1 by alveolar macrophages from

patients with chronic obstructive pulmonary disease. *Am J Respir Cell Mol Biol* 2002;26:602–9

104. Seersholm N, Wencker M, Banik N, Viskum K, Dirksen A, Kok-Jensen A, *et al.* Does alpha1-antitrypsin augmentation therapy slow the annual decline in FEV1 in patients with severe hereditary alpha1-antitrypsin deficiency? Wissenschaftliche Arbeitsgemeinschaft zur Therapie von Lungenerkrankungen (WATL) alpha1-AT study group. *Eur Respir J* 1997;10:2260–3

105. Hubbard RC, Crystal RG. Strategies for aerosol therapy of alpha 1-antitrypsin deficiency by the aerosol route. *Lung* 1990;168:565–78

106. Hubbard RC, Brantly ML, Sellers SE, Mitchell ME, Crystal RG. Anti-neutrophil-elastase defenses of the lower respiratory tract in alpha 1-antitrypsin deficiency directly augmented with an aerosol of alpha 1-antitrypsin. *Ann Intern Med* 1989;111:206–12

107. Dhami R, Gilks B, Xie C, Zay K, Wright JL, Churg A. Acute cigarette smoke-induced connective tissue breakdown is mediated by neutrophils and prevented by alpha1-antitrypsin. *Am J Respir Cell Mol Biol* 2000;22:244–52

108. Wallaert B, Gressier B, Marquette CH, Gosset P, Remy-Jardin M, Mizon J, *et al.* Inactivation of alpha 1-proteinase inhibitor by alveolar inflammatory cells from smoking patients with or without emphysema. *Am Rev Respir Dis* 1993;147:1537–43

109. Stockley RA, Bayley DL, Unsal I, Dowson LJ. The effect of augmentation therapy on bronchial inflammation in alpha1-antitrypsin deficiency. *Am J Respir Crit Care Med* 2002;165:1494–8

110. Forteza R, Botvinnikova Y, Ahmed A, Cortes A, Gundel RH, Wanner A, *et al.* The interaction of alpha 1-proteinase inhibitor and tissue kallikrein in controlling allergic ovine airway hyperresponsiveness. *Am J Respir Crit Care Med* 1996;154:36–42

111. Sallenave JM, Shulmann J, Crossley J, Jordana M, Gauldie J. Regulation of secretory leukocyte proteinase inhibitor (SLPI) and elastase-specific inhibitor (ESI/elafin) in human airway epithelial cells by cytokines and neutrophilic enzymes. *Am J Respir Cell Mol Biol* 1994;11:733–41

112. Llewellyn-Jones CG, Lomas DA, Stockley RA. Potential role of recombinant secretory leucoprotease inhibitor in the prevention of neutrophil mediated matrix degradation. *Thorax* 1994;49:567–72

113. McElvaney NG, Doujaiji B, Moan MJ, Burnham MR, Wu MC, Crystal RG. Pharmacokinetics of recombinant secretory leukoprotease inhibitor aerosolized to normals and individuals with cystic fibrosis. *Am Rev Respir Dis* 1993;148:1056–60

114. Vestbo J, Prescott E, Lange P. Association of chronic mucus hypersecretion with FEV1 decline and chronic obstructive pulmonary disease morbidity. *Am J Respir Crit Care Med* 1996;153:1530–5

115. Vestbo J, Lange P. Can GOLD Stage 0 provide information of prognostic value in chronic obstructive pulmonary disease? *Am J Respir Crit Care Med* 2002;166:329–32

116. Kuo HP, Barnes PJ, Rogers DF. Cigarette smoke-induced airway goblet cell secretion: dose dependent differential nerve activation. *Am J Physiol* 1992;7:L161–L167

117. Barnes PJ, Belvisi MG, Rogers DF. Modulation of neurogenic inflammation: novel approaches to inflammatory disease. *Trends Pharmacol Sci* 1990;11:185–9

118. Rogers DF, Barnes PJ. Opioid inhibition of neurally mediated mucus secretion in human bronchi. *Lancet* 1989;1:930–2

119. Kuo HP, Rohde JA, Barnes PJ, Rogers DF. K+ channel activator inhibition of neurogenic goblet cell secretion in guinea pig trachea. *Eur J Pharmacol* 1992;221:385–8

120. Perez-Vilar J, Sheehan JK, Randell SH. Making more MUCS. *Am J Respir Cell Mol Biol* 2003;28:267–70

121. Tamaoki J, Chiyotani A, Kobayashi K, Sakai N, Kanemura T, Takizawa T. Effect of indomethacin on bronchorrhea in patients with chronic bronchitis, diffuse panbronchiolitis, or bronchiectasis. *Am Rev Respir Dis* 1992;145:548–52

122. Reid CJ, Gould S, Harris A. Developmental expression of mucin genes in the human respiratory tract. *Am J Respir Cell Mol Biol* 1997;17:592–8

123. Kai H, Yoshitake K, Hisatsune A, Kido T, Isohama Y, Takahama K, *et al.* Dexamethasone suppresses mucus production and MUC-2 and MUC-5AC gene expression by NCI-H292 cells. *Am J Physiol* 1996;271:L484–8

124. Goswami SK, Kivity S, Marom Z. Erythromycin inhibits respiratory glycoconjugate secretion from human airways *in vitro*. *Am Rev Respir Dis* 1990;141:72–8

125. Takeyama K, Dabbagh K, Lee HM, Agusti C, Lausier JA, Ueki IF, *et al.* Epidermal growth factor system regulates mucin production in airways. *Proc Natl Acad Sci USA* 1999;96:3081–6

126. Takeyama K, Dabbagh K, Jeong SJ, Dao-Pick T, Ueki IF, Nadel JA. Oxidative stress causes mucin synthesis via transactivation of epidermal growth factor receptor: role of neutrophils. *J Immunol* 2000;164: 1546–52

127. Massaro GD, Massaro D. Retinoic acid treatment abrogates elastase-induced pulmonary emphysema in rats. *Nat Med* 1997;3:675–7

128. Belloni PN, Garvin L, Mao CP, Bailey-Healy I, Leaffer D. Effects of all-trans-retinoic acid in promoting alveolar repair. *Chest* 2000;117:235–41S

129. Brooks AD, Tong W, Benedetti F, Kaneda Y, Miller V, Warrell RP, Jr. Inhaled aerosolization of all-trans-retinoic acid for targeted pulmonary delivery. *Cancer Chemother Pharmacol* 2000;46:313–18

130. Massaro D, De Carlo MG. Retinoids, alveolus formation, and alveolar deficiency: clinical implications. *Am J Respir Cell Mol Biol* 2003;28:271–4

131. Nakajoh M, Fukushima T, Suzuki T, Yamaya M, Nakayama K, Sekizawa K, et al. Retinoic acid inhibits elastase-induced injury in human lung epithelial cell lines. *Am J Respir Cell Mol Biol* 2003;28:296–304

132. Mao JT, Goldin JG, Dermand J, Ibrahim G, Brown MS, Emerick A, et al. A pilot study of all-trans-retinoic acid for the treatment of human emphysema. *Am J Respir Crit Care Med* 2002;165:718–23

133. Ohmichi H, Koshimizu U, Matsumoto K, Nakamura T. Hepatocyte growth factor (HGF) acts as a mesenchyme-derived morphogenic factor during fetal lung development. *Development* 1998;125: 1315–24

134. Drazen JM, Takebayashi T, Long NC, De Sanctis GT, Shore SA. Animal models of asthma and chronic bronchitis. *Clin Exp Allergy* 1999;29:37–47

135. Shapiro SD. Animal models for chronic obstructive pulmonary disease: age of klotho and marlboro mice. *Am J Respir Cell Mol Biol* 2000;22:4–7

136. Dawkins PA, Stockley RA. Animal models of chronic obstructive pulmonary disease. *Thorax* 2001;56: 972–7

137. Mahadeva R, Shapiro SD. Chronic obstructive pulmonary disease. 3. Experimental animal models of pulmonary emphysema. *Thorax* 2002;57:908–14

138. Plant PK, Owen JL, Elliott MW. Early use of non-invasive ventilation for acute exacerbations of chronic obstructive pulmonary disease on general respiratory wards: a multicentre randomised controlled trial. *Lancet* 2000;355:1931–5

139. Sandford AJ, Silverman EK. Chronic obstructive pulmonary disease. 1. Susceptibility factors for COPD the genotype-environment interaction. *Thorax* 2002;57:736–41

140. Hoidal JR. Genetics of COPD: present and future. *Eur Respir J* 2001;18:741–3

141. Barnes PJ. Molecular genetics of chronic obstructive pulmonary disease. *Thorax* 1999;54:245–52

142. Sandford AJ, Chagani T, Weir TD, Connett JE, Anthonisen NR, Pare PD. Susceptibility genes for rapid decline of lung function in the lung health study. *Am J Respir Crit Care Med* 2001;163:469–73

143. Roses AD. Pharmacogenetics and the practice of medicine. *Nature* 2000;405:857–65

144. Brightling CE, Monterio W, Green RH, Parker D, Morgan MD, Wardlaw AJ, et al. Induced sputum and other outcome measures in chronic obstructive pulmonary disease: safety and repeatability. *Respir Med* 2001;95:999–1002

145. Bhowmik A, Seemungal TAR, Sapsford RJ, Devalia JL, Wedzicha JA. Comparison of spontaneous and induced sputum for investigation of airway inflammation in chronic obstructive pulmonary disease. *Thorax* 1998;53:953–6

146. Kharitonov SA, Barnes PJ. Exhaled markers of pulmonary disease. *Am J Respir Crit Care Med* 2001; 163:1693–722

147. Hunt J. Exhaled breath condensate: an evolving tool for noninvasive evaluation of lung disease. *J Allergy Clin Immunol* 2002;110:28–34

148. Barbato A, Magarotto M, Crivellaro M, Novello A, Jr, Cracco A, de Blic J, et al. Use of the paediatric bronchoscope, flexible and rigid, in 51 European centres. *Eur Respir J* 1997;10:1761–6

149. Jones PW, Mahler DA. Key outcomes in COPD: health-related quality of life. Proceedings of an expert round table held July 20–22, 2001 in Boston, Massachusetts, USA. *Eur Respir Rev* 2002;12

150. ATS statement: guidelines for the six-minute walk test. *Am J Respir Crit Care Med* 2002;166:111–17

151. Singh SJ, Morgan MD, Scott S, Walters D, Hardman AE. Development of a shuttle walking test of disability in patients with chronic airways obstruction. *Thorax* 1992;47:1019–24

152. Schols AM. Pulmonary cachexia. *Int J Cardiol* 2002; 85:101–10

153. ATS/ERS Statement on respiratory muscle testing. *Am J Respir Crit Care Med* 2002;166:518–624

154. Muller NL, Coxson H. Chronic obstructive pulmonary disease. 4. Imaging the lungs in patients with chronic obstructive pulmonary disease. *Thorax* 2002;57:982–5

Index